Non-motor Disorders in Parkinson Disease: Basic Science and Advances in Treatment

Non-motor Disorders in Parkinson Disease: Basic Science and Advances in Treatment

Editors

Patricia Martinez-Sanchez
Francisco Nieto-Escamez

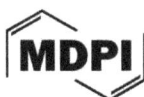

Basel • Beijing • Wuhan • Barcelona • Belgrade • Novi Sad • Cluj • Manchester

Editors

Patricia Martinez-Sanchez
Neurology
Torrecárdenas University Hospital
Almería
Spain

Francisco Nieto-Escamez
Psychology
University of Almeria
Almeria
Spain

Editorial Office
MDPI
St. Alban-Anlage 66
4052 Basel, Switzerland

This is a reprint of articles from the Special Issue published online in the open access journal *Brain Sciences* (ISSN 2076-3425) (available at: www.mdpi.com/journal/brainsci/special_issues/Non_Motor_Disorders_Parkinson).

For citation purposes, cite each article independently as indicated on the article page online and as indicated below:

Lastname, A.A.; Lastname, B.B. Article Title. *Journal Name* **Year**, *Volume Number*, Page Range.

ISBN 978-3-7258-0004-9 (Hbk)
ISBN 978-3-7258-0003-2 (PDF)
doi.org/10.3390/books978-3-7258-0003-2

© 2024 by the authors. Articles in this book are Open Access and distributed under the Creative Commons Attribution (CC BY) license. The book as a whole is distributed by MDPI under the terms and conditions of the Creative Commons Attribution-NonCommercial-NoDerivs (CC BY-NC-ND) license.

Contents

About the Editors vii

Preface ix

Francisco Nieto-Escamez, Esteban Obrero-Gaitán, Héctor García-López and Irene Cortés-Pérez
Unveiling the Hidden Challenges: Non-Motor Disorders in Parkinson's Disease
Reprinted from: *Brain Sci.* 2023, *13*, 1710, doi:10.3390/brainsci13121710 1

Francisco Nieto-Escamez, Esteban Obrero-Gaitán and Irene Cortés-Pérez
Visual Dysfunction in Parkinson's Disease
Reprinted from: *Brain Sci.* 2023, *13*, 1173, doi:10.3390/brainsci13081173 6

Fulvio Lauretani, Crescenzo Testa, Marco Salvi, Irene Zucchini, Francesco Giallauria and Marcello Maggio
Clinical Evaluation of Sleep Disorders in Parkinson's Disease
Reprinted from: *Brain Sci.* 2023, *13*, 609, doi:10.3390/brainsci13040609 29

Cristina del Toro-Pérez, Eva Guevara-Sánchez and Patricia Martínez-Sánchez
Treatment of Vascular Parkinsonism: A Systematic Review
Reprinted from: *Brain Sci.* 2023, *13*, 489, doi:10.3390/brainsci13030489 46

Ségolène De Waele, Patrick Cras and David Crosiers
Apathy in Parkinson's Disease: Defining the Park Apathy Subtype
Reprinted from: *Brain Sci.* 2022, *12*, 923, doi:10.3390/brainsci12070923 63

Ovidiu-Dumitru Ilie, Raluca Duta, Roxana Jijie, Ilinca-Bianca Nita, Mircea Nicoara and Caterina Faggio et al.
Assessing Anti-Social and Aggressive Behavior in a Zebrafish (*Danio rerio*) Model of Parkinson's Disease Chronically Exposed to Rotenone
Reprinted from: *Brain Sci.* 2022, *12*, 898, doi:10.3390/brainsci12070898 82

Diego Santos García, Gustavo Fernández Pajarín, Juan Manuel Oropesa-Ruiz, Francisco Escamilla Sevilla, Raúl Rashid Abdul Rahim López and José Guillermo Muñoz Enríquez
Opicapone Improves Global Non-Motor Symptoms Burden in Parkinson's Disease: An Open-Label Prospective Study
Reprinted from: *Brain Sci.* 2022, *12*, 383, doi:10.3390/brainsci12030383 94

Reinhard Janssen-Aguilar, Patricia Rojas, Elizabeth Ruiz-Sánchez, Mayela Rodriguez-Violante, Yessica M. Alcántara-Flores and Daniel Crail-Meléndez et al.
Naturalistic Study of Depression Associated with Parkinson's Disease in a National Public Neurological Referral Center in Mexico
Reprinted from: *Brain Sci.* 2022, *12*, 326, doi:10.3390/brainsci12030326 108

Satoshi Tada, Mohammed E. Choudhury, Madoka Kubo, Rina Ando, Junya Tanaka and Masahiro Nagai
Zonisamide Ameliorates Microglial Mitochondriopathy in Parkinson's Disease Models
Reprinted from: *Brain Sci.* 2022, *12*, 268, doi:10.3390/brainsci12020268 119

Héctor García-López, Esteban Obrero-Gaitán, Adelaida María Castro-Sánchez, Inmaculada Carmen Lara-Palomo, Francisco Antonio Nieto-Escamez and Irene Cortés-Pérez
Non-Immersive Virtual Reality to Improve Balance and Reduce Risk of Falls in People Diagnosed with Parkinson's Disease: A Systematic Review
Reprinted from: *Brain Sci.* 2021, *11*, 1435, doi:10.3390/brainsci11111435 129

Heithem Soliman, Benoit Coffin and Guillaume Gourcerol
Gastroparesis in Parkinson Disease: Pathophysiology, and Clinical Management
Reprinted from: *Brain Sci.* **2021**, *11*, 831, doi:10.3390/brainsci11070831 . . . . **143**

Cristina del Toro Pérez, Laura Amaya Pascasio, Antonio Arjona Padillo, Jesús Olivares Romero, María Victoria Mejías Olmedo and Javier Fernández Pérez et al.
Neurosonological Findings Related to Non-Motor Features of Parkinson's Disease: A Systematic Review
Reprinted from: *Brain Sci.* **2021**, *11*, 776, doi:10.3390/brainsci11060776 . . . . **153**

About the Editors

Patricia Martinez-Sanchez

Dr. Patricia Martínez-Sánchez currently works as a neurologist and a neuroscientist at the Department of Neurology at Torrecárdenas University Hospital, Almeria (Spain). Dr. Martínez-Sánchez is also an associate professor at the University of Almeria. Her current research project is 'Epidemiology and Predictive models in Stroke Mortality'.

Francisco Nieto-Escamez

Dr. Francisco Nieto-Escamez currently works at the Department of Psychology, Universidad de Almería. Dr. Nieto-Escamez conducts research in biological psychology, behavioural science, and neuropsychology, and is currently working on new projects devoted to the neurorehabilitiation of acquired brain damage, including neurodegeneration and neurodevelopmental pathologies using virtual reality technologies.

Preface

It is our pleasure to introduce a Special Issue of *Brain Science* dedicated to basic neuroscience and clinical research about the neurobiology of non-motor symptoms (NMSs) of Parkinson's disease and potential treatment strategies.

Parkinson's disease (PD) is the second most common neurodegenerative disorder, and although it is usually considered as a disorder that only affects movement, a broad spectrum of NMS can be observed in PD patients. Although the realities of the disease vary enormously from patient to patient, almost all of them have one or more NMS. In fact, a wide range of behavioural, neuropsychiatric, and physical symptoms frequently play a primary role in managing the disorder and constitute a major disease burden for patients and caregivers. Unfortunately, there is very little existing data about NMS, their neurobiology, and their treatment. It is therefore essential that researchers and practitioners comprehensively address the factors related to NMS if we want to achieve the best quality of life for PD patients.

The aim of this Special Issue is to provide an overview of evidence from clinical and basic research perspectives about Parkinson's NMS. A non-exhaustive list of potential papers may include research involving the use of neurophysiology techniques, genetics, pharmacological therapy, physical therapy, psychological intervention in clinical populations, as well as preclinical studies with animal models.

Patricia Martinez-Sanchez and Francisco Nieto-Escamez
Editors

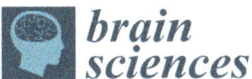

Editorial

Unveiling the Hidden Challenges: Non-Motor Disorders in Parkinson's Disease

Francisco Nieto-Escamez [1,2,*], Esteban Obrero-Gaitán [3,*], Héctor García-López [4] and Irene Cortés-Pérez [3]

1. Department of Psychology, University of Almeria, 04120 Almeria, Spain
2. CIBIS Research Center (Centro de Investigación para el Bienestar y la Inclusión Social), University of Almeria, 04120 Almeria, Spain
3. Department of Health Sciences, University of Jaen, Paraje Las Lagunillas s/n, 23071 Jaen, Spain; icortes@ujaen.es
4. Department of Nursing, Physical Therapy and Medicine, University of Almeria, Road Sacramento s/n, 04120 Almeria, Spain; hector.garcia@ual.es
* Correspondence: pnieto@ual.es (F.N.-E.); eobrero@ujaen.es (E.O.-G.)

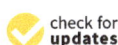

Citation: Nieto-Escamez, F.; Obrero-Gaitán, E.; García-López, H.; Cortés-Pérez, I. Unveiling the Hidden Challenges: Non-Motor Disorders in Parkinson's Disease. *Brain Sci.* 2023, 13, 1710. https://doi.org/10.3390/brainsci13121710

Received: 27 October 2023
Accepted: 7 November 2023
Published: 12 December 2023

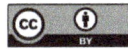

Copyright: © 2023 by the authors. Licensee MDPI, Basel, Switzerland. This article is an open access article distributed under the terms and conditions of the Creative Commons Attribution (CC BY) license (https://creativecommons.org/licenses/by/4.0/).

Parkinson's disease (PD) is not just a motor disorder, it is a complex condition that affects every aspect of a patient's life, from cognitive impairment and psychiatric disturbances to autonomic dysfunction and sleep disturbances [1]. Recognizing and addressing the non-motor aspects of PD is crucial for improving the overall well-being and quality of life for those living with the disease. Recent advances in our understanding of these non-motor disorders, and the development of innovative treatment approaches, offer hope for a better future for PD patients [2].

While the exact cause of Parkinson's disease remains the subject of extensive research, emerging evidence suggests a significant role of neurotoxic compounds in its pathogenesis [3]. Understanding the intricate relationships between neurotoxic compounds and PD is crucial to unraveling its origins and developing effective strategies for its prevention and treatment. Thus, in one of articles included in this Special Issue, Ilie et al. [4] observed that rotenone, a dopaminergic antagonistic that crosses the blood–brain barrier (BBB) and directly enters the central nervous system, and also other agents like valproic acid, levodopa/carbidopa, a probiotic supplement of lactobacillus, or a mixture of these compounds, impact zebrafish behavior, particularly in terms of sociability and aggression. However, probiotics had a positive impact, reducing the aggressive behaviors. Even the control group showed some behavioral impairments, although they were less pronounced than in the experimental groups. This research, focusing on animal behavior, marks the initial stage of a potentially promising research direction, particularly regarding the understanding of aggression and social dysfunction, which could have implications for PD patients. The study's approach, involving immunohistochemistry and assessing neuroinflammation and antioxidant enzyme impairment, holds substantial potential for further insights into this area.

Microglial cells are implicated in the progressive loss of dopaminergic neurons in PD through the release of potentially harmful substances. Excessive microglial phagocytosis of dopaminergic neurons in the substantia nigra is a key pathological event in PD [5]. In their article, Tada et al. [6] studied the impact of zonisamide (ZNS) on mitochondrial reactive oxygen species in microglial cells in a mouse PD model induced by two neurotoxins, MPTP and LPS. ZNS was found to inhibit the phagocytic activity and mitochondrial reactive oxygen species generation in LPS-treated microglial cells, potentially making it an effective antiparkinsonian drug that protects neurons in inflamed PD brains. These findings suggest that ZNS may modify the risk of rapid PD progression by influencing mitochondrial effects on microglial dysfunction.

Among the challenges in managing PD is addressing the fluctuations in the effectiveness of levodopa, a key medication used to alleviate motor symptoms. To tackle this issue,

Opicapone, a third-generation catechol-O-methyltransferase (COMT) inhibitor, prolongs the half-life of levodopa and maintains stable plasma levels of the drug, emerging as a promising therapeutic option [7]. In a groundbreaking multicenter, prospective study, Santos García et al. [8] evaluated the impact of Opicapone on non-motor symptoms (NMS) in PD patients. This research, conducted in Spain, focused on the global NMS burden in PD patients treated with Opicapone. Opicapone demonstrated remarkable efficacy in reducing the NMS total score, particularly in domains related to sleep, fatigue, mood, gastrointestinal symptoms, and pain. Notably, Opicapone was well-tolerated and safe, with a drug maintenance rate exceeding 90% after six months of treatment, even though dyskinesia was the most common adverse event reported. This study sheds light on Opicapone's potential as a therapeutic option for managing both motor and non-motor symptoms in PD, offering hope for improved patient outcomes and a better quality of life.

Psychiatric disturbances, such as depression, anxiety, and psychosis, are common in PD. These NMS not only contribute to the overall burden of the disease, but can also exacerbate motor symptoms [9]. Depression, for example, can lead to increased physical disability and decreased response to dopaminergic therapy [10]. Therefore, identifying and addressing these psychiatric symptoms is essential for improving patients' well-being and overall outcomes. In the study by Janssen-Aguilar et al. [11], the authors aimed to investigate the clinical and sociodemographic factors associated with major depressive disorder (MDD) in PD patients in a neurological referral center in Mexico. While the severity of MDD was higher in females than in males, there were no statistically significant differences between them. Marital status and educational level did not show a significant association with MDD severity. The study also explored the prevalence of arterial hypertension as a potential risk factor, and examined the relationship between rigidity, gait disturbances, and MDD. Patients with moderate to severe MDD exhibited more rigidity at the onset of PD, fewer gait alterations, and a higher prevalence of left-side disease onset. Additionally, cognitive assessments revealed mild cognitive impairment, with females scoring lower on the MMSE. These findings shed light on the complex factors contributing to MDD in PD patients and underscore the importance of considering these variables in clinical practice and research.

In recent years, transcranial sonography (TCS) has seen increased use as a supplementary tool for diagnosing PD by examining brainstem and subcortical structures [12]. Del Toro-Perez et al.'s [13] systematic review delves into ultrasound findings related to NMS in PD patients. The authors emphasize a link between brainstem raphe (BR) hypoechogenicity and depressive states in PD, potentially indicating structural BR disruption. They also note that substantia nigra (SN) hyperechogenicity is associated with a higher risk of depression, and may serve as a marker for PD development. The co-occurrence of SN hyperechogenicity and BR hypoechogenicity is connected to a history of depression preceding PD. Furthermore, the study explores the role of the vagus nerve in PD progression, with varying results in its relation to NMS, while also acknowledging the limitations of ultrasound evaluation protocols and the examination process.

Sleep disturbances in PD encompass a wide range of complexities, posing challenges in the development of clear treatment recommendations [14]. With the exception of rapid eye movement sleep behavior disorder (RBD), which can manifest as an early symptom, many sleep disorders tend to emerge in the later phases of the disease, frequently evading detection by affected individuals. This underscores the difficulty in effectively addressing these conditions within the framework of PD management. In Lauretani et al.'s [15] article, the authors detail sleep-related issues linked to PD, available medications, and the current status of treatment. The authors emphasize the need to consider sleep disturbances in PD patients from a multifaceted standpoint. It is crucial to recommend therapeutic interventions that align with the disease's stage, especially when dealing with elderly patients. These recommendations should be carefully weighed alongside other medications and the patient's existing health conditions to prevent potential risks like sedation and other detrimental side effects.

The term vascular parkinsonism (VP) is one of the most controversial in neurology, given the heterogeneity of the clinical picture that defines it. VP has also been termed "lower body parkinsonism", because it can manifest as predominant parkinsonism of the lower extremities, with difficulty walking, the absence of tremors, and minimal or no response to levodopa treatment. The studies reviewed by Del Toro-Pérez et al. [16] suggest that VP is a heterogeneous entity that should be properly subclassified to identify those patients with a response to levodopa. On the other hand, new therapies such as vitamin D, repetitive transcranial magnetic stimulation (rTMS), and intracerebral transcatheter laser photobiomodulation therapy (PBMT) warrant further studies to demonstrate their efficacy.

Virtual Reality has been utilized alongside medication in Parkinson's Disease treatment, offering the flexibility to tailor intervention plans by adjusting the content, duration, intensity, and feedback as required [17]. García-López et al. [18] discuss the use of non-immersive virtual reality (NIVR) in the rehabilitation of patients with PD to improve balance and reduce the risk of falls. These authors have conducted a systematic review that includes ten studies, highlighting the positive impact of NIVR on static and dynamic balance, along with a decrease in fall rates. This work also mentions that NIVR appears to be more effective than conventional physical therapy, and can be combined with other therapeutic methods to enhance results. However, the studies exhibit certain limitations, such as sample size variations and a lack of blinding, and therefore more research is needed in this area. Overall, this article concludes that NIVR has emerged as a promising tool in PD rehabilitation, offering potential benefits for balance and fall prevention.

Gastrointestinal (GI) issues can manifest in the initial stages of PD and, in certain instances, may appear years before motor symptoms [19], significantly impacting patients' quality of life [20]. Specifically, gastroparesis plays a role in the malnutrition and weight loss frequently observed in PD patients. In their study, Soliman et al. [21] explore the underlying physiological changes contributing to gastrointestinal dysfunction in PD. They also delve into the clinical symptoms associated with impaired stomach movement, particularly gastroparesis, outlining the diagnostic criteria for this condition and discussing its contemporary management based on recent findings. The authors suggest that correlating histological findings, assessments using novel endoscopic techniques, and treatment outcomes could assist in tailoring personalized treatment approaches.

Subclassifying PD based on NMS offers a promising and more precise approach for individualized treatment. Recent research suggests that apathy may serve as a specific indicator of a non-motor subtype known as the Park Apathy subtype [22]. Apathy manifests itself in all disease stages, and may serve as a prodromal symptom in some [23]. In their article, De Waele et al. [24] highlight the intricate pathophysiology of apathy in PD, indicating that distinct neural networks contribute to separate dimensions of apathy. They suggest that the LARS questionnaire can assess these dimensions, potentially aiding in personalized therapy, since each dimension corresponds to specific neurotransmitter deficiencies. However, further research is required to understand how these apathy dimensions manifest in PD patients, their progression, and their response to treatment.

NMS in PD encompass ocular, visuoperceptive, and visuospatial impairments linked to the neurodegenerative process. These symptoms include a range of visual issues, such as dry eyes, blink rate reduction, abnormal eye movements, contrast sensitivity and acuity problems, visuospatial challenges, attention difficulties, and perceptual disturbances, often leading to visual hallucinations. Nieto-Escámez et al.'s [25] review aims to provide a comprehensive understanding of these visual disruptions, exploring their neuroanatomical, functional, and neurochemical underpinnings, including the structural and functional changes in cortical and subcortical regions and their connections to neuropsychological findings, while also considering the involvement of various neurotransmitter systems like dopamine, acetylcholine, and serotonin.

In summary, addressing NMS in PD is critical for enhancing patient well-being. The studies in this Special Issue present promising avenues for understanding the disease's origin and developing effective therapies. These include exploring the impact of different compounds on behavior [4], identifying the role of microglial cells in disease progression [6], and assessing the effectiveness of drugs like Opicapone in managing both motor and non-motor symptoms [8]. Clinical and sociodemographic factors related to psychiatric disturbances are discussed [11]. Del Toro-Pérez et al. [13] show how the advancements in diagnostics like transcranial sonography provide valuable insights, whereas innovative approaches such as virtual reality demonstrate potential benefits [18]. Additionally, the articles by Soliman et al. [21], De Waele et al. [24], and Lauretani et al. [15] describe clinical and neurobiological characteristics of gastrointestinal, emotional, and sleep-related issues, respectively, proposing tailored therapies for each case. Furthermore, Del Toro-Pérez et al. [16] propose a personalized approach by subclassifying VP based on non-motor symptoms. Finally, Nieto-Escamez et al. [25] review ocular and visual impairments, offering a comprehensive understanding of these symptoms and their management. In conclusion, ongoing research efforts are enhancing our understanding of PD's non-motor aspects, raising hope for improved patient outcomes and a better quality of life.

Author Contributions: Conceptualization, F.N.-E., E.O.-G., H.G.-L. and I.C.-P.; writing—original draft preparation, F.N.-E. and E.O.-G.; writing—review and editing, F.N.-E., E.O.-G., H.G.-L. and I.C.-P. All authors have read and agreed to the published version of the manuscript.

Conflicts of Interest: The authors declare no conflict of interest.

References

1. Lee, H.M.; Koh, S.-B. Many Faces of Parkinson's Disease: Non-Motor Symptoms of Parkinson's Disease. *J. Mov. Disord.* **2015**, *8*, 92–97. [CrossRef] [PubMed]
2. Gupta, S.; Shukla, S. Non-Motor Symptoms in Parkinson's Disease: Opening New Avenues in Treatment. *Curr. Res. Behav. Sci.* **2021**, *2*, 100049. [CrossRef]
3. Drechsel, D.A.; Patel, M. Role of Reactive Oxygen Species in the Neurotoxicity of Environmental Agents Implicated in Parkinson's Disease. *Free Radic. Biol. Med.* **2008**, *44*, 1873–1886. [CrossRef] [PubMed]
4. Ilie, O.-D.; Duta, R.; Jijie, R.; Nita, I.-B.; Nicoara, M.; Faggio, C.; Dobrin, R.; Mavroudis, I.; Ciobica, A.; Doroftei, B. Assessing Anti-Social and Aggressive Behavior in a Zebrafish (Danio Rerio) Model of Parkinson's Disease Chronically Exposed to Rotenone. *Brain Sci.* **2022**, *12*, 898. [CrossRef] [PubMed]
5. Fu, R.; Shen, Q.; Xu, P.; Luo, J.J.; Tang, Y. Phagocytosis of Microglia in the Central Nervous System Diseases. *Mol. Neurobiol.* **2014**, *49*, 1422–1434. [CrossRef]
6. Tada, S.; Choudhury, M.E.; Kubo, M.; Ando, R.; Tanaka, J.; Nagai, M. Zonisamide Ameliorates Microglial Mitochondriopathy in Parkinson's Disease Models. *Brain Sci.* **2022**, *12*, 268. [CrossRef]
7. Scott, L.J. Opicapone: A Review in Parkinson's Disease. *CNS Drugs* **2021**, *35*, 121–131. [CrossRef]
8. Santos García, D.; Fernández Pajarín, G.; Oropesa-Ruiz, J.M.; Escamilla Sevilla, F.; Rahim López, R.R.A.; Muñoz Enríquez, J.G. Opicapone Improves Global Non-Motor Symptoms Burden in Parkinson's Disease: An Open-Label Prospective Study. *Brain Sci.* **2022**, *12*, 383. [CrossRef]
9. Han, J.W.; Ahn, Y.D.; Kim, W.-S.; Shin, C.M.; Jeong, S.J.; Song, Y.S.; Bae, Y.J.; Kim, J.-M. Psychiatric Manifestation in Patients with Parkinson's Disease. *J. Korean Med. Sci.* **2018**, *33*, e300. [CrossRef]
10. Marsh, L. Depression and Parkinson's Disease: Current Knowledge. *Curr. Neurol. Neurosci. Rep.* **2013**, *13*, 409. [CrossRef]
11. Janssen-Aguilar, R.; Rojas, P.; Ruiz-Sánchez, E.; Rodriguez-Violante, M.; Alcántara-Flores, Y.M.; Crail-Meléndez, D.; Cervantes-Arriaga, A.; Sánchez-Escandón, Ó.; Ruiz-Chow, Á.A. Naturalistic Study of Depression Associated with Parkinson's Disease in a National Public Neurological Referral Center in Mexico. *Brain Sci.* **2022**, *12*, 326. [CrossRef] [PubMed]
12. Li, D.-H.; He, Y.-C.; Liu, J.; Chen, S.-D. Diagnostic Accuracy of Transcranial Sonography of the Substantia Nigra in Parkinson's Disease: A Systematic Review and Meta-Analysis. *Sci. Rep.* **2016**, *6*, 20863. [CrossRef] [PubMed]
13. del Toro Pérez, C.; Amaya Pascasio, L.; Arjona Padillo, A.; Olivares Romero, J.; Mejías Olmedo, M.V.; Fernández Pérez, J.; Payán Ortiz, M.; Martínez-Sánchez, P. Neurosonological Findings Related to Non-Motor Features of Parkinson's Disease: A Systematic Review. *Brain Sci.* **2021**, *11*, 776. [CrossRef] [PubMed]
14. Albers, J.A.; Chand, P.; Anch, A.M. Multifactorial Sleep Disturbance in Parkinson's Disease. *Sleep Med.* **2017**, *35*, 41–48. [CrossRef]
15. Lauretani, F.; Testa, C.; Salvi, M.; Zucchini, I.; Giallauria, F.; Maggio, M. Clinical Evaluation of Sleep Disorders in Parkinson's Disease. *Brain Sci.* **2023**, *13*, 609. [CrossRef]
16. del Toro-Pérez, C.; Guevara-Sánchez, E.; Martínez-Sánchez, P. Treatment of Vascular Parkinsonism: A Systematic Review. *Brain Sci.* **2023**, *13*, 489. [CrossRef]
17. Nieto-Escamez, F.; Cortés-Pérez, I.; Obrero-Gaitán, E.; Fusco, A. Virtual Reality Applications in Neurorehabilitation: Current Panorama and Challenges. *Brain Sci.* **2023**, *13*, 819. [CrossRef]

18. García-López, H.; Obrero-Gaitán, E.; Castro-Sánchez, A.M.; Lara-Palomo, I.C.; Nieto-Escamez, F.A.; Cortés-Pérez, I. Non-Immersive Virtual Reality to Improve Balance and Reduce Risk of Falls in People Diagnosed with Parkinson's Disease: A Systematic Review. *Brain Sci.* **2021**, *11*, 1435. [CrossRef]
19. Cersosimo, M.G.; Raina, G.B.; Pecci, C.; Pellene, A.; Calandra, C.R.; Gutiérrez, C.; Micheli, F.E.; Benarroch, E.E. Gastrointestinal Manifestations in Parkinson's Disease: Prevalence and Occurrence before Motor Symptoms. *J. Neurol.* **2013**, *260*, 1332–1338. [CrossRef]
20. Kenna, J.E.; Bakeberg, M.C.; Abonnel, M.Y.; Mastaglia, F.L.; Anderton, R.S. Impact of Gastrointestinal Symptoms on Health-Related Quality of Life in an Australian Parkinson's Disease Cohort. *Park. Dis.* **2022**, *2022*, 4053665. [CrossRef]
21. Soliman, H.; Coffin, B.; Gourcerol, G. Gastroparesis in Parkinson Disease: Pathophysiology, and Clinical Management. *Brain Sci.* **2021**, *11*, 831. [CrossRef] [PubMed]
22. Sauerbier, A.; Jenner, P.; Todorova, A.; Chaudhuri, K.R. Non Motor Subtypes and Parkinson's Disease. *Park. Relat. Disord.* **2016**, *22* (Suppl. S1), S41–S46. [CrossRef] [PubMed]
23. Terashi, H.; Ueta, Y.; Kato, H.; Mitoma, H.; Aizawa, H. Characteristics of Apathy in Treatment-Naïve Patients with Parkinson's Disease. *Int. J. Neurosci.* **2019**, *129*, 16–21. [CrossRef] [PubMed]
24. De Waele, S.; Cras, P.; Crosiers, D. Apathy in Parkinson's Disease: Defining the Park Apathy Subtype. *Brain Sci.* **2022**, *12*, 923. [CrossRef]
25. Nieto-Escamez, F.; Obrero-Gaitán, E.; Cortés-Pérez, I. Visual Dysfunction in Parkinson's Disease. *Brain Sci.* **2023**, *13*, 1173. [CrossRef]

Disclaimer/Publisher's Note: The statements, opinions and data contained in all publications are solely those of the individual author(s) and contributor(s) and not of MDPI and/or the editor(s). MDPI and/or the editor(s) disclaim responsibility for any injury to people or property resulting from any ideas, methods, instructions or products referred to in the content.

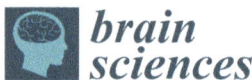

Review

Visual Dysfunction in Parkinson's Disease

Francisco Nieto-Escamez [1,2,*], Esteban Obrero-Gaitán [3,*] and Irene Cortés-Pérez [3]

1. Department of Psychology, University of Almeria, 04120 Almeria, Spain
2. Center for Neuropsychological Assessment and Rehabilitation (CERNEP), 04120 Almeria, Spain
3. Department of Health Sciences, University of Jaen, Paraje Las Lagunillas s/n, 23071 Jaen, Spain; icortes@ujaen.es
* Correspondence: pnieto@ual.es (F.N.-E.); eobrero@ujaen.es (E.O.-G.)

Abstract: Non-motor symptoms in Parkinson's disease (PD) include ocular, visuoperceptive, and visuospatial impairments, which can occur as a result of the underlying neurodegenerative process. Ocular impairments can affect various aspects of vision and eye movement. Thus, patients can show dry eyes, blepharospasm, reduced blink rate, saccadic eye movement abnormalities, smooth pursuit deficits, and impaired voluntary and reflexive eye movements. Furthermore, visuoperceptive impairments affect the ability to perceive and recognize visual stimuli accurately, including impaired contrast sensitivity and reduced visual acuity, color discrimination, and object recognition. Visuospatial impairments are also remarkable, including difficulties perceiving and interpreting spatial relationships between objects and difficulties judging distances or navigating through the environment. Moreover, PD patients can present visuospatial attention problems, with difficulties attending to visual stimuli in a spatially organized manner. Moreover, PD patients also show perceptual disturbances affecting their ability to interpret and determine meaning from visual stimuli. And, for instance, visual hallucinations are common in PD patients. Nevertheless, the neurobiological bases of visual-related disorders in PD are complex and not fully understood. This review intends to provide a comprehensive description of visual disturbances in PD, from sensory to perceptual alterations, addressing their neuroanatomical, functional, and neurochemical correlates. Structural changes, particularly in posterior cortical regions, are described, as well as functional alterations, both in cortical and subcortical regions, which are shown in relation to specific neuropsychological results. Similarly, although the involvement of different neurotransmitter systems is controversial, data about neurochemical alterations related to visual impairments are presented, especially dopaminergic, cholinergic, and serotoninergic systems.

Keywords: Parkinson's disease; visual impairment; visuoperceptive deficit; visuospatial deficit; visual hallucinations; dopamine

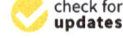

Citation: Nieto-Escamez, F.; Obrero-Gaitán, E.; Cortés-Pérez, I. Visual Dysfunction in Parkinson's Disease. *Brain Sci.* **2023**, *13*, 1173. https://doi.org/10.3390/brainsci13081173

Academic Editors: George B. Stefano and Abdelaziz M. Hussein

Received: 5 June 2023
Revised: 11 July 2023
Accepted: 3 August 2023
Published: 7 August 2023

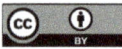

Copyright: © 2023 by the authors. Licensee MDPI, Basel, Switzerland. This article is an open access article distributed under the terms and conditions of the Creative Commons Attribution (CC BY) license (https://creativecommons.org/licenses/by/4.0/).

1. Introduction

Parkinson's disease (PD) is the second most common neurodegenerative disorder after Alzheimer's disease, with an estimated prevalence for industrialized countries of 1% of the population over 60 years and 3% in people older than 80 years [1]. PD is characterized by the loss of dopaminergic neurons in substantia nigra pars compacta, which modulate the fronto–thalamo–striatal circuit, leading to a wide range of motor and non-motor symptoms (NMSs). Thus, NMS is a broad spectrum of symptoms, including mood disorders [4], sensory and perceptual dysfunction [5], and cognitive disturbances [6], with visuospatial processing impairments among the NMSs having accumulated the most interest in the last years [7,8].

Basic visual processes are affected in PD, including reduced spatial contrast sensitivity and impaired color discrimination [9], oculomotor control defects and diplopia [10,11], dry eyes disease [12], glaucoma [13], and visual hallucinations even in the absence of dementia [14]. Furthermore, visual pathologies are accompanied by a poor performance in tasks requiring high-order processing capabilities, such as object mental rotation [15], perception of space [16], spatial maps representation, visuospatial working memory, effective navigation, and target localization [17–19], which can be considered as preclinical markers and predictors of disease development [20].

Impaired visual and visuospatial functions can affect a broad range of essential daily living skills, such as driving, reading, writing, or walking [21,22]. These problems have been reported to be increased throughout the progress of the illness, resulting in a reduction of self-efficacy and quality of life.

This review aims to provide a comprehensive review of ocular, visuoperceptive, and visuospatial disturbances in PD, as well as the consequences of integration deficits between high-level perceptual and cognitive processes. For that purpose, published research employing specific neuropsychological tasks have been included, and the disease's effects on their performance have been examined, even in different phases of the disease. The neurobiological substrates, including structural and functional alterations, and neurochemical mechanisms will be revised for each condition. Until now, some papers reviewing visual disturbances in PD have been published. Some time ago, an outstanding paper by Weil et al. [20] revised changes in visual function at different stages of visual processing, paying special attention to genetic factors, and the relation between clinical features of PD and visuoperceptual alterations as a biomarker of the disease. And, more recently, another remarkable review by Ghazi-Saidi [23] has analyzed the relation between visuospatial and executive deficits in PD. Our work is an attempt to provide an actual and comprehensive picture of visual dysfunctions in PD.

2. Ocular and Visual Impairments in Parkinson's Disease

PD patients show a number of ocular and visual impairments resulting from pathological processes or consequences of medication, and usually get worse during disease progression [24], with up to 70% of patients reporting recurrent visual complaints [25]. Thus, a panoply of oculomotor issues have been described in PD patients [10,26], including poor binocular convergence, double vision (diplopia), bradykinesia and hypokinesia of ocular pursuit, impaired vertical upward and downward glaze, defective saccadic movements with longer reaction times, hypometria, and square wave jerks [24,27–29]. These problems have direct consequences on patients' abilities to perform daily tasks, such as reading, writing, driving, or navigating [5]. Furthermore, visual deficits can even be found in the prodromal stages of PD, as early as decades before the onset of motor symptoms [30].

2.1. Retinal Changes

In the PD population, the main structures that make up the eyeball and the optic nerve are quantitatively and qualitatively affected. High-resolution structural imaging approaches by optical coherence tomography (OCT) of the retina show a decrease of the macular retinal thickness, macular volume, average retinal nerve fiber layer (RNFL), retinal ganglion cell layer (RGC), inner plexiform layer (IPL), inner nuclear layer (INL), outer plexiform layer (OPL), outer nuclear layer (ONL), retinal pigment epithelium, and photoreceptor layer in PD patients [31–34] (See Figure 1). However, macular thickness or volume are not always reduced [33,35].

Some authors have attempted to correlate retinal layer thinning with clinical scales scores. It has been reported that RNFL thickness reduction correlated to duration and severity of disease [35,36]. However, other authors could not confirm this alteration [37–39] nor its relation with disease duration or severity [40]. The RGCIPL layer thickness in the parafovea has been the parameter most frequently correlated with visual outcomes in PD patients [40–42].

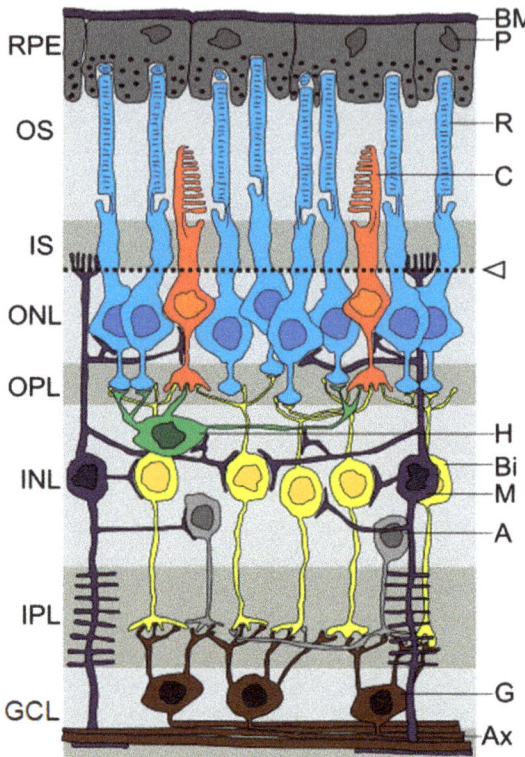

Figure 1. Portion of a human retina. A: Amacrine cell; Bi: Bipolar cell; BM: Bruch's membrane; C: Cone; GCL: Ganglion cell layer; H: Horizontal cell; INL: Inner nuclear layer; IPL: Inner plexiform layer; IS: Inner segment; M: Muller cell; ONL: Outer nuclear layer; OPL: Outer plexiform layer; OS: Outer Segment; P: Pigment epithelial cell; R: Rod; RPE: Retinal pigment epithelium; G: Ganglion cell; AX: Axons. Adapted from Hartmann and Schmid [43]. Image licensed under GFDL by the author. https://de.wikipedia.org/wiki/Datei:Retina.jpg (accessed on 19 June 2023).

Along with structural alterations, functional changes assessed through the visual evoked response (VER) and the electroretinogram (ERG) have also been shown to correlate with PD duration and severity [35]. It has also been proposed that electrophysiological alterations begin years before structural changes are observable [44].

Retinal degeneration may be caused by progressive dopamine depletion and α-synuclein-mediated axonal degeneration [13]. Dopamine is a key neurotransmitter in the retina, and its depletion results in a reduced electrical response under different light conditions [45]. IPL and GCL thinning observed in PD has been linked to dopaminergic loss in the left substantia and disease severity [46]. Furthermore, dopamine also influences other retinal neurotransmitters involved in retinal processing, such as glutamate, GABA, and glycine, disrupting these neurotransmission pathways [44].

Moreover, misfolded α-synuclein [47] and phosphorilated α-synuclein [48] have been reported in the inner retinal layer, and retinal α-synucleinopathy density scores positively correlate with brain α-synucleinopathy density scores, pathology stage, and the UPDRS-III motor sub-score [49].

Retinal and macula nerve fiber layer thinning is also linked with minor hallucinations [50] and disease duration and severity [51]. Moreover, retinal layer thinning correlates with frontal and occipital cortex thickness and is linked to lower scores in the Poppelreuter-Ghent overlapping figures test and the RPMT in a visually impaired PD sample [52].

Recently, Hannaway et al. [53] have reported that visual dysfunction is a better predictor than retinal thickness for dementia in PD.

2.2. Glaucomatous Disturbances

There is also a higher incidence of glaucoma and glaucomatous-like visual field defects, with the majority of cases related to open-angle glaucoma [54,55]. However, epidemiological data are scarce, and the evidence regarding these deficits is low [56,57].

2.3. Pupil Reactivity

Alterations in pupil reactivity have been observed in PD patients. PD patients show a significantly lager pupil diameter, with unequal pupil size after light adaptation and longer light reflex latencies and constriction times, along with reduced contraction amplitude [26,58]. Some studies suggest that pupil changes could be independent from dopaminergic deficiency [59], and dopaminergic treatment has no effect on the pupil light reflex [60]. Alhassan et al. [59] suggest that both parasympathetic (cholinergic) and sympathetic (adrenergic) autonomic systems are altered in PD, but the parasympathetic pathway is more affected. The parasympathetic imbalance is considered an early manifestation of PD [61]. You et al. [62] point out that pupillary parasympathetic dysfunction advances with the progression of PD, whereas pupillary sympathetic dysfunction changes slowly.

Pupil reactivity alterations may also reflect a sensory deficit due to impaired retinal or optic nerve function, but it has also been suggested they could be due to the degeneration of subcortical regions, such as the locus coeruleus in the brain stem [59].

Finally, cognitively impaired PD patients show more pupil constriction deficits than those with normal cognitive functions, similarly to pupil dysfunction reported in Alzheimer's disease [63]. Kahya et al. [64] have reported an increased pupillary response with increased postural demand in PD.

2.4. Eyelid and Blink Reflex

Eyelid impairments, including a reduction of blink rate, apraxia in the opening of the eyelid, blepharospasm, and ptosis of the upper and Meibomian gland disease have been reported [26,65–67]. Three types of eyelid movement abnormalities are notable in the experimental models of PD: blink hyperreflexia, impaired blink reflex plasticity, and reduced rate and impaired rhythm of the spontaneous blinks [68].

Blepharospasm (BSP) is a form of focal dystonia that manifests with spasms of the eyelids, involuntary closure of the eye, and enhanced spontaneous blinking, or any combination of the previous ones [69].

Armstrong [70] reported that blink duration and excitability appear to be increased, which may be related to a loss of dopaminergic neurons. Furthermore, many PD patients show a reduced habituation response of the blink reflex, which may improve after treatment with levodopa or amantidine [70], although other authors reported no positive relationship between blink rate and dopamine synthesis capacity [71].

A reduced corneal sensitivity has been reported in PD by Reddy et al. [72]. And, some authors have shown that the lens can show defects in PD [12], with an increased prevalence of marked nuclear cataracts and a higher intensity of subscapular cataracts.

One of the most usual oculo-visual conditions is dry eye disease, affecting up to 60% of PD patients [12,67]. Dry eye disease in PD can be the result of corneal hypoesthesia, decreasing blinking rate and reflex lacrimation, autonomic neuropathy leading to decreased tear secretion, increased tear osmolarity, decreased tear mucin, and lipid layer disruption secondary to meibomian gland dysfunction [67].

2.5. Visual Acuity, Contrast Sensitivity, and Color Vision in PD

PD patients often complain of poor vision. This deficit can result from, besides other reasons, impaired visual acuity, with low-contrast acuity particularly affected [73]. A reduction of contrast sensitivity has been reported, particularly for intermediate and high frequencies [27] in central (foveal) and peripheral locations [74]. Loss of color vision has also been described [75]. Cross-sectional studies show that PD patients self-report poor eyesight [76] and have poorer objectively measured visual function parameters [77].

Polo et al. [77] found that parameters corresponding to visual acuity at different contrast levels and all contrast sensitivity test results were altered in patients with PD in comparison with healthy participants, with contrast sensitivity the most affected variable. These authors also reported that patients had a tendency to protanomaly.

Polo et al. [77] also proposed that RGC loss could be the cause of contrast and color deficiencies in PD, with dopaminergic D1 and D2 receptors playing a role in color vision and contrast sensitivity alterations [32]. And, reduced macular thickness and volume have been associated with poor visual acuity, contrast sensitivity, and color vision [77].

Although a retinal dopamine deficit might be related to contrast sensitivity deficits, the orientation-specific impairment points to cerebral cortex involvement [20]. Contrast sensitivity deficits can be partially reversed with levodopa, and apomorphine has been shown to improve contrast perception at all spatial frequencies [78].

Color discrimination deficits may be an early dopaminergic symptom in PD and a disease-specific feature [75]. Red–green color blindness (protan–deutan axis) produces blurred vision, with reduced perception of monochromatic contours, especially for dark green, light blue, and dark red stimuli [20]. Color vision dysfunction is observed even at early stages of the disease and progresses with the disease [79], affecting the motor speed and core region of the body performance [73].

Recently, dysfunction across all aspects of vision, including visual acuity, contrast sensitivity, color vision, and higher-order visual processes, have been linked with a higher risk of dementia in PD [80].

2.6. Visual Hallucinations

Visual hallucinations (VHs) are the most common manifestation of psychosis in PD, and have been be associated with rapid cognitive decline in PD patients. Their occurrence takes place in up to 75% of PD patients [81]. Moreover, the pathogenesis of VHs in patients with PD is not well understood. Over the course of the disease, minor hallucinations may first evolve into VHs with retained insight and, subsequently, into multimodality hallucinations with loss of insight and delusions. These usually consist of vividly perceived scenes, including people and animals. Passage hallucinations with objects passing across the peripheral visual field, extracampine hallucinations, and a sense of presence have also been described [81].

VHs in PD have been explained as a result of dysfunction of attentional networks in combination with ambiguous visual input, which may lead to VHs when remembered images intrude into consciousness [82]. Abnormal levels of the default mode network (DMN), a large-scale network that activates during rest, and in daydreaming and musing are observed in PD patients with VHs [83]. According to Weil and Reeves [81], VHs are due to over interpretation of visual input. These authors describe a reduction of white matter in posterior thalamic projections, which may play an important role for network shifting and releasing DMN inhibition [84].

Regarding the contribution of neurotransmitter systems in VHs, it has proved difficult to disentangle, due to the overlapping functional networks involved. It is known that levodopa treatment and dopamine agonists produce VHs [85,86]. It has also been proposed that hypersensitization of nigrostriatal dopaminergic neurons by anti-Parkinson's drugs contribute to VHs [87]. The early disturbance of serotonergic and cholinergic pathways occurring in PD and glutamatergic and GABAergic changes affecting the overall balance between excitatory and inhibitory signaling may also play a role in the decoupling of the DMN [88]. It results in the perception of priors stored in the unconscious memory and the uncontrolled emergence of intrinsic narratives produced by the DMN [88].

VHs predict a range of poor outcomes, including more rapid cognitive decline and the development of dementia [89,90] and an increased likelihood of a move from independent living to a care home [91].

3. Visual Cognition Impairments in Parkinson's Disease

Visual cognition deficits have been commonly reported in PD, although there is no consensus regarding frequency, characteristics, and relationships with other variables. Nevertheless, although many authors agree that visual cognition is not the most affected domain in PD [92,93], the majority of studies report a significant decline in visuospatial, visuoperceptive, visuoconstructive, and visual memory functions [94–96].

Some authors state that visual cognition deficits in PD are the consequence of central processing dysfunction rather than specific visuospatial impairments, particularly low-level perceptual deficits and executive function impairment [97,98]. Low-level visual dysfunction has important implications for understanding cognitive deterioration, as visual input is required for most of the standard neuropsychological tests. But, visual scenery generation and perception are simultaneously coupled with cognitive processes [99]. Thus, it has been reported that PD patients' performance in a wide range of neuropsychological tests involving visual cognition can be attributed to abnormalities in low-level visual functions, especially low- and high-contrast visual acuity [96]. And, it has been suggested that lower-level vision acts as a confounder in object identification or in the time needed to interpret visual sceneries [96].

3.1. Visuospatial Impairment

Visuospatial deficits in PD patients have commonly been assessed with the Judgement of Line Orientation test (JLO), a tool that evaluates the ability to estimate angular relationships between line segments. Several studies have reported significant decreases in JLO scores [96,100–102], particularly in cognitively impaired PD patients [103]. PD patients are prone to confound oblique lines by two or more spacings [104], and show more severe intraquadrant and horizontal lines errors [105]. Some authors have reported that the interference of the visuospatial sketchpad (a component of working memory involved in the storage and manipulation of visual and spatial information) is relevant only in moderate to severe phases of the disease [106]. Recently, Kawashima et al. [107] showed that visuospatial recognition was impaired in the visuospatial o-back test, which does not involve a memory component. And, Kawabata et al. [8] have showed deficits in position discrimination in the Visual Object and Space Perception Battery (VOSP).

Mental rotation and three-dimensional and visual transformation processes have also been reported to be impaired in PD [15,108]. However, there is no consensus about mental rotation abilities in PD. Thus, some authors have documented impaired mental rotation and suggest a problem of the perception of extra-personal space [15], whereas other studies have reported spared mental rotation abilities in PD [109]. It can be argued that each mode of mental transformation is associated with a distinct network of brain regions, and these networks are likely affected differentially by the neuropathology of PD. Amick et al. [110] reported that PD patients showed an impaired ability to mentally rotate hands, but not objects. According to these authors, frontostriatal motor systems and the parietal lobes would play a necessary role for integrating visuospatial cognition with motor imagery during the mental rotation of hands. And, recently, Bek et al. [111] have proposed that PD patients would present difficulties integrating visual and kinesthetic elements of motor imagery.

3.2. Visuoperceptive Impairment

The Facial Recognition Test (FRT) has been used to assess the ability to recognize faces in PD patients without involving a memory component. Some PD patients, even cognitively unimpaired ones, present more difficulties on this test than on the JLO [103,112,113]. Another test, the Visual Form Discrimination Test (VFDT), has been used to evaluate visual recognition impairment in PD. Raskin et al. [114] showed a gradual impairment of visuospatial functions, and other authors have demonstrated that non-demented PD patients fail in this test [101,112]. Some authors have shown that PD patients have difficulties identifying objects embedded in complex figures and are less accurate and make more mistakes in perceptual judgements on a bistable percept paradigm (BPP) [115]. PD patients also show problems in semantical categorization of visual stimuli [116].

Kawabata et al. [8] investigated the features of visuoperceptual disturbances in PD using the battery VOSP. The authors found that one-third of patients exhibited impaired identification of incomplete letters and showed a reduction of functional connectivity in the primary visual network.

Difficulties in the perception of space and depth have also been observed in PD patients. Stereopsis impairment has been observed in some studies [117–119]. It has been explained as a result of basic visual perception alterations, such as color vision and contrast sensitivity deficits [118], and oculomotor behavior [120], which appear linked to the degree of disease deterioration and motor impairment [119].

Difficulties in the detection of motion are also observable in PD [121,122]. This deficit is independent of gait dysfunction and low-level vision changes, and may arise from difficulty perceptually integrating form and motion cues in posterior superior temporal sulcus [121]. These authors reported that PD patients perform significantly worse for human motion than the object motion task.

3.3. Visuoconstructive Impairment

Visuoconstructive impairment in the block design subtest from the Wechsler Adult Intelligence Scale (WAIS) has been related to worsening of other cognitive domains, and motor and severity in PD [123]. In the Clock Drawing Test (CDT), drawing and copy scores are significantly lower in PD, with the last correlated with high-contrast visual acuity measures [96]. Visuoconstructive abilities have also been assessed using more complex copy tests, such as the Rey–Osterrieth Copy Figure (ROCF) [123,124]. Patients show impaired visual cognition, particularly judgement of line orientation and rotation [124].

PD patients, with or without dementia, show a tendency to copy figures very close to the model, a phenomenon called "closing-in" [125]. Initially, it has been explained as a form of constructional apraxia, and some authors have proposed patients have difficulty in the visuospatial analysis of the model and/or in holding this representation in visual working memory [126]. Others suggest that the closing-in phenomenon would be an extreme manifestation of a default tendency of the motor system, so that the actions would be performed toward the focus of attention [127]. De Lucia et al. [128] have proposed that the closing-in phenomenon is related to frontal-executive impairments in PD dementia.

4. Side-of-Onset and Type of Parkinson's Disease in Relation to Visual Symptoms

The side of motor symptom onset is an important consideration in the study of PD, as most patients initially present with symptoms on one side of the body, reflecting the loss of dopamine primarily in the contra-lateral hemisphere. The right hemisphere is more responsible than the left for many spatial abilities, and failure to distinguish patients with LPD from RPD may mean that visuospatial deficits that contribute to functional decline are missed in patients with LPD [129].

A factor that has been shown to influence visual processing in people with PD is the body hemifield where the first motor symptoms appeared [130] and their characteristics [131]. Thus, Verreyt et al. [130] reported that LPD patients more often perform worse on tasks of spatial attention and visuospatial orienting. Davidsdottir et al. [132] examined spatial navigation and visuospatial functioning. LPD patients were generally more visually dependent than RPD patients, who in turn were more visually dependent than the control group. Moreover, egocentric midpoint estimation was dependent on visual input biases, with the deviation increasing for LPD and decreasing for RPD. Schendan et al. [133] used a hierarchical perception task in PD, distinguishing between patients whose motor symptoms started on the left side of the body (LPDs) or the right side (RPDs). These authors observed that LPDs showed an abnormal perception of global elements, whereas RPDs perceived worse the local elements that make up an object. According to Schendan et al. [133], the link between the link side of motor symptoms and visuospatial abilities would rely on the contralateral temporoparietal junction.

On the other side, visual deficits have also been analyzed according to the type of motor symptoms that characterize the onset of the disease, defining two phenotypes: tremor dominant-phenotype (T-D) vs. bradykinesia and rigidity dominant-phenotype (B/R-D). The Visual Activities Questionnaire showed that only the B/R-D group scored significantly worse than controls in light/dark adaptation, visual acuity, depth perception, peripheral vision, and visual processing speed, whereas B/R-D only scored worse in depth perception and light/dark adaptation compared to T-D, suggesting the influence of the type of initial symptoms on visuospatial processing [134]. Other authors have noticed an increased risk of developing VHs in rigid-akinetic patients [135], whereas patients with postural instability and gait difficulty performed worse than those with T-D on visuospatial measures [131].

5. Gender Influence in Visuospatial Symptoms in Parkinson's Disease

Several studies have focused on the analysis of gender differences in the manifestation of cognitive damage in patients with PD and the affected sub-processes. Gender differences have been observed on the Road Map Test of Direction Sense, a right–left discrimination task that requires egocentric mental rotation in space, with men being superior [136]. Davidsdottir et al. [132] examined spatial navigation and visuospatial functioning. Gender differences were found in the navigation task, egocentric midline test, line bisection, and motion perception. Oltra et al. [137] observed that female patients had lower scores than males in the JLO. In the same line, Pasotti et al. [138] analyzed 306 patients of both sexes, observing gender differences in the execution of cognitive tasks, with males superior in visuospatial tasks. These differences were more noticeable in the initial stages of the disease, with the presence of estrogens in dopaminergic neurons being a possible protective factor against cognitive deterioration in this disease. In this line, Crucian et al. [108] reported that men with PD demonstrated significantly lower scores on the Mental Rotations Test than men of similar age and education, whereas PD and control women performed at a similar low level.

Nevertheless, recent research has reported that there was no interaction between sex and Parkinson's diagnosis (with or without mild cognitive impairment) for visuospatial function [139]. Other studies have reported no male–female differences, including Cronin-Golomb and Braun [140] on visuospatial problem solving using Raven's Coloured Progressive Matrices; Amick et al. [110] on mental rotation; and Schendan et al. [133] on hierarchical pattern perception, a test of global and local visual pattern processing. The latter two studies reported LPD-RPD effects. Thus, several studies suggest that gender differences pertain to some, but not all, visuospatial abilities, and may interact with the side of disease onset [129].

6. Neuroanatomical Correlates of Visuospatial and Visuoperceptive Deficits in Parkinson's Disease

Visuospatial (VS) and visuoperceptive (VP) deficits in PD have been related to cortical thinning in the parieto-occipital and fronto-temporal networks, along with structural disturbances in antero-posterior white matter pathways (Table 1). Moreover, as brain degeneration progresses, there is a worsening in VS/VP performance, reaching its worst level with the onset of cognitive impairment [141,142] (Table 2).

Table 1. Neuroanatomical substrate of visuoperceptual, visuospatial, and visuoconstructive impairment in PD.

Domain	Task	Cortical Region
Visuoperceptual	Facial Recognition Test (FRT) [112,141] Visual Form Discrimination Test (VFDT) [112]	Fusiform Gyrus (BA 19, 36) Parahippocampal Middle Occipital Gyrus Inferior Frontal Gyrus (BA 47) Left Lateral Occipital Bilateral Superior Parietal (BA 7, 40) Superior Occipital (BA 19) Inferior Frontal Gyrus (BA 47)
Visuospatial	Judgement Line Orientation Task (JLO) [143]	Bilateral Superior Temporal Right Lateral Occipital
Visuoconstructive	Pentagon Copy Test (PCT) [143]	Right Supplementary Motor Left Rostral Middle Frontal Pars Triangularis Left Cuneus

Table 2. Neuroanatomical substrate of cortical thinning as a possible biomarker of evolution to dementia [141].

Domain	Task	Cortical Region
Visuoperceptual	Facial Recognition Test (FRT) Symbol Digit Modalities Test (SDMT)	Left Lingual Gyrus Left Superior Temporal Left Parahippocampal Left Lingual Gyrus Right Parahippocampal
Visuospatial	Judgement Line Orientation Task (JLO)	Left Insula Inferior Temporal Superior Temporal Right Fusiform Gyrus
Visuoconstruction	Pentagon Copy Test (PCT)	Left Entorhinal Middle and Inferior Temporal Gyri Medial Temporal Pole Parahippocampal Fusiform Cortex Lingual Cortex Lateral Occipital Cortex

Several structural magnetic resonance image (sMRI) studies have found a correlation between neuropsychological test scores and cortical thinning in PD. Pereira et al. [112] found that the gray matter density in the superior parietal and superior occipital gyrus correlated with visuospatial performance in PD, whereas reduced gray matter in the fusiform, the parahippocampus, and the middle occipital gyrus was associated with poor performance on visuoperceptual tests. These authors described the relationship between facial recognition deficits using the FRT and gray matter thinning in the fusiform gyrus (BA 19, 36), and clusters in the parahippocampal region, the middle occipital gyrus (BA 19), and the inferior frontal gyrus (BA 47). Using the same task, Garcia-Diaz et al. [141] described correlated patients' performance with cortical thinning in the left lateral occipital area. On the other side, using the visual form discrimination test (VFDT), Pereira et al. [112] observed that performance correlated with gray matter reductions in the bilateral superior parietal lobes (BA 7, 40) and the superior occipital (BA 19), the middle frontal (BA 9), and the inferior frontal gyrus (BA 47). These results would indicate different patterns in gray matter reduction in visual associative areas for facial recognition and visual form discrimination. Facial recognition would be related to gray matter reductions in areas of the ventral occipitotemporal cortex, whereas visual form discrimination would involve dorsal parietal areas. According to the authors, facial recognition impairment would correlate with the medial temporal lobe, and impaired visual form discrimination with superior parietal regions. Occipitotemporal and occipitoparietal pathways send projections to the prefrontal cortex, where spatial information is maintained "online".

Filoteo et al. [143] have reported a decreased volume bilaterally in the superior temporal cortex and the right lateral occipital cortex (both in the object-based system), with poorer performance in the JLO.

Poorer visuoconstructive performance on the Pentagon Copy test (PCT) has been correlated with decreased volume in the frontal regions (right Supplementary Motor Area, left rostral middle frontal cortex, and pars triangularis), as well as in the object-based system (left Cuneus) [143].

Cognitively impaired PD patients show a more pronounced and extended pattern of cortical atrophy. Rektorova et al. [144] observed gray matter volume reductions in the hippocampus, amygdala, and neocortical temporal regions related to impairment in visuospatial abilities in demented PD patients. More recently, Garcia-Diaz et al. [141] found that MCI-PD patients exhibit significantly greater progressive cortical thinning in left lateral occipital and inferior parietal regions, and in right medial temporal regions. The authors reported that scores on the PCT correlated with a cluster in the left entorhinal region that included the middle and inferior temporal gyri, the medial temporal pole, and the parahippocampal, fusiform, lingual, and lateral occipital cortices. Their performance on the JLO was related to cortical atrophy in clusters in the left insula, inferior, and superior temporal areas, and the right fusiform gyrus, which extended to the left temporal pole, entorhinal, fusiform, and lingual cortices. FRT scores correlated with cortical thinning in the left lingual gyrus. Similarly, the Symbol Digit Modalities Test (SDMT) correlated with a diminution in the left superior temporal, parahippocampal, and lingual, and the right parahippocampal cortices. According to the authors, this anatomical pattern of cortical atrophy was valid when only patients with sustained cognitive impairment at the 4-year follow-up were included. Lee et al. [145] have also described different patterns between amnestic MCI-PD patients (the most common MCI subtype) and non-amnestic MCI-PD patients. The authors reported that visuospatial impairment was more severe in the amnestic group, and a direct comparison between both groups showed a decreased gray matter density in the bilateral precuneus, left primary motor, and right parietal areas.

The side-of-onset also influences the gray matter density pattern in relation to visuospatial alterations. Thus, left PD patients have greater visuospatial impairments compared to right PD patients and lower gray matter volume in the right Dorsolateral Prefrontal Cortex, regardless of other variables, such as age or premorbid cognitive status [146].

Another marker of cortical degeneration in PD related to VS/VP impairment is brain asymmetry. Segura et al. [101] described an initial deterioration of right temporo-parietal regions, followed by a progressive bilateral hemisphere degeneration in PD. As mentioned above, lateralized motor symptoms onset has been studied as a variable that modulates visuospatial skills deterioration.

White matter loss also contributes to worsening visuospatial performance in PD [147]. In the study by García-Díaz et al. [7] on a sample of PD patients, with and without cognitive impairment, the authors reported correlations between VS/VP scores and white matter fractional anisotropy values in the corpus callosum, bilateral forceps minor, uncinate fasciculus, inferior frontooccipital fasciculus, forceps major, and inferior longitudinal fasciculus. All the VS/VP tests studied showed significant correlations between their scored and fractional anisometropia values, but it was larger for the SDMT.

7. Functional Neuroimage Correlates of VS/VP Deficits in Parkinsons' Disease

Most functional neuroimaging studies (functional MRI, positron emission tomography PET, and single-photon emission computerized tomography SPECT) have reported altered activation, altered blood flow, or reduced metabolism in both dorsal and ventral visual pathways, which probably indicates an alteration in the normal bottom–top visual processing and the presence of aberrant top–down visual processing [148].

Early studies based on PET imaging by Eberling et al. [149] and Bohnen et al. [150] showed a clear reduction of cerebral glucose metabolism in visual association, primary visual, and right parietal cortices in non-cognitively affected patients. Furthermore, lower performance in visuospatial tasks has been associated with fluoro-deoxyglucose hypometabolism or hypoperfusion in occipital and frontal cortices of non-cognitively impaired subjects [151], along with lower levels of 123I-iodoamphetamine single-photon emission computed tomography-based assessment in right hemisphere posterior-frontal cortices [152].

With disease progression, incident dementia in idiopathic PD is announced by metabolic changes within visual association (BA 18) and posterior cingulate cortices. Findings indicate that incident dementia preferentially involves BA18, whereas reductions in the primary visual cortex (BA 17) can be seen in PD without dementia. The Benton Visual Retention test, which assesses visuospatial perception, visuomotor and visuoconstructive abilities, and visual memory, best correlates with BA 18 metabolism [153]. Extension of occipital hypometabolism from the primary to the visual association cortices, together with precuneus hypometabolism, may be the early cortical metabolic "signature" of incident dementia in PD, with visual association cortex hypometabolism linked to the presence of VHs in more advanced PD [153].

Using functional magnetic resonance (fMRI), Caproni et al. [154] found that PD patients had reduced activation of the right insula, left putamen, bilateral caudate (in particular, in the right hemisphere), and right hippocampus, together with greater activation of the right dorso-lateral prefrontal cortex (DLPFC) and bilateral posterior parietal cortex (PPC) during visuospatial judgement. The authors propose that the DLPFC activation reflex is a compensatory mechanism, through continuous control by the top–down visual processing system.

Alteration in PD brain function related to VS/VP deficits has also been observed via non-invasive resting state fMRI, supporting the idea of a marked fronto-occipital-parietal dysfunction in the right hemisphere [155], which is more noticeable as the disease progresses [156], and is responsible for VS/VP impairments [157]. Although such reduction of right-hemisphere functional connectivity is observable in early stages, it progresses and affects bilateral prefrontal and frontoparietal networks when mild cognitive impairment (MCI) and/or dementia appear [158], accompanied by increased Regional Homogeneity (ReHo) in the medial-superior occipital gyrus compared to healthy controls [159].

8. Neuroanatomical Correlates of Parkinson's Disease Visual Hallucinations

Imaging studies of VHs in PD to date have been based on relatively small samples and have used different designs to control for the degree of cognitive decline, stage of PD, and dopamine medication, showing little consistency across studies [160].

A number of structural neuroimaging studies have analyzed the cerebral basis of VHs in PD. Gray matter atrophy has been described in multiple regions of the brain, such as the primary visual and visual association cortices; limbic regions, and cholinergic structures, such as the pedunculopontine nucleus and substantia innominata, which are involved in visuospatial-perception, attention control, and memory [148].

Widespread reductions in the cortical thickness of PD patients with hallucinations have been identified in the occipital, parietal, temporal, frontal, and limbic lobes of PD patients with VHs. However, not all regions are equally affected, and, notably, there appears to be a posterior asymmetry, with relative sparing of the left ventral visual stream (ventral occipitotemporal cortex) compared to the homologous region in the right hemisphere [161]. Of these, the cuneus and superior frontal gyrus bilaterally emerged as the dominant components.

Ramírez-Ruiz et al. [162], in a VBM study, reported reduced GM volume in the left lingual gyrus and bilateral superior parietal lobule in PD patients with VHs compared to those without VHs. Pagonabarraga et al. [163] have proposed a progressive volume reduction from the unilateral left superior parietal in minor hallucinations (mHs) to the bilateral superior parietal in VHs. A significant reduction of GM volume has been observed in the right inferior frontal, left temporal, and thalamic areas [164]; the left opercula frontal gyrus and left superior frontal gyrus [165]; the cingulate [166]; and in the bilateral dorsolateral prefrontal cortex, rostral part of prefrontal cortex, bilateral primary visual cortex, and regions corresponding to the secondary visual cortex, such as the left inferior occipital gyrus, right lingual cortex, right supramarginal gyrus, and left fusiform gyrus [167]. Vignando et al. [161] report that regions with reduced thickness for higher severity scores (negative correlation) were found in the posterior parietal, posterior cingulate, and superior temporal cortex. It has also been observed a degenerative process in the head of the hippocampus in hallucinating PD patients [168] that would involve the whole hippocampus and cause dementia in hallucinating PD patients. The atrophy of cholinergic structures, such as the pedunculopontine nucleus (PPN) and its thalamic projections, has also been associated with VHs in PD [169], the substantia innominata (SI) [164]. Finally, reduced volume in cerebellar lobules VIII, IX/VII, and Crus 1 has been associated with VHs in PD [170].

Goldman et al. [166] observed that gray matter atrophy occurred both in the ventral (what) and dorsal (where) pathways, responsible for object and facial recognition and identification of the spatial locations of objects. Thus, those patients who experienced VHs exhibited gray matter atrophy in the cuneus, lingual, and fusiform gyri; middle occipital lobe; inferior parietal lobe; and cingulate, paracentral, and precentral gyri. These structural changes were not related to the presence of dementia.

9. Functional Neuroimage Correlates of Parkinsons' Disease Visual Hallucinations

A seminal fMRI study by Stebbins et al. [171] reported that VHs in PD patients reflect an abnormally increased activation in anterior cortical regions, such as the inferior frontal cortex and caudate nucleus, accompanied with reduced activation in the parietal lobe and cingulate gyrus, which has been explained as a shifting of attentional visual circuitry from posterior (down–top) to anterior (top–down) regions. More recently, Yao et al. [83] reported an increased functional connectivity in the default mode network (DMN) in the right middle frontal gyrus and bilateral posterior cingulate gyrus/precuneus of VH PD patients in comparison to non-VH patients. These data support the hypothesis of an excessive and aberrant top–down processing.

PET studies have reported an increased glucose metabolism in frontal regions (the left superior frontal gyrus) in hallucinating PD patients [172], and a decreased metabolism in the occipito-parieto-temporal region (sparing the occipital pole) that included both dorsal and ventral visual streams [173]. Park et al. [174] has reported a reduced metabolism in both visual streams of hallucinating PD patients, but predominantly in the ventral one. In the same line, a SPECT study by Oishi et al. [175] reported increased perfusion in the right superior and middle temporal gyri in hallucinating PD patients. The increased perfusion of the superior temporal gyrus is in line with the hypothesis of prevalent top–down visual processing. Also, the fronto–striatal circuit involved in the dorsal attention network has been involved in the pathogenesis of VHs in PD [176]. Kiferle et al. [177] have suggested that frontal impairment observed in PD patients with VHs may be due to a right caudate dysfunction, reflecting an impairment of cortico–subcortical circuits.

Dysregulation of the ventral attentional network (VAN), dorsal attentional network (DAN), and default mode network (DMN) have been implicated in models of VHs in PD [178] with reduced activity in the DAN [82]. PD patients with hallucinations show widespread disruption in structural connections, which particularly affect highly connected brain regions or "hubs" required for brain transitions between different cognitive states [179,180] (See Figure 2). Zarkali et al. [181] found that PD patients with hallucinations show impaired temporal dynamics, with a predisposition towards a predominantly segregated state of functional connectivity, and require less energy to transition from the integrated to the segregated state. Moreover, the thalamus and regions within the DMN are critically involved in the network imbalance in PD hallucinations.

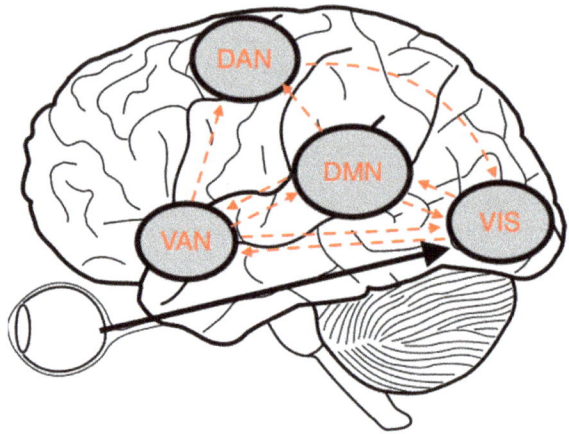

Figure 2. The van Ommen [182] model of visual hallucinations. Complex VHs are the result of a dissociation of higher-order visual processing areas from the primary visual cortex. Simultaneously, a looping of brain activity across the outside-world-focused DAN, the inner-world-focused and memory-related DMN, and the saliency-focused VAN, bias conscious visual perception away from information coming from the outer world and towards internally generated percepts. Visual network (VIS). Modified from "Human Brain sketch with eyes and cerebrellum.svg", work released into the public domain by Hankem. https://commons.wikimedia.org/wiki/File:Human_Brain_sketch_with_eyes_and_cerebrellum.svg (accessed on 11 July 2023).

10. Neurochemistry of VS/VP Deficits in Parkinsons' Disease

Dopaminergic neurons are diffusely present within the retina. Dopamine is present in the retina in amacrine cells of the inner border of the inner nuclear layer and in interplexiform cells, influencing the activity of photoreceptors, ganglion cells, and bipolar cell receptive fields [183,184]. The role of dopaminergic reduction in the basal ganglia and the impact on the arterial walls of the frontal cortex would explain the appearance of problems in eye movements and in pupil reactivity in PD [27,185]. Reductions in dopamine levels in the basal ganglia and frontal cortex may also deplete levels in the superior colliculus and, therefore, could be a factor in the production of defective saccades [186]. Furthermore, it has been observed that dopaminergic medication adversely impacts visuoperceptual performance, with it worse in the *on* compared to the *off* medication state. Thus, dopaminergic medication can ameliorate movement deficits, but reduces visuoperceptual accuracy because of overdosing [187]. Finally, it must be also noted that although all dopaminergic drugs have been associated with incident VHs, this association has been shown contradictory [163], and other factors could be considered responsible [188].

The imbalance of the pedunculopontine cholinergic projections on the visual cortex produces aberrant visuospatial processing [123]. Moreover, the appearance of abnormal VP phenomena, such as hallucinations in people with PD, has been associated with degeneration of the nucleus basalis of Meynert and its cholinergic projections between the brainstem and the frontal cortex, also affecting the execution of visuospatial tasks [189,190].

In addition to the dopaminergic–cholinergic balance, VHs have been associated with decreased occipital GABA in PD [191]. Whether this system is affected in the retina and visual cortex of all PD patients, and from early stages, remains to be determined.

Regarding other neurotransmission systems, the serotonergic system also seems to play a key role in the manifestation of VHs and visuoperceptual function in PD. Thus, VHs and other visual-perceptual dysfunctions have been observed in PD associated with a decrease of the serotonergic receptor 5-HT2A in the right insula, bilateral dorsolateral prefrontal cortex, right orbitofrontal cortex, right middle temporal gyrus, and right fusiform gyrus (Cho et al., 2017). Vignando et al. [161] reported an association for 5-HT2A and 5-HT1A confined to regions linked to VHs, rather than the cortex as a whole, suggesting the neurotransmitter effects were specific to VHs, suggesting the possibility that degeneration in these neurotransmitter systems in PD underlies synaptic loss and cortical thinning. Cho et al. [192] have also reported that 5-HT2A correlated with visuoperceptual function. In particular, the FRT score was related to receptor binding in the right anterior cingulate cortex (ACC), left DLPFC, and inferior temporal gyrus. A reduced binding in ACC and other prefrontal regions was related to a lower VOSP total score. The author also described negative correlations between 5-HT2A in the middle/inferior temporal gyrus and Rey Complex Figure copy scores, as well as between the occipital BA 18 and JLO scores. These regions are part of the ventral visual system within the bottom–up network.

11. Genetic Factors of VS/VP Deficits in Parkinsons' Disease

Although genetic factors are only implicated in a minority of cases of PD, genetic approaches could contribute to understanding the etiology and manifestation of VS/VP impairments in PD. Mutations in the leucine-rich repeat kinase 2 (LRRK2) and parkin RBR E3 ubiquitin protein ligase genes are thought to be protective against cognitive impairment and ocular disturbances [193]. Moreover, lysosomal enzyme glucocerebrosidase (GBA) mutation carriers show poor visuospatial performance [194,195] and a higher frequency of hallucinations [196]. Moreover, it has been reported that microtubule-associated protein tau (MAPT) H1 haplotype carriers present a higher risk of dementia, are less accurate with difficult spatial rotations, and show lower activity in the parietal cortex and caudate nuclei [197].

12. Conclusions

Numerous visual and perceptual problems have been observed in patients with PD. However, these problems are usually under-recognized and poorly understood, leading to a lack of appropriate treatment.

Different structures and networks have been involved in visual deficits in PD, from lower-level structures, such as the retina, to visual pathways involved in higher-level visual cognition. Thus, low-level visual dysfunction, like visual acuity and contrast sensitivity impairment, has been extensively observed in PD. And, as most of the standard neuropsychological measures rely on visual input for assessing cognitive functions, it is observed that lower mechanisms' deficits also affect higher cognitive capabilities. Moreover, visual scenery generation and perception are also limited by cognitive processes that are deteriorated in PD, such as attention [99]. As result, the incoming visual information is constantly regulated and tuned by top–down processes [154].

One of the main approaches to study the causes of VS/VP deficits in PD has been the structural neuroimage. Studies have shown alterations in the cortical thickness of bilateral temporo–parietal–occipital areas and widespread posterior–anterior white matter microstructure alterations [7,198]. In addition, bilateral degeneration of posterior cortical regions is associated with a progressive worsening in VS/VP performance. And, it is also observed a progressive cortical volume reduction in posterior parieto-temporal regions of PD-MCI in comparison with cognitively unimpaired PD subjects [141].

Functional alterations in both cortical areas and subcortical regions involved in VS/VP have been also observed in PD. In particular, a reduced activation in the right insula, left putamen, bilateral caudate, and right hippocampus, as well as an over-activation of the right dorso-lateral prefrontal and the posterior parietal cortices, particularly in the right hemisphere, have been observed in PD. Moreover, a loss of cortical efficiency and compensatory mechanisms during visual processing have also been observed in PD patients [143,154]. It has been observed that PD patients showed greater activations of right DLPFC and bilateral PPC. Both of these regions, together with frontal–striatal circuits, are known to be part of the "Top–Down" visual processing system, which is involved in the selection and organization of complex visual information. DLPFC greater activation has been considered a compensatory response in PD patients, involving a continuous control by "Top–Down" mechanisms associated with visual working memory. Moreover, the greater activation of bilateral PPC could be necessary to overcome the initial impairment of the network [154].

Some authors have also suggested a role for lateralization of the basal ganglia circuits in stimuli perception, associated with a different clinical manifestation in left- and right-side PD onset [133]. Thus, right-sided onset PD is characterized by impairment in local-level processing, a consequence of left frontal and parietal deficits, whereas left-sided onset PD is characterized by an alteration of global-level processing, due to right parietal dysfunction [110,133].

Research about neurochemical alterations associated with VS/VP disturbances in PD is scarce, and many times the results have been contradictory. Different studies have reported the dopaminergic basis of retinal and other neurodegenerative pathologies in PD related to visual and ocular alterations [27,185], whereas visuoperceptive and visuospatial impairments correlate with abnormalities in several interrelated neurotransmitter systems, mainly the dopaminergic, noradrenergic, serotonergic, and cholinergic systems [189,199].

Visuoperceptual and visuospatial deficits in PD correlate to disease progression and have been proposed as an early marker of cognitive deterioration [132]. For instance, cross-sectional correlational studies have established a relationship between the degree of atrophy in posterior brain regions and VS/VP impairment [141]. Moreover, visuoperceptual deficits have also been associated with VHs, which are also considered predictive of disease progression.

VHs are part of the syndrome of PD psychosis, and one of the most debilitating symptoms for patients' quality of life. Although, the precise pathophysiology of VHs in PD remains unclear, neuropathological and structural imaging studies have provided some insight [199]. Thus, neuroimaging studies have revealed gray matter atrophy in multiple regions, with the most prominent changes across areas involved in visual perception (including the ventral 'what' and dorsal 'where' pathways), the hippocampus, and several cholinergic brain structures, such as the substantia innominata and pedunculopontine nucleus [164,166]. It has been considered that dentification of brain structures associated with VHs in PD may permit earlier detection of at-risk patients and ultimately development of new therapies for targeting hallucinations and visuoperceptive functions [166].

As detailed above, the etiology and neurobiological bases of visual and perceptual impairments in PD are complex and multifaceted, and the same could be said with regard to their association with motor symptoms. Ocular, visual, visuoperceptive, and visuospatial deficits can occur independently in PD and may depend on multiple factors. Thus, each individual with PD may present a unique combination of these impairments, with variable symptomatology. Moreover, these alterations are hypothesized to play a role in the etiology of the main motor signs of PD, such as the freezing of gait [200]. Therefore, to reveal the particular mechanisms behind visual symptomatology and the potential therapeutic strategies poses a tremendous challenge for future research. The combination of genetics and functional neuroimaging can provide a promising strategy for classification and identification of potential biomarkers, which can be tested in future clinical trials designed to fight and prevent PD.

Author Contributions: Conceptualization, F.N.-E. and I.C.-P.; writing—original draft preparation, F.N.-E. and E.O.-G.; writing—review and editing, F.N.-E., E.O.-G. and I.C.-P. All authors have read and agreed to the published version of the manuscript.

Funding: This research received no external funding.

Institutional Review Board Statement: Not applicable.

Informed Consent Statement: Not applicable.

Data Availability Statement: No new data were created.

Conflicts of Interest: The authors declare no conflict of interest.

References

1. Lee, A.; Gilbert, R.M. Epidemiology of Parkinson Disease. *Neurol. Clin.* **2016**, *34*, 955–965. [CrossRef]
2. Poewe, W.; Seppi, K.; Tanner, C.M.; Halliday, G.M.; Brundin, P.; Volkmann, J.; Schrag, A.-E.; Lang, A.E. Parkinson disease. *Nat. Rev. Dis. Primer* **2017**, *3*, 17013. [CrossRef] [PubMed]
3. Zhai, S.; Tanimura, A.; Graves, S.M.; Shen, W.; Surmeier, D.J. Striatal synapses, circuits, and Parkinson's disease. *Curr. Opin. Neurobiol.* **2018**, *48*, 9–16. [CrossRef] [PubMed]
4. Lemke, M.R.; Fuchs, G.; Gemende, I.; Herting, B.; Oehlwein, C.; Reichmann, H.; Rieke, J.; Volkmann, J. Depression and Parkinson's disease. *J. Neurol.* **2004**, *251* (Suppl. S6), vi24–vi27. [CrossRef]
5. Davidsdottir, S.; Cronin-Golomb, A.; Lee, A. Visual and spatial symptoms in Parkinson's disease. *Vision Res.* **2005**, *45*, 1285–1296. [CrossRef]
6. Janvin, C.C.; Larsen, J.P.; Salmon, D.P.; Galasko, D.; Hugdahl, K.; Aarsland, D. Cognitive profiles of individual patients with Parkinson's disease and dementia: Comparison with dementia with lewy bodies and Alzheimer's disease. *Mov. Disord.* **2006**, *21*, 337–342. [CrossRef]
7. Garcia-Diaz, A.I.; Segura, B.; Baggio, H.C.; Marti, M.J.; Valldeoriola, F.; Compta, Y.; Bargallo, N.; Uribe, C.; Campabadal, A.; Abos, A.; et al. Structural Brain Correlations of Visuospatial and Visuoperceptual Tests in Parkinson's Disease. *J. Int. Neuropsychol. Soc.* **2018**, *24*, 33–44. [CrossRef] [PubMed]
8. Kawabata, K.; Ohdake, R.; Watanabe, H.; Bagarinao, E.; Hara, K.; Ogura, A.; Masuda, M.; Kato, T.; Yokoi, T.; Katsuno, M.; et al. Visuoperceptual disturbances in Parkinson's disease. *Clin. Park. Relat. Disord.* **2020**, *3*, 100036. [CrossRef]
9. Pieri, V.; Diederich, N.J.; Raman, R.; Goetz, C.G. Decreased color discrimination and contrast sensitivity in Parkinson's disease. *J. Neurol. Sci.* **2000**, *172*, 7–11. [CrossRef]
10. Almer, Z.; Klein, K.S.; Marsh, L.; Gerstenhaber, M.; Repka, M.X. Ocular motor and sensory function in Parkinson's disease. *Ophthalmology* **2012**, *119*, 178–182. [CrossRef]
11. Antoniades, C.A.; Kennard, C. Ocular motor abnormalities in neurodegenerative disorders. *Eye* **2015**, *29*, 200–207. [CrossRef]
12. Nowacka, B.; Lubinski, W.; Honczarenko, K.; Potemkowski, A.; Safranow, K. Ophthalmological features of Parkinson disease. *Med. Sci. Monit. Int. Med. J. Exp. Clin. Res.* **2014**, *20*, 2243–2249. [CrossRef]
13. Nucci, C.; Martucci, A.; Cesareo, M.; Garaci, F.; Morrone, L.A.; Russo, R.; Corasaniti, M.T.; Bagetta, G.; Mancino, R. Links among glaucoma, neurodegenerative, and vascular diseases of the central nervous system. *Prog. Brain Res.* **2015**, *221*, 49–65. [CrossRef]
14. Gibson, G.; Mottram, P.G.; Burn, D.J.; Hindle, J.V.; Landau, S.; Samuel, M.; Hurt, C.S.; Brown, R.G.; M Wilson, K.C. Frequency, prevalence, incidence and risk factors associated with visual hallucinations in a sample of patients with Parkinson's disease: A longitudinal 4-year study. *Int. J. Geriatr. Psychiatry* **2013**, *28*, 626–631. [CrossRef] [PubMed]
15. Lee, A.C.; Harris, J.P.; Calvert, J.E. Impairments of mental rotation in Parkinson's disease. *Neuropsychologia* **1998**, *36*, 109–114. [CrossRef] [PubMed]
16. Harris, J.P.; Atkinson, E.A.; Lee, A.C.; Nithi, K.; Fowler, M.S. Hemispace differences in the visual perception of size in left hemiParkinson's disease. *Neuropsychologia* **2003**, *41*, 795–807. [CrossRef] [PubMed]
17. Owen, A.M.; Beksinska, M.; James, M.; Leigh, P.N.; Summers, B.A.; Marsden, C.D.; Quinn, N.P.; Sahakian, B.J.; Robbins, T.W. Visuospatial memory deficits at different stages of Parkinson's disease. *Neuropsychologia* **1993**, *31*, 627–644. [CrossRef] [PubMed]
18. Possin, K.L.; Filoteo, J.V.; Song, D.D.; Salmon, D.P. Spatial and Object Working Memory Deficits in Parkinson's Disease are Due to Impairment in Different Underlying Processes. *Neuropsychology* **2008**, *22*, 585–595. [CrossRef]
19. Possin, K.L. Visual Spatial Cognition in Neurodegenerative Disease. *Neurocase* **2010**, *16*, 466–487. [CrossRef]
20. Weil, R.S.; Schrag, A.E.; Warren, J.D.; Crutch, S.J.; Lees, A.J.; Morris, H.R. Visual dysfunction in Parkinson's disease. *Brain* **2016**, *139*, 2827–2843. [CrossRef]
21. Hertanti, A.; Retnawati, H.; Wutsqa, D.U. The role of spatial experience in mental rotation. *J. Phys. Conf. Ser.* **2019**, *1320*, 012043. [CrossRef]
22. Tinella, L.; Lopez, A.; Caffò, A.O.; Nardulli, F.; Grattagliano, I.; Bosco, A. Cognitive Efficiency and Fitness-to-Drive along the Lifespan: The Mediation Effect of Visuospatial Transformations. *Brain Sci.* **2021**, *11*, 1028. [CrossRef]
23. Ghazi-Saidi, L. Visuospatial and Executive Deficits in Parkinson's Disease: A Review. *Acta Sci. Neurol.* **2020**, *3*, 08–26. [CrossRef]
24. Ekker, M.S.; Janssen, S.; Seppi, K.; Poewe, W.; de Vries, N.M.; Theelen, T.; Nonnekes, J.; Bloem, B.R. Ocular and visual disorders in Parkinson's disease: Common but frequently overlooked. *Park. Relat. Disord.* **2017**, *40*, 1–10. [CrossRef] [PubMed]
25. Urwyler, P.; Nef, T.; Killen, A.; Collerton, D.; Thomas, A.; Burn, D.; McKeith, I.; Mosimann, U.P. Visual complaints and visual hallucinations in Parkinson's disease. *Park. Relat. Disord.* **2014**, *20*, 318–322. [CrossRef]

26. Biousse, V.; Skibell, B.C.; Watts, R.L.; Loupe, D.N.; Drews-Botsch, C.; Newman, N.J. Ophthalmologic features of Parkinson's disease. *Neurology* **2004**, *62*, 177–180. [CrossRef]
27. Armstrong, R.A. Oculo-Visual Dysfunction in Parkinson's Disease. *J. Park. Dis.* **2015**, *5*, 715–726. [CrossRef] [PubMed]
28. Buhmann, C.; Kraft, S.; Hinkelmann, K.; Krause, S.; Gerloff, C.; Zangemeister, W.H. Visual Attention and Saccadic Oculomotor Control in Parkinson's Disease. *Eur. Neurol.* **2015**, *73*, 283–293. [CrossRef]
29. Tomsak, R.L.; Daroff, R.B. Ophthalmologic features of Parkinson's disease. *Neurology* **2004**, *63*, 940–941. [CrossRef]
30. Mahlknecht, P.; Seppi, K.; Poewe, W. The Concept of Prodromal Parkinson's Disease. *J. Park. Dis.* **2015**, *5*, 681–697. [CrossRef]
31. Chrysou, A.; Jansonius, N.M.; van Laar, T. Retinal layers in Parkinson's disease: A meta-analysis of spectral-domain optical coherence tomography studies. *Park. Relat. Disord.* **2019**, *64*, 40–49. [CrossRef] [PubMed]
32. Hajee, M.E.; March, W.F.; Lazzaro, D.R.; Wolintz, A.H.; Shrier, E.M.; Glazman, S.; Bodis-Wollner, I.G. Inner retinal layer thinning in Parkinson disease. *Arch. Ophthalmol.* **2009**, *127*, 737–741. [CrossRef]
33. Huang, J.; Li, Y.; Xiao, J.; Zhang, Q.; Xu, G.; Wu, G.; Liu, T.; Luo, W. Combination of Multifocal Electroretinogram and Spectral-Domain OCT Can Increase Diagnostic Efficacy of Parkinson's Disease. *Park. Dis.* **2018**, *2018*, 4163239. [CrossRef] [PubMed]
34. Unlu, M.; Gulmez Sevim, D.; Gultekin, M.; Karaca, C. Correlations among multifocal electroretinography and optical coherence tomography findings in patients with Parkinson's disease. *Neurol. Sci.* **2018**, *39*, 533–541. [CrossRef] [PubMed]
35. Kaur, M.; Saxena, R.; Singh, D.; Behari, M.; Sharma, P.; Menon, V. Correlation Between Structural and Functional Retinal Changes in Parkinson Disease. *J. Neuro-Ophthalmol.* **2015**, *35*, 254–258. [CrossRef]
36. Garcia-Martin, E.; Rodriguez-Mena, D.; Satue, M.; Almarcegui, C.; Dolz, I.; Alarcia, R.; Seral, M.; Polo, V.; Larrosa, J.M.; Pablo, L.E. Electrophysiology and optical coherence tomography to evaluate Parkinson disease severity. *Investig. Ophthalmol. Vis. Sci.* **2014**, *55*, 696–705. [CrossRef]
37. Moschos, M.M.; Tagaris, G.; Markopoulos, I.; Margetis, I.; Tsapakis, S.; Kanakis, M.; Koutsandrea, C. Morphologic changes and functional retinal impairment in patients with Parkinson disease without visual loss. *Eur. J. Ophthalmol.* **2011**, *21*, 24–29. [CrossRef]
38. Archibald, N.K.; Clarke, M.P.; Mosimann, U.P.; Burn, D.J. Retinal thickness in Parkinson's disease. *Park. Relat. Disord.* **2011**, *17*, 431–436. [CrossRef]
39. Tsironi, E.E.; Dastiridou, A.; Katsanos, A.; Dardiotis, E.; Veliki, S.; Patramani, G.; Zacharaki, F.; Ralli, S.; Hadjigeorgiou, G.M. Perimetric and retinal nerve fiber layer findings in patients with Parkinson's disease. *BMC Ophthalmol.* **2012**, *12*, 54. [CrossRef]
40. Sari, E.S.; Koc, R.; Yazici, A.; Sahin, G.; Ermis, S.S. Ganglion cell-inner plexiform layer thickness in patients with Parkinson disease and association with disease severity and duration. *J. Neuro-Ophthalmol.* **2015**, *35*, 117–121. [CrossRef]
41. Liu, L.; Jia, Y.; Takusagawa, H.L.; Pechauer, A.D.; Edmunds, B.; Lombardi, L.; Davis, E.; Morrison, J.C.; Huang, D. Optical Coherence Tomography Angiography of the Peripapillary Retina in Glaucoma. *JAMA Ophthalmol.* **2015**, *133*, 1045–1052. [CrossRef] [PubMed]
42. Sung, M.S.; Choi, S.-M.; Kim, J.; Ha, J.Y.; Kim, B.-C.; Heo, H.; Park, S.W. Inner retinal thinning as a biomarker for cognitive impairment in de novo Parkinson's disease. *Sci. Rep.* **2019**, *9*, 11832. [CrossRef] [PubMed]
43. Hartmann, P.; Schmid, M.G. Retina Layers. Available online: https://de.wikipedia.org/wiki/Datei:Retina.jpg (accessed on 19 July 2023).
44. Alves, J.N.; Westner, B.U.; Højlund, A.; Weil, R.S.; Dalal, S.S. Structural and functional changes in the retina in Parkinson's disease. *J. Neurol. Neurosurg. Psychiatry* **2023**, *94*, 448–456. [CrossRef]
45. Bodis-Wollner, I. Neuropsychological and perceptual defects in Parkinson's disease. *Park. Relat. Disord.* **2003**, *9* (Suppl. S2), S83–S89. [CrossRef]
46. Ahn, J.; Lee, J.-Y.; Kim, T.W.; Yoon, E.J.; Oh, S.; Kim, Y.K.; Kim, J.-M.; Woo, S.J.; Kim, K.W.; Jeon, B. Retinal thinning associates with nigral dopaminergic loss in de novo Parkinson disease. *Neurology* **2018**, *91*, e1003–e1012. [CrossRef] [PubMed]
47. Bodis-Wollner, I.; Kozlowski, P.B.; Glazman, S.; Miri, S. α-synuclein in the inner retina in parkinson disease. *Ann. Neurol.* **2014**, *75*, 964–966. [CrossRef]
48. Beach, T.G.; Carew, J.; Serrano, G.; Adler, C.H.; Shill, H.A.; Sue, L.I.; Sabbagh, M.N.; Akiyama, H.; Cuenca, N.; Arizona Parkinson's Disease Consortium. Phosphorylated α-synuclein-immunoreactive retinal neuronal elements in Parkinson's disease subjects. *Neurosci. Lett.* **2014**, *571*, 34–38. [CrossRef]
49. Ortuño-Lizarán, I.; Beach, T.G.; Serrano, G.E.; Walker, D.G.; Adler, C.H.; Cuenca, N. Phosphorylated α-synuclein in the retina is a biomarker of Parkinson's disease pathology severity. *Mov. Disord.* **2018**, *33*, 1315–1324. [CrossRef]
50. Lee, J.-Y.; Kim, J.M.; Ahn, J.; Kim, H.-J.; Jeon, B.S.; Kim, T.W. Retinal nerve fiber layer thickness and visual hallucinations in Parkinson's Disease. *Mov. Disord.* **2014**, *29*, 61–67. [CrossRef]
51. Miri, S.; Shrier, E.M.; Glazman, S.; Ding, Y.; Selesnick, I.; Kozlowski, P.B.; Bodis-Wollner, I. The avascular zone and neuronal remodeling of the fovea in Parkinson disease. *Ann. Clin. Transl. Neurol.* **2015**, *2*, 196–201. [CrossRef]
52. Litvinenko, I.V.; Boyko, E.V.; Kulikov, A.N.; Dynin, P.S.; Trufanov, A.G.; Mal'tsev, D.S.; Yurin, A.A. The Relationship between Visuospatial Impairments and Retinal and Cortical Thickness in Parkinson's Disease. *Hum. Physiol.* **2017**, *43*, 863–869. [CrossRef]
53. Hannaway, N.; Zarkali, A.; Leyland, L.-A.; Bremner, F.; Nicholas, J.M.; Wagner, S.K.; Roig, M.; Keane, P.A.; Toosy, A.; Chataway, J.; et al. Visual dysfunction is a better predictor than retinal thickness for dementia in Parkinson's disease. *J. Neurol. Neurosurg. Psychiatry* **2023**, *0*, 1–9. [CrossRef]

54. Bayer, A.U.; Keller, O.N.; Ferrari, F.; Maag, K.-P. Association of glaucoma with neurodegenerative diseases with apoptotic cell death: Alzheimer's disease and Parkinson's disease. *Am. J. Ophthalmol.* **2002**, *133*, 135–137. [CrossRef] [PubMed]
55. Yenice, O.; Onal, S.; Midi, I.; Ozcan, E.; Temel, A.; I-Gunal, D. Visual field analysis in patients with Parkinson's disease. *Park. Relat. Disord.* **2008**, *14*, 193–198. [CrossRef]
56. Ture, S.; Inci, I.; Gedizlioglu, M. Abnormalities of contrast sensitivity, visual fields and visual evoked potentials in Parkinson's disease and effect of dopaminergic treatment. *J. Neurol.* **2007**, *254* (Suppl. S3). [CrossRef]
57. Zhao, L.; Li, J.; Feng, L.; Zhang, C.; Zhang, W.; Wang, C.; He, Y.; Wen, D.; Song, W. Depicting Developing Trend and Core Knowledge of Primary Open-Angle Glaucoma: A Bibliometric and Visualized Analysis. *Front. Med.* **2022**, *9*, 922527. [CrossRef] [PubMed]
58. Micieli, G.; Tassorelli, C.; Martignoni, E.; Pacchetti, C.; Bruggi, P.; Magri, M.; Nappi, G. Disordered pupil reactivity in Parkinson's disease. *Clin. Auton. Res.* **1991**, *1*, 55–58. [CrossRef] [PubMed]
59. Alhassan, M.; Hovis, J.K.; Almeida, Q.J. Pupil light reflex in Parkinson's disease patients with and without freezing of gait symptoms. *Saudi J. Ophthalmol.* **2021**, *35*, 332. [CrossRef]
60. Hori, N.; Takamori, M.; Hirayama, M.; Watanabe, H.; Nakamura, T.; Yamashita, F.; Ito, H.; Mabuchi, N.; Sobue, G. Pupillary supersensitivity and visual disturbance in Parkinson's disease. *Clin. Auton. Res.* **2008**, *18*, 20–27. [CrossRef]
61. Postuma, R.B.; Gagnon, J.-F.; Pelletier, A.; Montplaisir, J. Prodromal autonomic symptoms and signs in Parkinson's disease and dementia with Lewy bodies. *Mov. Disord.* **2013**, *28*, 597–604. [CrossRef]
62. You, S.; Hong, J.-H.; Yoo, J. Analysis of pupillometer results according to disease stage in patients with Parkinson's disease. *Sci. Rep.* **2021**, *11*, 17880. [CrossRef]
63. Fotiou, D.F.; Stergiou, V.; Tsiptsios, D.; Lithari, C.; Nakou, M.; Karlovasitou, A. Cholinergic deficiency in Alzheimer's and Parkinson's disease: Evaluation with pupillometry. *Int. J. Psychophysiol.* **2009**, *73*, 143–149. [CrossRef] [PubMed]
64. Kahya, M.; Lyons, K.E.; Pahwa, R.; Akinwuntan, A.E.; He, J.; Devos, H. Pupillary Response to Postural Demand in Parkinson's Disease. *Front. Bioeng. Biotechnol.* **2021**, *9*, 617028. [CrossRef]
65. Agostino, R.; Bologna, M.; Dinapoli, L.; Gregori, B.; Fabbrini, G.; Accornero, N.; Berardelli, A. Voluntary, spontaneous, and reflex blinking in Parkinson's disease. *Mov. Disord.* **2008**, *23*, 669–675. [CrossRef] [PubMed]
66. Lamberti, P.; De Mari, M.; Zenzola, A.; Aniello, M.S.; Defazio, G. Frequency of apraxia of eyelid opening in the general population and in patients with extrapyramidal disorders. *Neurol. Sci.* **2002**, *23* (Suppl. S2), S81–S82. [CrossRef]
67. Nagino, K.; Sung, J.; Oyama, G.; Hayano, M.; Hattori, N.; Okumura, Y.; Fujio, K.; Akasaki, Y.; Huang, T.; Midorikawa-Inomata, A.; et al. Prevalence and characteristics of dry eye disease in Parkinson's disease: A systematic review and meta-analysis. *Sci. Rep.* **2022**, *12*, 18348. [CrossRef] [PubMed]
68. Shaikh, A.G. Translational neurophysiology of Parkinson's disease: Can't blink on an eye blink. *J. Neurophysiol.* **2015**, *114*, 761–762. [CrossRef]
69. Valls-Sole, J.; Defazio, G. Blepharospasm: Update on Epidemiology, Clinical Aspects, and Pathophysiology. *Front. Neurol.* **2016**, *7*, 45. [CrossRef]
70. Armstrong, R.A. Visual signs and symptoms of Parkinson's disease. *Clin. Exp. Optom.* **2008**, *91*, 129–138. [CrossRef]
71. Sescousse, G.; Ligneul, R.; van Holst, R.J.; Janssen, L.K.; de Boer, F.; Janssen, M.; Berry, A.S.; Jagust, W.J.; Cools, R. Spontaneous eye blink rate and dopamine synthesis capacity: Preliminary evidence for an absence of positive correlation. *Eur. J. Neurosci.* **2018**, *47*, 1081–1086. [CrossRef]
72. Reddy, V.C.; Patel, S.V.; Hodge, D.O.; Leavitt, J.A. Corneal sensitivity, blink rate, and corneal nerve density in progressive supranuclear palsy and Parkinson disease. *Cornea* **2013**, *32*, 631–635. [CrossRef] [PubMed]
73. Armstrong, R.A. Visual Symptoms in Parkinson's Disease. *Park. Dis.* **2011**, *2011*, 908306. [CrossRef] [PubMed]
74. Silva, M.F.; Faria, P.; Regateiro, F.S.; Forjaz, V.; Januário, C.; Freire, A.; Castelo-Branco, M. Independent patterns of damage within magno-, parvo- and koniocellular pathways in Parkinson's disease. *Brain* **2005**, *128*, 2260–2271. [CrossRef]
75. Piro, A.; Tagarelli, A.; Nicoletti, G.; Fletcher, R.; Quattrone, A. Color vision impairment in Parkinson's disease. *J. Park. Dis.* **2014**, *4*, 317–319. [CrossRef] [PubMed]
76. Hamedani, A.G.; Willis, A.W. Self-reported visual dysfunction in Parkinson disease: The Survey of Health, Ageing and Retirement in Europe. *Eur. J. Neurol.* **2020**, *27*, 484–489. [CrossRef]
77. Polo, V.; Satue, M.; Rodrigo, M.J.; Otin, S.; Alarcia, R.; Bambo, M.P.; Fuertes, M.I.; Larrosa, J.M.; Pablo, L.E.; Garcia-Martin, E. Visual dysfunction and its correlation with retinal changes in patients with Parkinson's disease: An observational cross-sectional study. *BMJ Open* **2016**, *6*, e009658. [CrossRef]
78. Büttner, T.; Müller, T.; Kuhn, W. Effects of apomorphine on visual functions in Parkinson's disease. *J. Neural Transm.* **2000**, *107*, 87–94. [CrossRef]
79. Diederich, N.J.; Raman, R.; Leurgans, S.; Goetz, C.G. Progressive worsening of spatial and chromatic processing deficits in Parkinson disease. *Arch. Neurol.* **2002**, *59*, 1249–1252. [CrossRef]
80. Leyland, L.-A.; Bremner, F.D.; Mahmood, R.; Hewitt, S.; Durteste, M.; Cartlidge, M.R.E.; Lai, M.M.-M.; Miller, L.E.; Saygin, A.P.; Keane, P.A.; et al. Visual tests predict dementia risk in Parkinson disease. *Neurol. Clin. Pract.* **2020**, *10*, 29–39. [CrossRef]
81. Weil, R.S.; Reeves, S. Hallucinations in Parkinson's disease: New insights into mechanisms and treatments. *Adv. Clin. Neurosci. Rehabil.* **2020**, *19*, ONNS5189. [CrossRef]

82. Shine, J.M.; O'Callaghan, C.; Halliday, G.M.; Lewis, S.J.G. Tricks of the mind: Visual hallucinations as disorders of attention. *Prog. Neurobiol.* **2014**, *116*, 58–65. [CrossRef] [PubMed]
83. Yao, N.; Shek-Kwan Chang, R.; Cheung, C.; Pang, S.; Lau, K.K.; Suckling, J.; Rowe, J.B.; Yu, K.; Ka-Fung Mak, H.; Chua, S.; et al. The default mode network is disrupted in parkinson's disease with visual hallucinations. *Hum. Brain Mapp.* **2014**, *35*, 5658–5666. [CrossRef] [PubMed]
84. Onofrj, M.; Carrozzino, D.; D'Amico, A.; Di Giacomo, R.; Delli Pizzi, S.; Thomas, A.; Onofrj, V.; Taylor, J.-P.; Bonanni, L. Psychosis in parkinsonism: An unorthodox approach. *Neuropsychiatr. Dis. Treat.* **2017**, *13*, 1313–1330. [CrossRef] [PubMed]
85. Sweet, R.D.; McDowell, F.H.; Feigenson, J.S.; Loranger, A.W.; Goodell, H. Mental symptoms in Parkinson's disease during chronic treatment with levodopa. *Neurology* **1976**, *26*, 305–310. [CrossRef]
86. Poewe, W. Psychosis in Parkinson's disease. *Mov. Disord.* **2003**, *18* (Suppl. S6), S80–S87. [CrossRef] [PubMed]
87. Zahodne, L.B.; Fernandez, H.H. Pathophysiology and treatment of psychosis in Parkinson's disease: A review. *Drugs Aging* **2008**, *25*, 665–682. [CrossRef]
88. Russo, M.; Carrarini, C.; Dono, F.; Rispoli, M.G.; Di Pietro, M.; Di Stefano, V.; Ferri, L.; Bonanni, L.; Sensi, S.L.; Onofrj, M. The Pharmacology of Visual Hallucinations in Synucleinopathies. *Front. Pharmacol.* **2019**, *10*, 1379. [CrossRef]
89. Anang, J.B.M.; Gagnon, J.-F.; Bertrand, J.-A.; Romenets, S.R.; Latreille, V.; Panisset, M.; Montplaisir, J.; Postuma, R.B. Predictors of dementia in Parkinson disease. *Neurology* **2014**, *83*, 1253–1260. [CrossRef]
90. Uc, E.Y.; McDermott, M.P.; Marder, K.S.; Anderson, S.W.; Litvan, I.; Como, P.G.; Auinger, P.; Chou, K.L.; Growdon, J.C.; Parkinson Study Group DATATOP Investigators. Incidence of and risk factors for cognitive impairment in an early Parkinson disease clinical trial cohort. *Neurology* **2009**, *73*, 1469–1477. [CrossRef]
91. Aarsland, D.; Larsen, J.P.; Tandberg, E.; Laake, K. Predictors of nursing home placement in Parkinson's disease: A population-based, prospective study. *J. Am. Geriatr. Soc.* **2000**, *48*, 938–942. [CrossRef]
92. Kalbe, E.; Rehberg, S.P.; Heber, I.; Kronenbuerger, M.; Schulz, J.B.; Storch, A.; Linse, K.; Schneider, C.; Gräber, S.; Liepelt-Scarfone, I.; et al. Subtypes of mild cognitive impairment in patients with Parkinson's disease: Evidence from the LANDSCAPE study. *J. Neurol. Neurosurg. Psychiatry* **2016**, *87*, 1099–1105. [CrossRef]
93. Lawrence, B.J.; Gasson, N.; Loftus, A.M. Prevalence and Subtypes of Mild Cognitive Impairment in Parkinson's Disease. *Sci. Rep.* **2016**, *6*, 33929. [CrossRef] [PubMed]
94. Johnson, D.K.; Langford, Z.; Garnier-Villarreal, M.; Morris, J.C.; Galvin, J.E. Onset of Mild Cognitive Impairment in Parkinson Disease. *Alzheimer Dis. Assoc. Disord.* **2016**, *30*, 127–133. [CrossRef] [PubMed]
95. Caspell-Garcia, C.; Simuni, T.; Tosun-Turgut, D.; Wu, I.-W.; Zhang, Y.; Nalls, M.; Singleton, A.; Shaw, L.A.; Kang, J.-H.; Trojanowski, J.Q.; et al. Multiple modality biomarker prediction of cognitive impairment in prospectively followed de novo Parkinson disease. *PLoS ONE* **2017**, *12*, e0175674. [CrossRef]
96. Pino, R.D.; Acera, M.; Murueta-Goyena, A.; Lucas-Jiménez, O.; Ojeda, N.; Ibarretxe-Bilbao, N.; Peña, J.; Reyero, P.; Cortés, J.; Tijero, B.; et al. Visual dysfunction is associated with cognitive impairment in Parkinson's disease. *Park. Relat. Disord.* **2021**, *92*, 22–25. [CrossRef]
97. Dubois, B.; Pillon, B. Cognitive deficits in Parkinson's disease. *J. Neurol.* **1997**, *244*, 2–8. [CrossRef]
98. Waterfall, M.L.; Crowe, S.F. Meta-analytic comparison of the components of visual cognition in Parkinson's disease. *J. Clin. Exp. Neuropsychol.* **1995**, *17*, 759–772. [CrossRef] [PubMed]
99. Norton, D.J.; Nguyen, V.A.; Lewis, M.F.; Reynolds, G.O.; Somers, D.C.; Cronin-Golomb, A. Visuospatial Attention to Single and Multiple Objects Is Independently Impaired in Parkinson's Disease. *PLoS ONE* **2016**, *11*, e0150013. [CrossRef]
100. Gullett, J.M.; Price, C.C.; Nguyen, P.; Okun, M.S.; Bauer, R.M.; Bowers, D. Reliability of three Benton Judgment of Line Orientation short forms in idiopathic Parkinson's disease. *Clin. Neuropsychol.* **2013**, *27*, 1167–1178. [CrossRef]
101. Segura, B.; Baggio, H.C.; Marti, M.J.; Valldeoriola, F.; Compta, Y.; Garcia-Diaz, A.I.; Vendrell, P.; Bargallo, N.; Tolosa, E.; Junque, C. Cortical thinning associated with mild cognitive impairment in Parkinson's disease. *Mov. Disord.* **2014**, *29*, 1495–1503. [CrossRef]
102. Renfroe, J.B.; Turner, T.H.; Hinson, V.K. Assessing Visuospatial Skills in Parkinson's: Comparison of Neuropsychological Assessment Battery Visual Discrimination to the Judgment of Line Orientation. *Arch. Clin. Neuropsychol.* **2017**, *32*, 123–127. [CrossRef] [PubMed]
103. Levin, B.E.; Llabre, M.M.; Reisman, S.; Weiner, W.J.; Sanchez-Ramos, J.; Singer, C.; Brown, M.C. Visuospatial impairment in Parkinson's disease. *Neurology* **1991**, *41*, 365–369. [CrossRef] [PubMed]
104. Finton, M.J.; Lucas, J.A.; Graff-Radford, N.R.; Uitti, R.J. Analysis of visuospatial errors in patients with Alzheimer's disease or Parkinson's disease. *J. Clin. Exp. Neuropsychol.* **1998**, *20*, 186–193. [CrossRef] [PubMed]
105. Alegret, M.; Vendrell, P.; Junque, C.; Valldeoriola, F.; Tolosa, E. Visuospatial Deficits in Parkinsons Disease Assessed by Judgment of Line Orientation Test: Error Analyses and Practice Effects. *J. Clin. Exp. Neuropsychol.* **2001**, *23*, 592–598. [CrossRef]
106. Kemps, E.; Szmalec, A.; Vandierendonck, A.; Crevits, L. Visuo-spatial processing in Parkinson's disease: Evidence for diminished visuo-spatial sketch pad and central executive resources. *Park. Relat. Disord.* **2005**, *11*, 181–186. [CrossRef]
107. Kawashima, S.; Shimizu, Y.; Ueki, Y.; Matsukawa, N. Impairment of the visuospatial working memory in the patients with Parkinson's Disease: An fMRI study. *BMC Neurol.* **2021**, *21*, 335. [CrossRef]
108. Crucian, G.P.; Barrett, A.M.; Burks, D.W.; Riestra, A.R.; Roth, H.L.; Schwartz, R.L.; Triggs, W.J.; Bowers, D.; Friedman, W.; Greer, M.; et al. Mental object rotation in Parkinson's disease. *J. Int. Neuropsychol. Soc.* **2003**, *9*, 1078–1087. [CrossRef]

109. Duncombe, M.E.; Bradshaw, J.L.; Iansek, R.; Phillips, J.G. Parkinsonian patients without dementia or depression do not suffer from bradyphrenia as indexed by performance in mental rotation tasks with and without advance information. *Neuropsychologia* **1994**, *32*, 1383–1396. [CrossRef]
110. Amick, M.M.; Schendan, H.E.; Ganis, G.; Cronin-Golomb, A. Frontostriatal circuits are necessary for visuomotor transformation: Mental rotation in Parkinson's disease. *Neuropsychologia* **2006**, *44*, 339–349. [CrossRef]
111. Bek, J.; Humphries, S.; Poliakoff, E.; Brady, N. Mental rotation of hands and objects in ageing and Parkinson's disease: Differentiating motor imagery and visuospatial ability. *Exp. Brain Res.* **2022**, *240*, 1991–2004. [CrossRef]
112. Pereira, J.B.; Junqué, C.; Martí, M.-J.; Ramirez-Ruiz, B.; Bargalló, N.; Tolosa, E. Neuroanatomical substrate of visuospatial and visuoperceptual impairment in Parkinson's disease. *Mov. Disord.* **2009**, *24*, 1193–1199. [CrossRef]
113. Archibald, N.K.; Hutton, S.B.; Clarke, M.P.; Mosimann, U.P.; Burn, D.J. Visual exploration in Parkinson's disease and Parkinson's disease dementia. *Brain* **2013**, *136*, 739–750. [CrossRef] [PubMed]
114. Raskin, S.A.; Borod, J.C.; Wasserstein, J.; Bodis-Wollner, I.; Coscia, L.; Yahr, M.D. Visuospatial orientation in Parkinson's disease. *Int. J. Neurosci.* **1990**, *51*, 9–18. [CrossRef] [PubMed]
115. Shine, J.M.; Muller, A.J.; O'Callaghan, C.; Hornberger, M.; Halliday, G.M.; Lewis, S.J. Abnormal connectivity between the default mode and the visual system underlies the manifestation of visual hallucinations in Parkinson's disease: A task-based fMRI study. *NPJ Park. Dis.* **2015**, *1*, 15003. [CrossRef] [PubMed]
116. Laatu, S.; Revonsuo, A.; Pihko, L.; Portin, R.; Rinne, J.O. Visual object recognition deficits in early Parkinson's disease. *Park. Relat. Disord.* **2004**, *10*, 227–233. [CrossRef]
117. Koh, S.-B.; Suh, S.-I.; Kim, S.-H.; Kim, J.H. Stereopsis and extrastriate cortical atrophy in Parkinson's disease: A voxel-based morphometric study. *Neuroreport* **2013**, *24*, 229–232. [CrossRef]
118. Sun, L.; Zhang, H.; Gu, Z.; Cao, M.; Li, D.; Chan, P. Stereopsis impairment is associated with decreased color perception and worse motor performance in Parkinson's disease. *Eur. J. Med. Res.* **2014**, *19*, 29. [CrossRef]
119. Kim, S.-H.; Park, J.-H.; Kim, Y.H.; Koh, S.-B. Stereopsis in drug naïve Parkinson's disease patients. *Can. J. Neurol. Sci.* **2011**, *38*, 299–302. [CrossRef]
120. Ba, F.; Sang, T.T.; He, W.; Fatehi, J.; Mostofi, E.; Zheng, B. Stereopsis and Eye Movement Abnormalities in Parkinson's Disease and Their Clinical Implications. *Front. Aging Neurosci.* **2022**, *14*, 783773. [CrossRef]
121. Jaywant, A.; Shiffrar, M.; Roy, S.; Cronin-Golomb, A. Impaired perception of biological motion in Parkinson's disease. *Neuropsychologia* **2016**, *30*, 720–730. [CrossRef]
122. Kloeters, S.; Hartmann, C.J.; Pundmann, V.D.; Schnitzler, A.; Südmeyer, M.; Lange, J. Impaired perception of human movements in Parkinson's disease. *Behav. Brain Res.* **2017**, *317*, 88–94. [CrossRef] [PubMed]
123. Uc, E.Y.; Rizzo, M.; Anderson, S.W.; Qian, S.; Rodnitzky, R.L.; Dawson, J.D. Visual dysfunction in Parkinson disease without dementia. *Neurology* **2005**, *65*, 1907–1913. [CrossRef] [PubMed]
124. Scarpina, F.; Ambiel, E.; Albani, G.; Pradotto, L.G.; Mauro, A. Utility of Boston Qualitative Scoring System for Rey-Osterrieth Complex Figure: Evidence from a Parkinson's Diseases sample. *Neurol. Sci.* **2016**, *37*, 1603–1611. [CrossRef]
125. De Lucia, N.; Trojano, L.; Vitale, C.; Grossi, D.; Barone, P.; Santangelo, G. The closing-in phenomenon in Parkinson's disease. *Park. Relat. Disord.* **2015**, *21*, 793–796. [CrossRef] [PubMed]
126. Ambron, E.; Della Sala, S. A critical review of closing-in. *Neuropsychology* **2017**, *31*, 105–117. [CrossRef] [PubMed]
127. Ambron, E.; Piretti, L.; Lunardelli, A.; Coslett, H.B. Closing-in Behavior and Parietal Lobe Deficits: Three Single Cases Exhibiting Different Manifestations of the Same Behavior. *Front. Psychol.* **2018**, *9*, 1617. [CrossRef]
128. De Lucia, N.; Grossi, D.; Mauro, A.; Trojano, L. Closing-in in Parkinson's disease individuals with dementia: An experimental study. *J. Clin. Exp. Neuropsychol.* **2015**, *37*, 946–955. [CrossRef]
129. Miller, I.N.; Cronin-Golomb, A. Gender differences in Parkinson's disease: Clinical characteristics and cognition. *Mov. Disord.* **2010**, *25*, 2695–2703. [CrossRef]
130. Verreyt, N.; Nys, G.M.S.; Santens, P.; Vingerhoets, G. Cognitive Differences Between Patients with Left-sided and Right-sided Parkinson's Disease. A Review. *Neuropsychol. Rev.* **2011**, *21*, 405–424. [CrossRef]
131. Lally, H.; Hart, A.R.; Bay, A.A.; Kim, M.C.; Wolf, S.L.; Hackney, M.E. Association Between Motor Subtype and Visuospatial and Executive Function in Mild-Moderate Parkinson Disease. *Arch. Phys. Med. Rehabil.* **2020**, *101*, 1580–1589. [CrossRef]
132. Davidsdottir, S.; Wagenaar, R.; Young, D.; Cronin-Golomb, A. Impact of optic flow perception and egocentric coordinates on veering in Parkinson's disease. *Brain* **2008**, *131*, 2882–2893. [CrossRef]
133. Schendan, H.E.; Amick, M.M.; Cronin-Golomb, A. Role of a lateralized parietal-basal ganglia circuit in hierarchical pattern perception: Evidence from Parkinson's disease. *Behav. Neurosci.* **2009**, *123*, 125–136. [CrossRef]
134. Seichepine, D.R.; Neargarder, S.; Davidsdottir, S.; Reynolds, G.O.; Cronin-Golomb, A. Side and type of initial motor symptom influences visuospatial functioning in Parkinson's disease. *J. Park. Dis.* **2015**, *5*, 75–83. [CrossRef] [PubMed]
135. Baumann, C.R.; Held, U.; Valko, P.O.; Wienecke, M.; Waldvogel, D. Body side and predominant motor features at the onset of Parkinson's disease are linked to motor and nonmotor progression. *Mov. Disord.* **2014**, *29*, 207–213. [CrossRef] [PubMed]
136. Locascio, J.; Corkin, S.; Growdon, J. Relation Between Clinical Characteristics of Parkinson's Disease and Cognitive Decline. *J. Clin. Exp. Neuropsychol.* **2003**, *25*, 94–109. [CrossRef]

137. Oltra, J.; Uribe, C.; Campabadal, A.; Inguanzo, A.; Monté-Rubio, G.C.; Martí, M.J.; Compta, Y.; Valldeoriola, F.; Junque, C.; Segura, B. Sex Differences in Brain and Cognition in de novo Parkinson's Disease. *Front. Aging Neurosci.* **2022**, *13*, 791532. [CrossRef] [PubMed]
138. Passoti, C.; Zanzaglia, R.; Sinforiani, E.; Minafra, B.; Bertaina, I.; Pacchetti, C. Cognitive function in Parkinson's disease: The influence of gender. *Basal Ganglia* **2013**, *3*, 131–135. [CrossRef]
139. Bayram, E.; Banks, S.J.; Shan, G.; Kaplan, N.; Caldwell, J.Z.K. Sex Differences in Cognitive Changes in de Novo Parkinson's Disease. *J. Int. Neuropsychol. Soc.* **2020**, *26*, 241–249. [CrossRef]
140. Cronin-Golomb, A.; Braun, A.E. Visuospatial dysfunction and problem solving in Parkinson's disease. *Neuropsychology* **1997**, *11*, 44–52. [CrossRef]
141. Garcia-Diaz, A.I.; Segura, B.; Baggio, H.C.; Uribe, C.; Campabadal, A.; Abos, A.; Marti, M.J.; Valldeoriola, F.; Compta, Y.; Bargallo, N.; et al. Cortical thinning correlates of changes in visuospatial and visuoperceptual performance in Parkinson's disease: A 4-year follow-up. *Park. Relat. Disord.* **2018**, *46*, 62–68. [CrossRef]
142. Baggio, H.-C.; Segura, B.; Sala-Llonch, R.; Marti, M.-J.; Valldeoriola, F.; Compta, Y.; Tolosa, E.; Junqué, C. Cognitive impairment and resting-state network connectivity in Parkinson's disease. *Hum. Brain Mapp.* **2015**, *36*, 199–212. [CrossRef] [PubMed]
143. Filoteo, J.V.; Reed, J.D.; Litvan, I.; Harrington, D.L. Volumetric correlates of cognitive functioning in nondemented patients with Parkinson's disease. *Mov. Disord.* **2014**, *29*, 360–367. [CrossRef]
144. Rektorova, I.; Biundo, R.; Marecek, R.; Weis, L.; Aarsland, D.; Antonini, A. Grey Matter Changes in Cognitively Impaired Parkinson's Disease Patients. *PLoS ONE* **2014**, *9*, e85595. [CrossRef] [PubMed]
145. Lee, J.E.; Park, H.-J.; Song, S.K.; Sohn, Y.H.; Lee, J.D.; Lee, P.H. Neuroanatomic basis of amnestic MCI differs in patients with and without Parkinson disease. *Neurology* **2010**, *75*, 2009–2016. [CrossRef]
146. Foster, E.R.; Black, K.J.; Antenor-Dorsey, J.A.V.; Perlmutter, J.S.; Hershey, T. Motor asymmetry and substantia nigra volume are related to spatial delayed response performance in Parkinson disease. *Brain Cogn.* **2008**, *67*, 1–10. [CrossRef]
147. Hattori, T.; Orimo, S.; Aoki, S.; Ito, K.; Abe, O.; Amano, A.; Sato, R.; Sakai, K.; Mizusawa, H. Cognitive status correlates with white matter alteration in Parkinson's disease. *Hum. Brain Mapp.* **2012**, *33*, 727–739. [CrossRef]
148. Lenka, A.; Jhunjhunwala, K.R.; Saini, J.; Pal, P.K. Structural and functional neuroimaging in patients with Parkinson's disease and visual hallucinations: A critical review. *Park. Relat. Disord.* **2015**, *21*, 683–691. [CrossRef] [PubMed]
149. Eberling, J.L.; Richardson, B.C.; Reed, B.R.; Wolfe, N.; Jagust, W.J. Cortical glucose metabolism in Parkinson's disease without dementia. *Neurobiol. Aging* **1994**, *15*, 329–335. [CrossRef]
150. Bohnen, N.I.; Minoshima, S.; Giordani, B.; Frey, K.A.; Kuhl, D.E. Motor correlates of occipital glucose hypometabolism in Parkinson's disease without dementia. *Neurology* **1999**, *52*, 541–546. [CrossRef]
151. Hosokai, Y.; Nishio, Y.; Hirayama, K.; Takeda, A.; Ishioka, T.; Sawada, Y.; Suzuki, K.; Itoyama, Y.; Takahashi, S.; Fukuda, H.; et al. Distinct patterns of regional cerebral glucose metabolism in Parkinson's disease with and without mild cognitive impairment. *Mov. Disord.* **2009**, *24*, 854–862. [CrossRef]
152. Kawabata, K.; Tachibana, H.; Kasama, S. Cerebral blood flow and cognitive function in Parkinson's disease. *Int. Congr. Ser.* **2002**, *1232*, 583–586. [CrossRef]
153. Bohnen, N.I.; Koeppe, R.A.; Minoshima, S.; Giordani, B.; Albin, R.L.; Frey, K.A.; Kuhl, D.E. Cerebral Glucose Metabolic Features of Parkinson Disease and Incident Dementia: Longitudinal Study. *J. Nucl. Med.* **2011**, *52*, 848–855. [CrossRef] [PubMed]
154. Caproni, S.; Muti, M.; Renzo, A.D.; Principi, M.; Caputo, N.; Calabresi, P.; Tambasco, N. Subclinical Visuospatial Impairment in Parkinson's Disease: The Role of Basal Ganglia and Limbic System. *Front. Neurol.* **2014**, *5*, 152. [CrossRef]
155. Göttlich, M.; Münte, T.F.; Heldmann, M.; Kasten, M.; Hagenah, J.; Krämer, U.M. Altered Resting State Brain Networks in Parkinson's Disease. *PLoS ONE* **2013**, *8*, e77336. [CrossRef]
156. Pereira, J.B.; Aarsland, D.; Ginestet, C.E.; Lebedev, A.V.; Wahlund, L.-O.; Simmons, A.; Volpe, G.; Westman, E. Aberrant cerebral network topology and mild cognitive impairment in early Parkinson's disease. *Hum. Brain Mapp.* **2015**, *36*, 2980–2995. [CrossRef] [PubMed]
157. Lou, W.; Shi, L.; Wang, D.; Tam, C.W.C.; Chu, W.C.W.; Mok, V.C.T.; Cheng, S.-T.; Lam, L.C.W. Decreased activity with increased background network efficiency in amnestic MCI during a visuospatial working memory task. *Hum. Brain Mapp.* **2015**, *36*, 3387–3403. [CrossRef]
158. Amboni, M.; Tessitore, A.; Esposito, F.; Santangelo, G.; Picillo, M.; Vitale, C.; Giordano, A.; Erro, R.; de Micco, R.; Corbo, D.; et al. Resting-state functional connectivity associated with mild cognitive impairment in Parkinson's disease. *J. Neurol.* **2015**, *262*, 425–434. [CrossRef]
159. Li, Y.; Liang, P.; Jia, X.; Li, K. Abnormal regional homogeneity in Parkinson's disease: A resting state fMRI study. *Clin. Radiol.* **2016**, *71*, e28–e34. [CrossRef]
160. Weil, R.S.; Hsu, J.K.; Darby, R.R.; Soussand, L.; Fox, M.D. Neuroimaging in Parkinson's disease dementia: Connecting the dots. *Brain Commun.* **2019**, *1*, fcz006. [CrossRef]
161. Vignando, M.; Ffytche, D.; Lewis, S.J.G.; Lee, P.H.; Chung, S.J.; Weil, R.S.; Hu, M.T.; Mackay, C.E.; Griffanti, L.; Pins, D.; et al. Mapping brain structural differences and neuroreceptor correlates in Parkinson's disease visual hallucinations. *Nat. Commun.* **2022**, *13*, 519. [CrossRef]
162. Ramírez-Ruiz, B.; Martí, M.-J.; Tolosa, E.; Giménez, M.; Bargalló, N.; Valldeoriola, F.; Junqué, C. Cerebral atrophy in Parkinson's disease patients with visual hallucinations. *Eur. J. Neurol.* **2007**, *14*, 750–756. [CrossRef]

163. Pagonabarraga, J.; Soriano-Mas, C.; Llebaria, G.; López-Solà, M.; Pujol, J.; Kulisevsky, J. Neural correlates of minor hallucinations in non-demented patients with Parkinson's disease. *Park. Relat. Disord.* **2014**, *20*, 290–296. [CrossRef]
164. Shin, S.; Lee, J.; Hong, J.; Sunwoo, M.K.; Sohn, Y.; Lee, P. Neuroanatomical substrates of visual hallucinations in patients with non-demented Parkinson's disease. *J. Neurol. Neurosurg. Psychiatry* **2012**, *83*, 1155–1161. [CrossRef]
165. Gama, R.L.; Bruin, V.M.S.; Távora, D.G.F.; Duran, F.L.S.; Bittencourt, L.; Tufik, S. Structural brain abnormalities in patients with Parkinson's disease with visual hallucinations: A comparative voxel-based analysis. *Brain Cogn.* **2014**, *87*, 97–103. [CrossRef] [PubMed]
166. Goldman, J.G.; Stebbins, G.T.; Dinh, V.; Bernard, B.; Merkitch, D.; deToledo-Morrell, L.; Goetz, C.G. Visuoperceptive region atrophy independent of cognitive status in patients with Parkinson's disease with hallucinations. *Brain* **2014**, *137*, 849–859. [CrossRef] [PubMed]
167. Watanabe, H.; Senda, J.; Kato, S.; Ito, M.; Atsuta, N.; Hara, K.; Tsuboi, T.; Katsuno, M.; Nakamura, T.; Hirayama, M.; et al. Cortical and subcortical brain atrophy in Parkinson's disease with visual hallucination. *Mov. Disord.* **2013**, *28*, 1732–1736. [CrossRef] [PubMed]
168. Ibarretxe-Bilbao, N.; Ramírez-Ruiz, B.; Tolosa, E.; Marti, M.; Valldeoriola, F.; Bargalló, N.; Junqué, C. Hippocampal head atrophy predominance in Parkinson's disease with hallucinations and with dementia. *J. Neurol.* **2008**, *255*, 1324–1331. [CrossRef] [PubMed]
169. Janzen, J.; van 't Ent, D.; Lemstra, A.W.; Berendse, H.W.; Barkhof, F.; Foncke, E.M.J. The pedunculopontine nucleus is related to visual hallucinations in Parkinson's disease: Preliminary results of a voxel-based morphometry study. *J. Neurol.* **2012**, *259*, 147–154. [CrossRef]
170. Lawn, T.; Ffytche, D. Cerebellar correlates of visual hallucinations in Parkinson's disease and Charles Bonnet Syndrome. *Cortex* **2021**, *135*, 311–325. [CrossRef]
171. Stebbins, G.T.; Goetz, C.G.; Carrillo, M.C.; Bangen, K.J.; Turner, D.A.; Glover, G.H.; Gabrieli, J.D.E. Altered cortical visual processing in PD with hallucinations: An fMRI study. *Neurology* **2004**, *63*, 1409–1416. [CrossRef]
172. Nagano-Saito, A.; Washimi, Y.; Arahata, Y.; Iwai, K.; Kawatsu, S.; Ito, K.; Nakamura, A.; Abe, Y.; Yamada, T.; Kato, T.; et al. Visual hallucination in Parkinson's disease with FDG PET. *Mov. Disord.* **2004**, *19*, 801–806. [CrossRef] [PubMed]
173. Boecker, H.; Ceballos-Baumann, A.O.; Volk, D.; Conrad, B.; Forstl, H.; Haussermann, P. Metabolic alterations in patients with Parkinson disease and visual hallucinations. *Arch. Neurol.* **2007**, *64*, 984–988. [CrossRef] [PubMed]
174. Park, H.K.; Kim, J.S.; Im, K.C.; Kim, M.J.; Lee, J.-H.; Lee, M.C.; Kim, J.; Chung, S.J. Visual Hallucinations and Cognitive Impairment in Parkinson's Disease. *Can. J. Neurol. Sci.* **2013**, *40*, 657–662. [CrossRef] [PubMed]
175. Oishi, N.; Udaka, F.; Kameyama, M.; Sawamoto, N.; Hashikawa, K.; Fukuyama, H. Regional cerebral blood flow in Parkinson disease with nonpsychotic visual hallucinations. *Neurology* **2005**, *65*, 1708–1715. [CrossRef] [PubMed]
176. Shine, J.M.; Halliday, G.M.; Naismith, S.L.; Lewis, S.J.G. Visual misperceptions and hallucinations in Parkinson's disease: Dysfunction of attentional control networks? *Mov. Disord.* **2011**, *26*, 2154–2159. [CrossRef]
177. Kiferle, L.; Ceravolo, R.; Giuntini, M.; Linsalata, G.; Puccini, G.; Volterrani, D.; Bonuccelli, U. Caudate dopaminergic denervation and visual hallucinations: Evidence from a ^{123}I-FP-CIT SPECT study. *Park. Relat. Disord.* **2014**, *20*, 761–765. [CrossRef]
178. Shine, J.M.; Halliday, G.M.; Gilat, M.; Matar, E.; Bolitho, S.J.; Carlos, M.; Naismith, S.L.; Lewis, S.J.G. The role of dysfunctional attentional control networks in visual misperceptions in Parkinson's disease. *Hum. Brain Mapp.* **2014**, *35*, 2206–2219. [CrossRef]
179. Hall, J.M.; O'Callaghan, C.; Muller, A.J.; Ehgoetz Martens, K.A.; Phillips, J.R.; Moustafa, A.A.; Lewis, S.J.G.; Shine, J.M. Changes in structural network topology correlate with severity of hallucinatory behavior in Parkinson's disease. *Netw. Neurosci.* **2019**, *3*, 521–538. [CrossRef]
180. Zarkali, A.; McColgan, P.; Ryten, M.; Reynolds, R.; Leyland, L.-A.; Lees, A.J.; Rees, G.; Weil, R.S. Differences in network controllability and regional gene expression underlie hallucinations in Parkinson's disease. *Brain* **2020**, *143*, 3435–3448. [CrossRef]
181. Zarkali, A.; McColgan, P.; Leyland, L.A.; Lees, A.J.; Weil, R.S. Longitudinal thalamic white and grey matter changes associated with visual hallucinations in Parkinson's disease. *J. Neurol. Neurosurg. Psychiatry* **2022**, *93*, 169–179. [CrossRef]
182. van Ommen, M.M.; van Laar, T.; Renken, R.; Cornelissen, F.W.; Bruggeman, R. Visual Hallucinations in Psychosis: The Curious Absence of the Primary Visual Cortex. *Schizophr. Bull.* **2023**, *49*, S68–S81. [CrossRef] [PubMed]
183. Popova, E. Role of Dopamine in Retinal Function. In *Webvision: The Organization of the Retina and Visual System*; Kolb, H., Fernandez, E., Nelson, R., Eds.; University of Utah Health Sciences Center: Salt Lake City, UT, USA, 2020.
184. Warwick, R.A.; Heukamp, A.S.; Riccitelli, S.; Rivlin-Etzion, M. Dopamine differentially affects retinal circuits to shape the retinal code. *J. Physiol.* **2023**, *601*, 1265–1286. [CrossRef] [PubMed]
185. Railo, H.; Olkoniemi, H.; Eeronheimo, E.; Pääkkönen, O.; Joutsa, J.; Kaasinen, V. Dopamine and eye movement control in Parkinson's disease: Deficits in corollary discharge signals? *PeerJ* **2018**, *6*, e6038. [CrossRef] [PubMed]
186. Crawford, T.J.; Henderson, L.; Kennard, C. Abnormalities of nonvisually-guided eye movements in Parkinson's disease. *Brain* **1989**, *112*, 1573–1586. [CrossRef] [PubMed]
187. Hanna-Pladdy, B.; Pahwa, R.; Lyons, K.E. Dopaminergic Basis of Spatial Deficits in Early Parkinson's Disease. *Cereb. Cortex Commun.* **2021**, *2*, tgab042. [CrossRef]
188. Ravina, B.; Marder, K.; Fernandez, H.H.; Friedman, J.H.; McDonald, W.; Murphy, D.; Aarsland, D.; Babcock, D.; Cummings, J.; Endicott, J.; et al. Diagnostic criteria for psychosis in Parkinson's disease: Report of an NINDS, NIMH work group. *Mov. Disord.* **2007**, *22*, 1061–1068. [CrossRef]

189. Bohnen, N.I.; Kaufer, D.I.; Hendrickson, R.; Ivanco, L.S.; Lopresti, B.J.; Constantine, G.M.; Mathis, C.A.; Davis, J.G.; Moore, R.Y.; Dekosky, S.T. Cognitive correlates of cortical cholinergic denervation in Parkinson's disease and parkinsonian dementia. *J. Neurol.* **2006**, *253*, 242–247. [CrossRef]
190. Manganelli, F.; Vitale, C.; Santangelo, G.; Pisciotta, C.; Iodice, R.; Cozzolino, A.; Dubbioso, R.; Picillo, M.; Barone, P.; Santoro, L. Functional involvement of central cholinergic circuits and visual hallucinations in Parkinson's disease. *Brain* **2009**, *132*, 2350–2355. [CrossRef]
191. Firbank, M.J.; Parikh, J.; Murphy, N.; Killen, A.; Allan, C.L.; Collerton, D.; Blamire, A.M.; Taylor, J.-P. Reduced occipital GABA in Parkinson disease with visual hallucinations. *Neurology* **2018**, *91*, e675–e685. [CrossRef]
192. Cho, S.S.; Strafella, A.P.; Duff-Canning, S.; Zurowski, M.; Vijverman, A.; Bruno, V.; Aquino, C.C.; Criaud, M.; Rusjan, P.M.; Houle, S.; et al. The Relationship Between Serotonin-2A Receptor and Cognitive Functions in Nondemented Parkinson's Disease Patients with Visual Hallucinations. *Mov. Disord. Clin. Pract.* **2017**, *4*, 698–709. [CrossRef]
193. Marras, C.; Schüle, B.; Munhoz, R.P.; Rogaeva, E.; Langston, J.W.; Kasten, M.; Meaney, C.; Klein, C.; Wadia, P.M.; Lim, S.-Y.; et al. Phenotype in parkinsonian and nonparkinsonian LRRK2 G2019S mutation carriers. *Neurology* **2011**, *77*, 325–333. [CrossRef] [PubMed]
194. Alcalay, R.N.; Caccappolo, E.; Mejia-Santana, H.; Tang, M.-X.; Rosado, L.; Orbe Reilly, M.; Ruiz, D.; Ross, B.; Verbitsky, M.; Kisselev, S.; et al. Cognitive performance of GBA mutation carriers with early-onset PD: The CORE-PD study. *Neurology* **2012**, *78*, 1434–1440. [CrossRef] [PubMed]
195. Zokaei, N.; McNeill, A.; Proukakis, C.; Beavan, M.; Jarman, P.; Korlipara, P.; Hughes, D.; Mehta, A.; Hu, M.T.M.; Schapira, A.H.V.; et al. Visual short-term memory deficits associated with GBA mutation and Parkinson's disease. *Brain* **2014**, *137*, 2303–2311. [CrossRef]
196. Neumann, J.; Bras, J.; Deas, E.; O'Sullivan, S.S.; Parkkinen, L.; Lachmann, R.H.; Li, A.; Holton, J.; Guerreiro, R.; Paudel, R.; et al. Glucocerebrosidase mutations in clinical and pathologically proven Parkinson's disease. *Brain* **2009**, *132*, 1783–1794. [CrossRef]
197. Nombela, C.; Rowe, J.B.; Winder-Rhodes, S.E.; Hampshire, A.; Owen, A.M.; Breen, D.P.; Duncan, G.W.; Khoo, T.K.; Yarnall, A.J.; Firbank, M.J.; et al. Genetic impact on cognition and brain function in newly diagnosed Parkinson's disease: ICICLE-PD study. *Brain* **2014**, *137*, 2743–2758. [CrossRef]
198. Garcia-Diaz, A.I.; Segura, B.; Baggio, H.C.; Marti, M.J.; Valldeoriola, F.; Compta, Y.; Vendrell, P.; Bargallo, N.; Tolosa, E.; Junque, C. Structural MRI correlates of the MMSE and pentagon copying test in Parkinson's disease. *Park. Relat. Disord.* **2014**, *20*, 1405–1410. [CrossRef]
199. Powell, A.; Ireland, C.; Lewis, S.J.G. Visual Hallucinations and the Role of Medications in Parkinson's Disease: Triggers, Pathophysiology, and Management. *J. Neuropsychiatry Clin. Neurosci.* **2020**, *32*, 334–343. [CrossRef] [PubMed]
200. Nantel, J.; McDonald, J.C.; Tan, S.; Bronte-Stewart, H. Deficits in visuospatial processing contribute to quantitative measures of freezing of gait in Parkinson's disease. *Neuroscience* **2012**, *221*, 151–156. [CrossRef] [PubMed]

Disclaimer/Publisher's Note: The statements, opinions and data contained in all publications are solely those of the individual author(s) and contributor(s) and not of MDPI and/or the editor(s). MDPI and/or the editor(s) disclaim responsibility for any injury to people or property resulting from any ideas, methods, instructions or products referred to in the content.

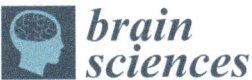
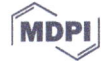

Systematic Review

Clinical Evaluation of Sleep Disorders in Parkinson's Disease

Fulvio Lauretani [1,2,*], Crescenzo Testa [1], Marco Salvi [1], Irene Zucchini [1], Francesco Giallauria [3] and Marcello Maggio [1,2]

1 Department of Medicine and Surgery, University of Parma, 43126 Parma, Italy
2 Clinic Geriatric Unit and Cognitive and Motor Center, Medicine and Geriatric-Rehabilitation Department, University-Hospital of Parma, 43126 Parma, Italy
3 Department of Translational Medical Sciences, "Federico II" University of Naples, Via S. Pansini 5, 80131 Naples, Italy
* Correspondence: fulvio.lauretani@unipr.it

Abstract: The paradigm of the framing of Parkinson's disease (PD) has undergone significant revision in recent years, making this neurodegenerative disease a multi-behavioral disorder rather than a purely motor disease. PD affects not only the "classic" substantia nigra at the subthalamic nuclei level but also the nerve nuclei, which are responsible for sleep regulation. Sleep disturbances are the clinical manifestations of Parkinson's disease that most negatively affect the quality of life of patients and their caregivers. First-choice treatments for Parkinson's disease determine amazing effects on improving motor functions. However, it is still little known whether they can affect the quantity and quality of sleep in these patients. In this perspective article, we will analyze the treatments available for this specific clinical setting, hypothesizing a therapeutic approach in relation to neurodegenerative disease state.

Keywords: Parkinson's disease; sleep disorders; Braak's stages; treatment; drugs

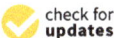
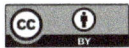

1. Introduction

Parkinson's disease affects 1–2% of the population over 60 years of age. Its incidence and prevalence are constantly increasing, especially in the last decades of life [1,2]. Due to the age of onset and the complexity and manifestation of symptoms, a comprehensive geriatric assessment is considered the best-suited approach for this disease.

Recently, Parkinson's disease has been recognized as a multisystemic disorder, and while the inflammatory pathogenesis for years was only the prerogative of the cardiovascular system [3], more and more evidence indicates that even neurodegeneration is secondary to genetic causes and to alterations of the inflammatory state [4,5].

This is an important upgrade in comparison with preexisting theories focusing only on the dopaminergic neurons of the substantia nigra [6–13]. Thus, in the absence of treatments attenuating or reverting neurodegeneration, the symptomatic management of the disease, targeting both motor and nonmotor symptoms, has become very important. Over the years, the therapeutic approach to motor symptoms has produced surprising results in patients who fully respond to dopamine replacement therapy [14].

However, more remains to be done for non-motor symptoms. Given the growing number of elderly and multimorbid patients and the increasingly demanding management of chronic and advanced stages of the disease, this approach is particularly relevant to the quality of life of patients and their caregivers [15].

Therefore, regarding the plethora of drugs available for the treatment of Parkinson's disease, the choice must be accurate and suited to the patient's needs. Any treatment worsening the quality of life of patients or their caregivers should be avoided [16].

Under the umbrella of non-motor symptoms, sleep disturbances are among the most common and those with the greatest impact on a patient's quality of life [17,18]. It is estimated that nearly half of the patients with Parkinson's disease suffer from sleep disturbances. Surprisingly, many patients underreport the symptom simply because they do not consider it as part of the disease [17–20]. Thus, the correct classification of sleep disorders in Parkinson's disease is relevant. The aim of this perspective article is to provide a correct framing of sleep disturbances in Parkinson's disease in relation to the Braak's scale. Finally, we will try to identify the most correct treatment in relation to the disease state.

2. Sleep Disorders in Parkinson's Disease: A Motley Melting Pot

Symptom-wise, sleep disturbances in Parkinson's occur in variegate ways. In this section, we will analyze the different ways in which sleep disorders can occur. Insomnia is the most frequent sleep disorder in Parkinson's disease with the prevalence, ranging from 30% to 80% of affected patients, increasing as the disease progresses [21,22]. Insomnia is difficulty in initiating or maintaining sleep. In patients with Parkinson's disease, difficulty in maintaining sleep (with early awakenings and sleep fragmentation) is more frequently described than difficulty in initiating sleep [23]. The sleep and circadian rhythm regulatory centers are affected by the neurodegeneration typical of Parkinson's disease, which lays the pathophysiological basis for the development of insomnia [24]. This substrate combined with the presence of the off symptoms contributes to the development and aggravation of insomnia as the disease progresses [25,26].

As for the diagnosis, in addition to an accurate medical history, clinicians have at their disposal a series of questionnaires, some of these specifically validated for Parkinson's disease (PDSS, PDSS-II, and SCOPA). In the most severe cases or the differential diagnosis of comorbidities, polysomnography is indicated [27,28]. Another way of presentation of sleep disturbances in Parkinson's disease is restless legs syndrome (RLS). A meta-analysis clearly shows that this syndrome affects about 15% of Parkinsonian patients [29]. This disorder occurs with the urge to move the legs and is usually associated with leg discomfort. Symptoms generally begin in the late afternoon or during the night, causing a great deal of discomfort to the patient and her/his partner. Regarding the etiology, there are three pathogenetic hypotheses: (one) in relation to the response to dopaminergic supplementation, Parkinson's disease and RLS share a common dopaminergic degeneration and a possible genetic connection [30]; (two) RLS in Parkinson's disease has a different etiology than idiopathic RLS; (three) RLS and Parkinson's disease are two different pathologies [31].

As evident from these hypotheses, there is also a type of RLS that occurs independently of Parkinson's disease [31]. The diagnostic criteria of RLS are described in the International Classification of Sleep Disorders [32]. Particular attention is needed in the diagnosis of this syndrome since it is capable of imitating other common symptoms, especially in elderly patients such as myalgia, leg cramps, and arthritis. Another sleep disorder typical of Parkinson's disease is rapid eye movement sleep behavior disorder (RBD). This disorder is parasomnia and consists of repeated vocalizations during sleep or complex motor behaviors during REM sleep. Polysomnographic studies have shown that the loss of muscle tone typical of the REM phase is lost in this disorder [32]. Approximately 24% of patients with Parkinson's disease are affected by this disorder, compared with 3.4% of affected individuals in the general population [33]. Similar rates were also found in another study [34]. It is important to highlight how idiopathic RBD is considered a strong predictor of synucleinopathies. A multicenter study reported a conversion rate from RBD to Parkinson's disease of approximately 6.3% annually and 73.5% after a 12-year follow-up period [35]. RBD precedes the onset of Parkinson's disease by about 13 years [36]. As far as pathophysiology is concerned, RBD has been associated with dysfunction in the pontomedullary and other structures regulating REM sleep, in particular, the locus coeruleus [37]. Also, in this case, in addition to the diagnostic criteria of the *International Classification of Sleep Disorders*, a specific diagnostic questionnaire was drawn up [38].

A consequence of sleep disturbances in patients with Parkinson's disease is excessive daytime sleepiness (EDS) which occurs in 20 to 75% of patients with Parkinson's disease [39–41]. This disorder consists of difficulty staying awake and alert during the day [32]. An accredited etiopathogenetic hypothesis ascribes this disorder to hypothalamic neurodegeneration and different nuclei of the brain stem responsible for the sleep–wake cycle [42]. As regards the diagnostic process, the Epworth sleepiness scale (ESS) is generally used as a screening tool. It is important to exclude other diseases that can cause daytime sleepiness such as RLS, OSA, and RBD. Finally, sleep disorders related to respiratory problems, in particular obstructive sleep apnea, should be accounted giving the prevalence of 20–60% of patients with Parkinson's disease [43,44]. In Parkinsonian patients, laryngopharyngeal motor dysfunction with occlusion of the upper respiratory tract is the cause of obstructive apneas [45]. As far as diagnosis is concerned, polysomnography is the gold standard exam, also validated in patients with Parkinson's disease [46,47]. Sleep disorders in Parkinson's disease are a heterogeneous melting pot of disorders. It is difficult to draw a guideline to guide clinicians in the treatment of these pathologies since many patients do not even ascribe the problem to Parkinson's disease. Except for RBD, which can be framed as a prodrome of Parkinson's disease, the rest of the sleep disorders generally present with a more advanced state of disease. It will be the task of the clinician who, with a careful history and a comprehensive assessment, will be able to diagnose and treat these disorders. An upgrade toward a comprehensive assessment of Parkinson's disease patients cannot be postponed. There is increasing evidence that sleep disturbances not only correlate with a worse quality of life but also trigger a pathophysiological mechanism that exacerbates major depressive states [20]. Especially in the later stages of life with Parkinson's disease, depression and nonmotor symptoms, rather than motor symptoms, have a greater impact on the quality of life of patients [48]. Therefore, patients with Parkinson's require a comprehensive assessment to stop this vicious circle (neurodegenerative disease -> depression -> neurodegenerative disease) that, in the long term, leads to disability [49]. It will be interesting in the future to try to identify the primum movens of this vicious circle, also in consideration of its pathogenetic affinity with sleep disorders.

3. The Braak Scale: An Old Staging with a New Awareness

For more than 20 years, Braak and colleagues [42] have postulated the hypothesis of progressive neurodegeneration in the etiology of sporadic Parkinson's disease, and although there are numerous scales for staging Parkinson's [50], the Braak scale is the one that best explains the pathophysiology of the disease. Regardless of the underlying etiological cause, over time, this hypothesis has been examined in various clinical and preclinical settings and was recently confirmed [51]. The concept of progressive neurodegeneration that inexorably advances and affects more and more brain areas is supported by the clinical manifestations of the disease. Six microscopically additive disease stages are described, with typical histological lesions (Lewy neurites and Lewy bodies): (one) lesions in the dorsal IX/X motor nucleus and/or intermediate reticular zone; (two) lesions in caudal raphe nuclei, gigantocellular reticular nucleus, and coeruleus—subcoeruleus complex; (three) midbrain lesions, particularly in the pars compacta of the substantia nigra; (four) prosencephalic lesions. Cortical involvement is confined to the temporal mesocortex (transentorhinal region) and allocortex (CA2-plexus). The neocortex is unaffected; (five) lesions in high-order sensory association areas of the neocortex and prefrontal neocortex; (six) lesions in first-order sensory association areas of the neocortex and premotor areas, occasionally mild changes in primary sensory areas and the primary motor field.

It should be emphasized that the motor symptoms appear during the late phase of the disease progression, Braak stages 3–4 (39). The long prodromal phase corresponds to a neurodegeneration that remains in the subclinical state. RBD, which by many authors is considered a prodrome of Parkinson's disease, is caused precisely by a degeneration at the level of the locus coeruleus which is affected in the initial stages of the disease (Braak stage two). Unlike RBD, other sleep disorders generally occur at or shortly after the onset of motor symptoms. The mode of presentation varies from patient to patient but with the progression of the disease and the worsening of motor symptoms less controlled by pharmacological treatment, there is a worsening presentation of sleep disturbances. This, almost schematic, trend must guide the clinical approach to stabilizing the sleep–wake cycle in the prodromal phases of the disease, to prevent dopaminergic neurodegeneration in the intermediate phases of the disease up to treatment with drugs that also target cognitive impairment associated-conditions during the final stages of the disease.

4. Clinical Implications and Available Treatments for Sleep Disorders in Parkinson's Disease

The main clinical implication of sleep disorders is the major negative impact on the quality of life of patients with Parkinson's disease. Reduced quality of life very often results in a greater tendency to develop a mood disorder. In recent years, clinicians have begun to focus their attention on treating non-motor symptoms, particularly depression. Recent evidence indicates that drugs such as SSRI and SNRI, in young subjects' tricyclic antidepressants, dopamine agonists, and behavioral therapy have good efficacy in the treatment of depression in patients with Parkinson's disease.

Insomnia and depression are closely related to Parkinson's disease [23]. Patients with insomnia usually have a more advanced state of disease and are more prone to symptoms due to the wearing-off of the levodopa effect. They also show problems such as autonomic dysfunction, hallucinations, and postural instability [23,52]. The correct treatment of insomnia in Parkinson's disease starts with the careful collection of patients' histories. Insomnia can occur during the night as an end-of-dose effect of dopamine. For this reason, the use of an additional tablet of levodopa, prolonged-release levodopa, or a dopamine agonist finds more and more space in this clinical setting. Recent evidence indicates that drugs such as eszopiclone and melatonin also find their place in the treatment of insomnia related to Parkinson's disease, especially in the early phase of the disease [53].

Related to insomnia or the underlying cause of insomnia, is restless leg syndrome (RLS). Dopamine agonists such as pramipexole, rotigotine, and ropinirole have their therapeutic rationale for treating it [54–56]. Careful attention is needed in the use of these drugs since, in some cases, they lead to a worsening of nocturnal symptoms after an initial benefit or could produce impulse compulsive disorders (ICDs) with nocturnal activity and sleep interruption [57]. In these cases, the treatment must be suspended and replaced either with a long-acting dopaminergic drug or with a drug acting beyond dopamine stimulation [58]. In this regard, good evidence of efficacy has been found with the use of gabapentin or pregabalin [59,60].

The clinical implications of rapid eye movement sleep behavior disorder (RBD) are very important because when this syndrome occurs as a comorbidity in Parkinson's disease, it is associated with increased motor dysfunction, hallucinations, cognitive impairment, and autonomic dysfunction, especially in the advanced phase of the disease [61,62]. There is still little evidence of an effective treatment for RBD, though some evidence of efficacy has been obtained with melatonin or clonazepam [63,64].

Older age is characterized by a worse presentation of disease symptoms and is also associated with excessive daytime sleepiness (EDS). EDS is often also the consequence of the breathing disorders associated with Parkinson's disease. Once again, a correct diagnosis is important since in OSAs independent of Parkinson's disease, the treatment of choice is C-PAP, while in OSAs caused by Parkinson's disease, the use of controlled release formulations of carbidopa/levodopa at bedtime may improve symptoms [65].

It is evident that there is a lack of effective treatments in most of the analyzed conditions. Furthermore, to set up a correct therapeutic procedure, a precise diagnosis is required, together with a good knowledge of the different ways in which sleep disorders can occur in relation to the degree of neurodegeneration. Finally, it is necessary to modulate the therapeutic treatments based on the caregiver's feedback, especially in the most advanced stages of the disease. The application of these procedures allows the avoidance of pharmacological overshooting that can lead to a decrease in alertness with very serious consequences such as inhalations of ingests and consequent pneumonia.

5. Available Drugs and State of Art of Treatment

Although sleep disorders in Parkinson's disease have been a clinical problem receiving interest from the scientific community for many years, no effective and lasting therapeutic approach has still been validated. Probably, the primary reason for the existing gap between clinical need and lack of adequate therapies is due to the heterogeneity, not only of the clinical manifestations but also of the type of patient in which these clinical manifestations appear. With the need to improve patients' symptoms, numerous therapeutic approaches have been attempted, whose clinical efficacy is substantially anecdotal and not evidence-based. The complexity of the patients and the heterogeneous responses to the different pharmacological treatments must direct clinicians to have an excellent knowledge of the numerous drugs available to avoid exposing the patient to the sedative actions of these drugs. In this clinical setting, there is no "one drug fits all", though only an adequate comprehensive assessment oriented to the patient and the living environment can help physicians towards a multidomain treatment, including prescribing or sometimes deprescribing certain medications.

Among the first drugs used in this clinical context are melatonin and its synthetic derivative (Ramelteon and Agomelatine), agonists of melatonin receptors. Melatonin is an agonist of the MT1, MT2, and MT3 receptors, has a half-life of about 4 h, and is one of the first drugs used in patients with insomnia. Experiences in patients with Parkinson's disease indicate that melatonin can improve the quality of sleep [66,67]. We have previously found that in patients with Parkinson's disease, insomnia does not manifest itself as difficulty falling asleep, but rather as difficulty staying asleep. In this regard, various therapeutic approaches are available, and one of these is the use of prolonged-release melatonin. In two recent studies, a 2 mg dose of prolonged-release melatonin was associated with significant improvements in night-time frequency and nocturnal voided volumes, and beneficial effects on sleep quality with improved nonmotor symptoms and quality of life in PD patients [68,69]. In patients in whom a coexistence between sleep disorder and depression of mood emerges at the visit, the use of agomelatine at a dosage of 12.5 mg, titrated up to 50 mg, could be useful [70]. Ramelteon is the synthetic derivative of melatonin mostly used in patients with Parkinson's disease. It acts as an MT1 and MT2 receptor agonist and has a half-life of approximately 2.5 h. At an 8 mg dose, ramelteon was effective in the treatment of sleep disorders in Parkinson's patients, particularly in RBD [71].

There is little data in the literature on the use of benzodiazepines in patients with Parkinson's disease, although in clinical practice they are often used above all for the relief of depressive symptoms and for their hypnotic action. These drugs act as positive allosteric modulators of the GABA receptor and differ substantially in the length of half-life. In light of the scarcity of significant evidence, the use of benzodiazepines in patients with Parkinson's disease should be weighed on a case-by-case basis, especially in relation to their side effects, one of which is inhalation pneumonia. A case-control study of over 550,000 patients found that benzodiazepine use is associated with an increased risk of pneumonia in elderly patients with Parkinson's disease [72]. It is therefore essential that the indication for the use of these drugs, in this particular setting, should be managed by expert physicians. Among the various benzodiazepines, more consistent data have emerged on the use of clonazepam for RBD. Clonazepam is a benzodiazepine with a long half-life (30–40 h) and is indicated by many as the first-line treatment in RBD. The evidence for the use of clonazepam in RBD is supported by studies with small sample sizes, some of which did not reach statistical significance when compared to a placebo [73–75]. Considering the long half-life and the possibility of accumulation phenomena, especially in elderly patients, the use of clonazepam in this clinical setting requires careful attention. Among the antidepressants, the one with the greatest sedative action, trazodone, is often used off label as a hypnotic inducer in elderly patients. This molecule acts as an antagonist of the serotonin 5HT2a/c receptor, the stimulation of which has a known antidopaminergic effect. In relation to this function, trazodone improved depressive symptoms and motor function in patients with Parkinson's disease [76]. In patients with Parkinson's, there are few data concerning the use of trazodone as a hypnotic inducer. However, a very recent experience conducted on 31 patients demonstrated its efficacy and tolerability at a sedative hypnotic dosage (50 mg) in this clinical setting [77]. The efficacy of trazodone as a hypnotic inducer is probably also due to its biphasic half-life with a first phase of 3–6 h and a second phase of 5–6 h. This biphasic effect is particularly welcome in Parkinsonian patients where insomnia is mainly due to difficulty staying asleep.

Among the nonbenzodiazepine allosteric modulators of the GABA receptor, z-compounds are often used in clinical practice as hypnotic agents due to their reduced sedative effects and therapeutic handling [53,78]. Randomized controlled trials on the use of these drugs in the setting of our interest are scarce. More significant experiences have been made with eszoplicone, which has demonstrated excellent tolerance and good clinical efficacy as a hypnoinducer in Parkinson's patients [79].

Among the nonbenzodiazepine allosteric modulators of the GABA receptor, drugs such as gabapentin and pregabalin have a more defined and codified therapeutic niche for sleep disorders in Parkinson's patients. In fact, there are numerous pieces of evidence, especially for the long-release pharmaceutical formulation of gabapentin, of their effectiveness in restless leg syndrome. In geriatric patients, these drugs are well-tolerated, though they require careful evaluation of renal function before starting and during treatment [80–82].

Few randomized controlled trials are available for the use of antipsychotic drugs in patients with sleep disorders and Parkinson's disease. The complexity of using these drugs is mainly due to the side effects, in particular sedation, and the need for clinical monitoring at the time of cardiac repolarization, exposing the patient to a greater risk of arrhythmias. There is no indication of these drugs in the initial stages of the disease, while their use will be more appropriate in the very advanced stage. Quetiapine is an atypical antipsychotic drug with low receptor specificity. Antagonized receptors include the histamine H1 receptor and serotonin 2A receptor. Consequently, sedation is intrinsic to the drug's activity. Due to this receptor specificity, attempts have been made to use quetiapine for the treatment of insomnia, regardless of the presence of Parkinson's disease, though the results due to the sedative effects, often in the presence of the other approved drugs for insomnia, are largely disappointing and the benefits of using quetiapine do not outweigh the risks [83]. The results of an open-label study have demonstrated that quetiapine can find its place in the treatment of insomnia in patients with Parkinson's [84]. However, these results need to be confirmed with an appropriate study design that includes the comparison with placebo control or with drugs already approved for insomnia and using an adequate sample size. The effects of quetiapine in improving visual hallucinations in Parkinson's patients are not related to a normalization of sleep architecture [85]. The effects of clozapine on sleep have not been specifically studied in patients with Parkinson's disease, though its use may consolidate sleep in psychiatric patients [86].

In patients with Parkinson's dementia, and consequent behavioral disturbances, low-dose clozapine may have a clinical indication, especially in patients where behavioral disturbances are particularly accentuated [87]. The use of other antipsychotic drugs in patients with sleep disorders and Parkinson's disease has very little evidence-based validation in the literature and, consequently, their use must be weighed on a case-by-case basis. The use of antipsychotics in Parkinson's disease is especially indicated in the treatment of psychosis in patients who have a very advanced state of the disease. However, compliance with therapy is low, and about one-third of patients prematurely terminate therapy due to both the side and antidopaminergic effects [88].

Pimavanserin is the most recently developed antipsychotic and has a peculiar mechanism of action that makes it substantially inactive on dopamine receptors. It acts as an antagonist and inverse agonist of serotonin 2A and 2C receptors. It finds indication above- all for hallucinations and delusions associated with psychoses related to Parkinson's dementia, a fact now corroborated in the literature [89]. Already in phase 1/2 studies, some evidence indicated that pimavanserin could have an effect objectively assessed on the sleep rhythm [90]. Recent findings indicate that this new treatment may improve the quality of sleep both in patients treated for major depressive disorder and in those with psychosis in Parkinson's disease [91,92].

Among the tricyclic antidepressants, doxepin has been shown to be effective in improving the quality of sleep in patients with Parkinson's disease, though its use in this setting is not widespread [93].

Despite its efficacy in the treatment of primary insomnia and the prevention of delirium in hospitalized patients [94], Suvorexant has not yet found a validated clinical indication in patients with sleep disorders and Parkinson's disease. Numerous scientific pieces of evidence justify the use of antidepressant drugs for Parkinson's disease. However, it is still difficult in this setting to identify a treatment that has independent effects on sleep disturbances alone, rather than depression, given the close relationship between these two conditions in Parkinson's disease. In addition to the drugs already highlighted, venlafaxine also seems to have a role in this clinical setting [95,96].

An off phase during the night can manifest itself as insomnia and modulation of dopaminergic therapy can be the best treatment. It is therefore essential to frame the sleep disorder presented by the patient with a correct medical history also detailed in the history of pharmacological therapy. There are numerous studies in the literature that have tried to endorse this therapeutic attitude. The use of a dose of levodopa upon awakening during the night as the main therapeutic action in insomnia linked to Parkinson's disease is an approach that has yet to be validated in the literature, though it is certainly supported by numerous indirect evidence, which indicates that more constant dopaminergic stimulation is effective in this regard. Treatment with a levodopa-carbidopa gastrointestinal gel that achieves a constant therapeutic drug plasma concentration was shown in one study to improve sleep disturbances together with other symptoms in Parkinson's disease [97].

Dopaminergic agonists are known to have a longer half-life and are less subject to change in pharmacokinetics than levodopa. A transdermal system for the release of rotigotine in patients complaining of sleep disturbances has shown how this treatment could improve the quality of sleep by reducing nocturnal awakenings and improving motor performance upon morning awakening [98]. In patients with advanced Parkinson's disease, both the immediate-release and prolonged-release pharmaceutical formulations of pramipexole have been shown to be effective in improving the subjective quality of sleep [99]. Ropinirole as an add on to levodopa therapy has also been shown to improve subjective symptoms in patients with Parkinson's disease, both with immediate-release pharmaceutical formulations and with prolonged-release pharmaceutical formulations in different disease stages [100,101]. Cabergoline therapy as an add on to levodopa monotherapy has also been shown to be effective in improving both polysomnographic parameters and the subjective quality of sleep in patients with idiopathic Parkinson's disease [102].

Dopaminergic stimulation has also been shown to be effective in treating sleep disorders in Parkinson's disease other than insomnia. In a randomized controlled study of over 300 patients, the efficacy of levodopa and cabergoline in the treatment of RLS was compared; the study showed a greater efficacy on symptoms for the cabergoline treatment, while patients in the levodopa treatment group reported better tolerability [103]. Pramipexole, rotigotine, and ropinirole have also shown good efficacy in controlling RLS symptoms [104–106]. Finally, both immediate-release and extended-release ropinirole have been shown to have a significant effect in mitigating daytime sleepiness episodes in EDS [107].

To support our hypothesis postulating the undertreatment of sleep disorder in Parkinson's disease, two authors (FL and CT) separately screened major medical databases in search of clinical randomized controlled trials conducted in the setting of our interest. The keywords "Parkinson's disease" and "sleep disorder" and all possible combinations were used to screen the Medline, EMBASE, and Scopus databases, and 5786 articles were screened. The article selection process is summarized in Figure 1 according to a PRISMA diagram. In Table 1 are summarized all the randomized controlled trial regard the setting of our interest.

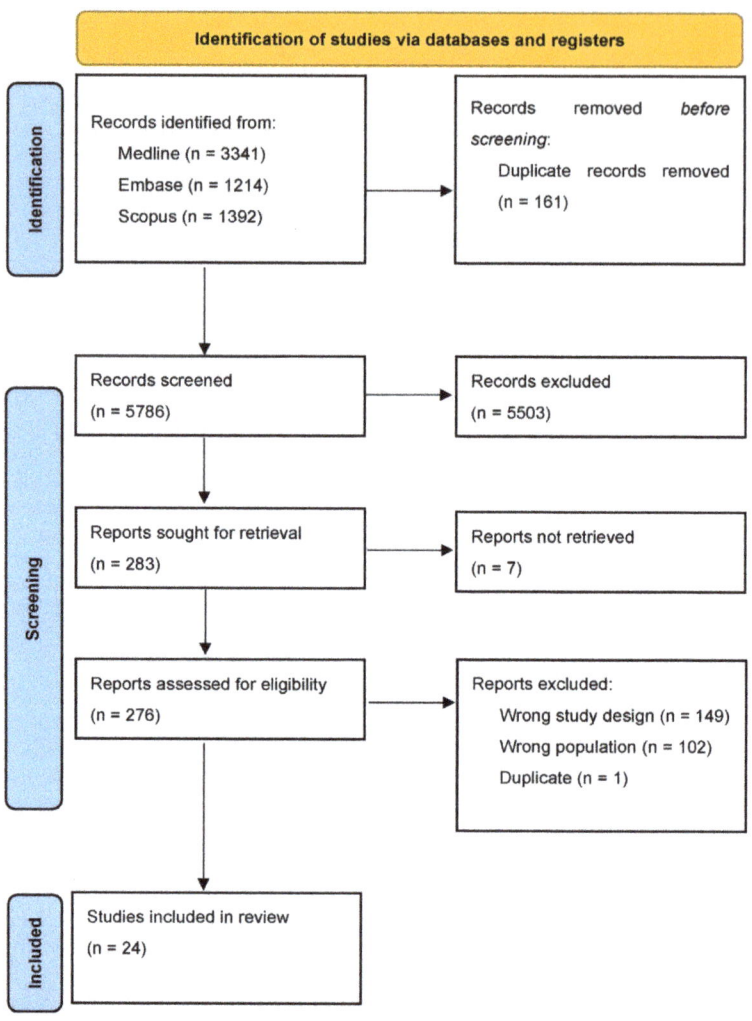

Figure 1. PRISMA diagram of selection process.

Table 1. Summary of the evidence currently available in the literature.

Authors	Parkinson's Disease Setting	Sleep Assessment	Mean Age (Years)	Design and Methods	Main Conclusion
Moran Gilat et al., 2020 [108]	REM sleep behavior disorder (RBD)	Weekly CIRUS-RBD Questionnaire Video Polisomnography	65	Randomized, double-blind, placebo-controlled, parallel-group trial with an 8-week intervention (melatonin RP 4 mg) and 4-week observation pre- and postintervention	Prolonged-release melatonin 4 mg did not reduce rapid eye movement sleep behavior disorder in PD
Amara et al., 2020 [109]	Subjective sleep quality	Polysomnography. Pittsburgh Sleep Quality Index (PSQI) Epworth Sleepiness Scale (ESS) Psychomotor vigilance task (PVT)	65	Persons with PD were randomized to exercise (supervised 3×/week for 16 weeks) (N = 27) or a sleep hygiene, no-exercise control (in-person discussion and monthly phone calls) (N = 28). Participants underwent polysomnography at baseline and post-intervention. Change in sleep efficiency was the primary outcome, measured from baseline to postintervention	High-intensity exercise rehabilitation improves objective sleep outcomes in PD
Meloni et al., 2021 [110]	REM sleep behavior disorder (RBD)	Video Polisomnography	67	Single-center, randomized, double-blind placebo-controlled crossover trial was performed in a selected population of 18 patients with PD and RBD. The patients received a placebo and 50 mg of 5-HTP daily in a crossover design over a period of 4 weeks	5-HTP is safe and effective in improving sleep stability in PD, contributing to ameliorating patients' global sleep quality

Table 1. Cont.

Authors	Parkinson's Disease Setting	Sleep Assessment	Mean Age (Years)	Design and Methods	Main Conclusion
Hadi et al., 2022 [76]	Subjective sleep quality	Pittsburgh Sleep Quality Index (PSQI) Epworth Sleepiness Scale (ESS) RBD screening questionnaire (RBDSQ)	66	Single-center, double-blind, randomized clinical trial conducted on PD patients with subjective sleep complaints. Eligible patients were randomized 1:1:1 to receive melatonin 3 mg/day, clonazepam 1 mg/day, or trazodone 50 mg/day for 4 weeks. 112 eligible patients were randomized, and 93 participants, melatonin ($n = 31$), trazodone ($n = 31$), and clonazepam ($n = 31$)	Trazodone 50 mg/day, clonazepam 1 mg/day, and melatonin 3 mg/day were all tolerable and effective in improving sleep quality in patients with PD
Peball et al., 2020 [111]	Nonmotor symptoms (NMS)	Epworth Sleepiness Scale (ESS)	65	Placebo-controlled, double-blind, parallel-group, enriched enrollment randomized withdrawal trial; 47 patients with PD with stable motor disease and disturbing NMS underwent open-label nabilone titration (0.25 mg once daily to 1 mg twice daily, phase I). Responders were randomized 1:1 to continue with nabilone or switch to placebo for 4 weeks (phase II)	Improvement of overall NMS burden with nabilone, especially reflected by amelioration of anxiety and sleeping problems
Shin et al., 2019 [74]	REM sleep behavior disorder (RBD)	Korean Epworth Sleepiness Scale (KESS) score 13-item self-reported RBD questionnaire (RBDQ-HK)	66	Four-week, randomized, double-blind, placebo-controlled, parallel group trial in patients with PD and RBD. A total of 40 patients were enrolled, with 20 assigned to receive clonazepam and 20 to receive the placebo	Both clonazepam and placebo tended toward improvement in pRBD symptoms in patients with PD
Stefani et al., 2021 [112]	REM-sleep behavior disorder (RBD)	Video Polisomnography	71	This was a phase 2 multicenter study in Dementia with Lewy Body or Parkinson's Disease Dementia (PDD) with video polysomnography (vPSG)-confirmed RBD. After a single-blind placebo run-in period, patients meeting eligibility criteria entered a 4-week double-blind treatment period (1:1 ratio with nelotanserin 80 mg/placebo); 8 Patients with PDD were included in the analyses	No difference between nelotanserin and placebo in RBD behaviors
Garcia-Borreguero et al., 2021 [113]	Restless leg syndrome (RLS)	Medical Outcomes Sleep Scale (MOS)	60	A 2-week double-blind, placebo-controlled crossover study assessed the efficacy of dipyridamole (possible up-titration to 300 mg) in untreated patients with idiopathic restless legs syndrome	Dipyridamole has significant therapeutic effects on both sensory and motor symptoms of restless legs syndrome and sleep
Pierantozzi et al., 2016 [114]	Sleep architecture	Polisomnography	63	Randomized, double-blind, placebo-controlled, parallel-group study to determine the efficacy of rotigotine vs. placebo on polysomnography parameters in moderately advanced PD patients	Rotigotine significantly increased sleep efficiency and reduced both wakefulness after sleep onset and sleep latency compared to the placebo
Schrempf et al., 2018 [115]	Sleep parameters	Polisomnography	69	Single-center, double-blind, baseline-controlled investigator-initiated clinical trial of rasagiline 1 mg/day over 8 weeks in PD patients with sleep disturbances	In PD patients with sleep disturbances rasagiline showed beneficial effects on sleep quality as measured by polysomnography
Trenkwalder et al., 2010 [116]	Early-morning motor function and nocturnal sleep disturbance	15-item Parkinson's Disease Sleep Scale (PDSS-2)	64	Multinational, double-blind, placebo-controlled trial where 287 subjects with Parkinson's disease (PD) and unsatisfactory early-morning motor symptom control were randomized 2:1 to receive rotigotine 2–16 mg/24 h (190) or placebo (97)	Twenty-four-hour transdermal delivery of rotigotine to PD patients with early-morning motor dysfunction resulted in significant benefits in the control of both motor function and nocturnal sleep disturbances
Silva-Batista et al., 2017 [117]	Sleep quality	Pittsburgh Sleep Quality Index (PSQI)	64	Randomized controlled trial where 22 subjects with moderate PD were randomly as- signed to a nonexercising control group ($n = 11$) or a resistance training group ($n = 11$)	Resistance training improves sleep quality
Larsson et al., 2010 [118]	Sleep disturbances in Parkinson's disease dementia (PDD)	Stavanger Sleep Questionnaire Epworth Sleepiness Scale (ESS)	76	Randomized controlled trial of 42 patients (20 memantine group, 22 placebo)	Memantine decreases probable REM sleep behaviour disorder in patients with PDD
Di Giacopo et al., 2011 [119]	REM-sleep behavior disorder (RBD)	RBD episodes were monitored by diaries of bed partners	67	Pilot trial	Rivastigmine was well tolerated in most patients, with minor side effects, mainly related to peripheral cholinergic action, and significantly reduced the mean frequency of RBD episodes during the observation time
Büchele et al., 2018 [120]	Excessive Daytime Sleepiness and Sleep Disturbance	Epworth Sleepiness Scale (ESS) Parkinson's Disease Sleep Scale-2	62	Double-blind, placebo-controlled crossover trial including 12 patients with Parkinson's disease	Sodium oxybate significantly improved sleepiness and disturbed nighttime sleep both subjectively and objectively
Chaudhuri et al., 2012 [121]	Nocturnal symptoms	Parkinson's Disease Sleep Scale	66	A 24-week, Phase III, randomized, double-blind, placebo-controlled, multicenter study	Once-daily ropinirole prolonged-release improves nocturnal symptoms in patients with advanced PD not optimally controlled with levodopa
Adler et al., 2004 [122]	Restless leg syndrome (RLS)	RLS rating scale Epworth Sleepiness Scale (ESS)	60	Double-blind, placebo-controlled, crossover study of ropinirole (0.5 to 6.0 mg/day) for restless legs syndrome (RLS)	Ropinirole was effective and well tolerated for treating the symptoms of RLS

Table 1. Cont.

Authors	Parkinson's Disease Setting	Sleep Assessment	Mean Age (Years)	Design and Methods	Main Conclusion
Adler et al., 2002 [123]	Subjective Daytime Sleepiness	Epworth Sleepiness Scale (ESS)	65	Single-site, randomized, double-blind, placebo-controlled crossover study of 21 PD patients. They received either a placebo or modafinil 200 mg/day for 3 weeks, followed by a washout week, then the alternate treatment for 3 weeks	Administration of 200 mg/day of modafinil is associated with few side effects and is modestly effective for the treatment of excessive daytime sleepiness in patients with PD
de Almeida et al., 2021 [124]	REM-sleep behavior disorder (RBD)	Video Polisomnography	57	Phase II/III, double-blind, placebo-controlled clinical trial in 33 patients with RBD and PD. Patients were randomized 1:1 to CBD in doses of 75 to 300 mg or matched capsules placebo and were followed up for 14 weeks	Cannabidiol, as an adjunct therapy, showed no reduction in RBD manifestations in PD patients
Plastino et al., 2021 [125]	REM-sleep behavior disorder (RBD)	RBD-screening questionnaire (RBDSQ) REM—sleep behavior disorder questionnaire-Hong Kong (RBDQ-HS) REM Sleep Behavior Disorder Severity scale (RBDSS) Video-Polisomnography	66	Pilot study of 30 patients with PD and RBD was randomized into two groups (15 subjects each), those that received for a period of 3 months safinamide (50 mg/die) in addition (Group A+) or in the absence (Group B) to the usual antiparkinsonian therapy	Safinamide is well tolerated and improves RBD-symptom in parkinsonian
De Cock et al., 2022 [126]	Insomnia	Parkinson's disease sleep scale (PDSS) Polysomnography	63	Randomised, multicentre, double-blind, placebo-controlled, crossover trial of 46 patients randomly assigned to receive apomorphine or placebo	Subcutaneous nighttime-only apomorphine infusion improved sleep disturbances according to differences on PDSS score, with an overall safety profile
Ahn etl al., 2020 [69]	Poor sleep quality	Pittsburgh Sleep Quality Index (PSQI) Epworth Sleepiness Scale (ESS)	66	Double-blind, placebo-controlled, multicenter trial to evaluate the efficacy and safety of prolonged-release melatonin (PRM) in Parkinson's disease (PD) patients with poor sleep quality	PRM is an effective and safe treatment option for subjective sleep quality in PD patients and beneficial effects on sleep quality are associated with improved nonmotor symptoms and quality of life in PD patients
Menza et al., 2010 [78]	Insomnia	Polysomnography	56	Six-week, randomized, controlled trial of eszopiclone and placebo in 30 patients with PD and insomnia	Eszopiclone did not increase total sleep time significantly but was superior to placebo in improving the quality of sleep and some measures of sleep maintenance which is the most common sleep difficulty experienced by patients with PD
Wailke et al., 2011 [127]	Microstructure of sleep in Parkinson's	Polysomnography	61	There were 32 patients with dopamine-responsive, akinetic-rigid PD, not taking neuroleptic medication, or suffering from dementia were randomized into two groups. Both groups had to withhold their usual dopaminergic medication until after noon. At bedtime, one group received 200 mg controlled-release (CR) levodopa/carbidopa, whilst the other group spent the night in the off state	Levodopa/carbidopa CR has no impact on the altered sleep structure in PD

6. Right Medication at Right Disease State

Figure 2 is the mainstay of our therapeutic proposal. It is essential to associate the correct treatment for sleep disturbance with a certain disease state. In the prodromal phases, there are medications such as melatonin or antidepressants such as trazodone or mirtazapine. In the symptomatic phases for motor disturbances, treatment with additional doses of levodopa in the night or with prolonged release formulations of levodopa or dopamine agonists may be useful, supporting the idea that the sleep disorder could be a "non-motor off state". Finally, in the final stages of the disease, in which modest cognitive impairment with behavior disorders can be present, the use of antipsychotics finds space. In this advanced phase of the disease, normally, many drugs affecting cognition, depression, anxiety, behavior symptoms, and mobility are prescribed with a tailored therapy that could be specific for each patient. This topic was recently emphasized in the context of psychosis, where authors underlined different sleep disorders throughout the course of the disease and different psychosis stages showed distinct abnormalities in sleep quality, architecture, and spindles [128]. These findings altogether suggest that sleep disorders could become a core treatment in different neurodegenerative diseases, such as psychosis, Parkinson's disease, and dementia [129,130]. In this clinical context, a correct pharmacological treatment can only take place after the comprehensive evaluation of the patient accompanied by a correct pharmacological history. Especially in elderly patient, drug treatment can itself be a cause of clinical worsening and hospitalizations that negatively impact the patient's prognosis.

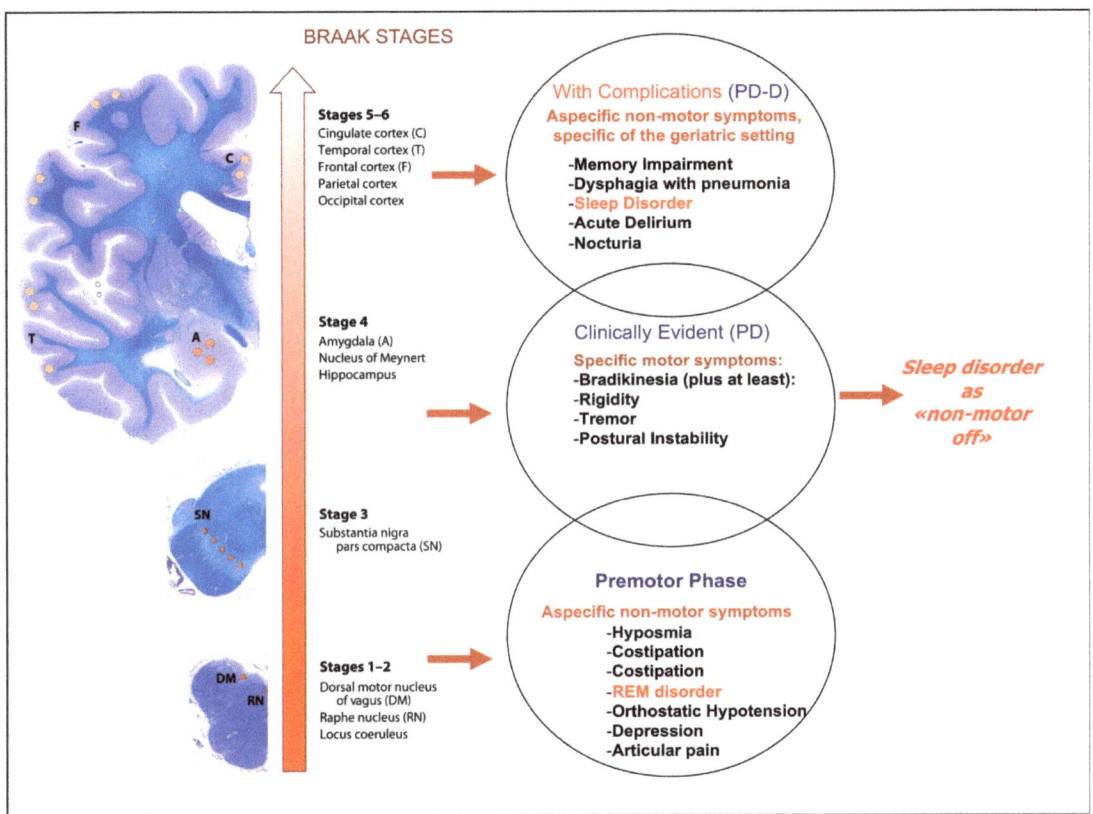

Figure 2. Correlation between the Braak scale in Parkinson's disease and symptom presentation. In sleep disorders, the indications for pharmacological therapy depend on the multidimensional evaluation of the patient.

In the advanced stage of neurodegenerative diseases, sleep disorders probably represent a challenge for physicians [131,132], especially geriatricians, where the balance between deprescribing or drug appropriateness could become the key element for maintaining a patient at home.

7. Conclusions

In the world of the geriatric population, polypharmacotherapy frequently occurs. Epidemiological trends indicate that more and more elderly patients are exposed to the risk of being overtreated without a real clinical benefit and to a greater risk of adverse clinical consequences. We have already described how the improper use of sedative drugs in Parkinson's disease such as benzodiazepines can expose patients to a greater risk of inhalation pneumonia, as reported for other drug classes such as antipsychotics and antidepressants. The treatment of sleep disorders in Parkinson's disease cannot benefit from dichotomous indications. This clinical problem is strictly dependent on factors such as the stage of the disease and the patient's insight into the problem. The scenario totally changes in the advanced stages of Parkinson's dementia. In light of the considerations made, and the available evidence, it is possible to make an indication of a therapeutic attitude rather than a therapeutic indication. The sleep disorders in a patient with Parkinson's disease must be viewed from a multidimensional perspective. It is essential to indicate therapeutic treatments that are biologically consistent with the stage of the disease. Especially in an elderly patient, the therapeutic indications must be balanced with other pharmacological treatments and the patient's comorbidities, avoiding the exposure of the patient to sedation and other relevant harmful side effects. In this setting, it will be important in the future to design randomized controlled trials that take into account the heterogeneity of the elderly population with Parkinson's disease and the different types and modalities of presentation of sleep disorders.

Author Contributions: Conceptualization, F.L., M.M. and C.T.; methodology, C.T. and F.G.; software, M.S.; validation, M.M., F.L. and I.Z.; investigation, F.L.; resources, F.G.; data curation, C.T.; writing—original draft preparation, F.L. and C.T.; writing—review and editing, M.M. and F.G.; visualization, I.Z. and M.S.; supervision, M.M. and F.L.; project administration, F.L. All authors have read and agreed to the published version of the manuscript.

Funding: This research received no external funding.

Institutional Review Board Statement: Not applicable.

Informed Consent Statement: Not applicable.

Data Availability Statement: Not applicable.

Conflicts of Interest: The authors declare no conflict of interest.

References

1. Zhang, S.; Smailagic, N.; Hyde, C.; Noel-Storr, A.H.; Takwoingi, Y.; McShane, R.; Feng, J. (11)C-PIB-PET for the early diagnosis of Alzheimer's disease dementia and other dementias in people with mild cognitive impairment (MCI). *Cochrane Database Syst. Rev.* **2014**, *7*, CD010386. [CrossRef]
2. Hou, Y.; Dan, X.; Babbar, M.; Wei, Y.; Hasselbalch, S.G.; Croteau, D.L.; Bohr, V.A. Ageing as a risk factor for neurodegenerative disease. *Nat. Rev. Neurol.* **2019**, *15*, 565–581. [CrossRef]
3. Testa, C.; DILorenzo, A.; Parlato, A.; D'Ambrosio, G.; Merolla, A.; Pacileo, M.; Iannuzzo, G.; Gentile, M.; Nugara, C.; Sarullo, F.M.; et al. Exercise for slowing the progression of atherosclerotic process: Effects on inflammatory markers. *Panminerva Med.* **2021**, *63*, 122–132. [CrossRef]
4. Madetko, N.; Migda, B.; Alster, P.; Turski, P.; Koziorowski, D.; Friedman, A. Platelet-to-lymphocyte ratio and neutrophil-tolymphocyte ratio may reflect differences in PD and MSA-P neuroinflammation patterns. *Neurol. Neurochir. Pol.* **2022**, *56*, 148–155. [CrossRef]
5. Dumbhare, O.; Gaurkar, S.S. A Review of Genetic and Gene Therapy for Parkinson's Disease. *Cureus* **2023**, *15*, e34657. [CrossRef]
6. Beach, T.G.; Adler, C.H.; Sue, L.I.; Vedders, L.; Lue, L.; White Iii, C.L.; Akiyama, H.; Caviness, J.N.; Shill, H.A.; Sabbagh, M.N.; et al. Multi-organ distribution of phosphorylated alpha-synuclein histopathology in subjects with Lewy body disorders. *Acta Neuropathol.* **2010**, *119*, 689–702. [CrossRef]
7. Dickson, D.W.; Braak, H.; Duda, J.E.; Duyckaerts, C.; Gasser, T.; Halliday, G.M.; Hardy, J.; Leverenz, J.B.; Del Tredici, K.; Wszolek, Z.K.; et al. Neuropathological assessment of Parkinson's disease: Refining the diagnostic criteria. *Lancet Neurol.* **2009**, *8*, 1150–1157. [CrossRef]
8. Lang, A.E.; Obeso, J.A. Challenges in Parkinson's disease: Restoration of the nigrostriatal dopamine system is not enough. *Lancet Neurol.* **2004**, *3*, 309–316. [CrossRef]
9. Langston, J.W. The Parkinson's complex: Parkinsonism is just the tip of the iceberg. *Ann. Neurol.* **2006**, *59*, 591–596. [CrossRef]
10. Ahlskog, J.E. Beating a dead horse: Dopamine and Parkinson disease. *Neurology* **2007**, *69*, 1701–1711. [CrossRef]
11. Adler, C.H.; Beach, T.G. Neuropathological basis of nonmotor manifestations of Parkinson's disease. *Mov. Disord.* **2016**, *31*, 1114–1119. [CrossRef]
12. Halliday, G.; Lees, A.; Stern, M. Milestones in Parkinson's disease—Clinical and pathologic features. *Mov. Disord.* **2011**, *26*, 1015–1021. [CrossRef] [PubMed]
13. Armstrong, M.J.; Okun, M.S. Diagnosis and Treatment of Parkinson Disease: A Review. *JAMA* **2020**, *323*, 548–560. [CrossRef]
14. Mosley, P.E.; Moodie, R.; Dissanayaka, N. Caregiver Burden in Parkinson Disease: A Critical Review of Recent Literature. *J. Geriatr. Psychiatry Neurol.* **2017**, *30*, 235–252. [CrossRef] [PubMed]
15. Lauretani, F.; Ruffini, L.; Testa, C.; Salvi, M.; Scarlattei, M.; Baldari, G.; Zucchini, I.; Lorenzi, B.; Cattabiani, C.; Maggio, M. Cognitive and Behavior Deficits in Parkinson's Disease with Alteration of FDG-PET Irrespective of Age. *Geriatrics* **2021**, *6*, 110. [CrossRef] [PubMed]
16. Chaudhuri, K.R.; Martinez-Martin, P.; Schapira, A.H.; Stocchi, F.; Sethi, K.; Odin, P.; Brown, R.G.; Koller, W.; Barone, P.; MacPhee, G.; et al. International multicenter pilot study of the first comprehensive self-completed nonmotor symptoms questionnaire for Parkinson's disease: The NMSQuest study. *Mov. Disord.* **2006**, *21*, 916–923. [CrossRef]

17. Martinez-Martin, P.; Schapira, A.H.; Stocchi, F.; Sethi, K.; Odin, P.; MacPhee, G.; Brown, R.G.; Naidu, Y.; Clayton, L.; Abe, K.; et al. Prevalence of nonmotor symptoms in Parkinson's disease in an international setting; study using nonmotor symptoms questionnaire in 545 patients. *Mov. Disord.* **2007**, *22*, 1623–1629. [CrossRef]
18. Karlsen, K.H.; Larsen, J.P.; Tandberg, E.; Maeland, J.G. Influence of clinical and demographic variables on quality of life in patients with Parkinson's disease. *J. Neurol. Neurosurg. Psychiatry* **1999**, *66*, 431–435. [CrossRef]
19. Tholfsen, L.K.; Larsen, J.P.; Schulz, J.; Tysnes, O.B.; Gjerstad, M.D. Changes in insomnia subtypes in early Parkinson disease. *Neurology* **2017**, *88*, 352–358. [CrossRef]
20. Kadastik-Eerme, L.; Rosenthal, M.; Paju, T.; Muldmaa, M.; Taba, P. Health-related quality of life in Parkinson's disease: A cross-sectional study focusing on non-motor symptoms. *Health Qual. Life Outcomes* **2015**, *13*, 83. [CrossRef]
21. Loddo, G.; Calandra-Buonaura, G.; Sambati, L.; Giannini, G.; Cecere, A.; Cortelli, P.; Provini, F. The Treatment of Sleep Disorders in Parkinson's Disease: From Research to Clinical Practice. *Front. Neurol.* **2017**, *8*, 42. [CrossRef] [PubMed]
22. Zhu, K.; van Hilten, J.J.; Marinus, J. The course of insomnia in Parkinson's disease. *Park. Relat. Disord.* **2016**, *33*, 51–57. [CrossRef]
23. Diederich, N.J.; Vaillant, M.; Mancuso, G.; Lyen, P.; Tiete, J. Progressive sleep 'destructuring' in Parkinson's disease. A polysomnographic study in 46 patients. *Sleep Med.* **2005**, *6*, 313–318. [CrossRef]
24. Louter, M.; van Sloun, R.J.; Pevernagie, D.A.; Arends, J.B.; Cluitmans, P.J.; Bloem, B.R.; Overeem, S. Subjectively impaired bed mobility in Parkinson disease affects sleep efficiency. *Sleep Med.* **2013**, *14*, 668–674. [CrossRef] [PubMed]
25. Gómez-Esteban, J.C.; Zarranz, J.J.; Lezcano, E.; Velasco, F.; Ciordia, R.; Rouco, I.; Losada, J.; Bilbao, I. Sleep complaints and their relation with drug treatment in patients suffering from Parkinson's disease. *Mov. Disord.* **2006**, *21*, 983. [CrossRef]
26. Schutte-Rodin, S.; Broch, L.; Buysse, D.; Dorsey, C.; Sateia, M. Clinical guideline for the evaluation and management of chronic insomnia in adults. *J. Clin. Sleep Med.* **2008**, *4*, 487–504. [CrossRef] [PubMed]
27. Högl, B.; Arnulf, I.; Comella, C.; Ferreira, J.; Iranzo, A.; Tilley, B.; Trenkwalder, C.; Poewe, W.; Rascol, O.; Sampaio, C.; et al. Scales to assess sleep impairment in Parkinson's disease: Critique and recommendations. *Mov. Disord.* **2010**, *25*, 2704–2716. [CrossRef]
28. Yang, X.; Liu, B.; Shen, H.; Li, S.; Zhao, Q.; An, R.; Hu, F.; Ren, H.; Xu, Y.; Xu, Z. Prevalence of restless legs syndrome in Parkinson's disease: A systematic review and meta-analysis of observational studies. *Sleep Med.* **2018**, *43*, 40–46. [CrossRef]
29. Alonso-Navarro, H.; García-Martín, E.; Agúndez, J.A.G.; Jiménez-Jiménez, F.J. Association between restless legs syndrome and other movement disorders. *Neurology* **2019**, *92*, 948–964. [CrossRef]
30. Ferini-Strambi, L.; Carli, G.; Casoni, F.; Galbiati, A. Restless Legs Syndrome and Parkinson Disease: A Causal Relationship Between the Two Disorders? *Front. Neurol.* **2018**, *9*, 551. [CrossRef]
31. Medicine AAoS. *The International Classification of Sleep Disorders: Diagnostic and Coding Manual American Academy of Sleep Medicine*, 3rd ed.; American Academy of Sleep Medicine: Darien, IL, USA, 2014.
32. Zhang, J.; Xu, C.Y.; Liu, J. Meta-analysis on the prevalence of REM sleep behavior disorder symptoms in Parkinson's disease. *BMC Neurol.* **2017**, *17*, 23. [CrossRef]
33. Mollenhauer, B.; Trautmann, E.; Sixel-Döring, F.; Wicke, T.; Ebentheuer, J.; Schaumburg, M.; Lang, E.; Focke, N.K.; Kumar, K.R.; Lohmann, K.; et al. Nonmotor and diagnostic findings in subjects with de novo Parkinson disease of the DeNoPa cohort. *Neurology* **2013**, *81*, 1226–1234. [CrossRef]
34. Postuma, R.B.; Iranzo, A.; Hu, M.; Högl, B.; Boeve, B.F.; Manni, R.; Oertel, W.H.; Arnulf, I.; Ferini-Strambi, L.; Puligheddu, M.; et al. Risk and predictors of dementia and parkinsonism in idiopathic REM sleep behaviour disorder: A multicentre study. *Brain* **2019**, *142*, 744–759. [CrossRef]
35. Postuma, R.B.; Berg, D. Advances in markers of prodromal Parkinson disease. *Nat. Rev. Neurol.* **2016**, *12*, 622–634. [CrossRef]
36. Boeve, B.F.; Silber, M.H.; Saper, C.B.; Ferman, T.J.; Dickson, D.W.; Parisi, J.E.; Benarroch, E.E.; Ahlskog, J.E.; Smith, G.E.; Caselli, R.C.; et al. Pathophysiology of REM sleep behaviour disorder and relevance to neurodegenerative disease. *Brain* **2007**, *130 Pt 11*, 2770–2788. [CrossRef]
37. Stiasny-Kolster, K.; Mayer, G.; Schäfer, S.; Möller, J.C.; Heinzel-Gutenbrunner, M.; Oertel, W.H. The REM sleep behavior disorder screening questionnaire—A new diagnostic instrument. *Mov. Disord.* **2007**, *22*, 2386–2393. [CrossRef] [PubMed]
38. O'Suilleabhain, P.E.; Dewey, R.B., Jr. Contributions of dopaminergic drugs and disease severity to daytime sleepiness in Parkinson disease. *Arch. Neurol.* **2002**, *59*, 986–989. [CrossRef]
39. Suzuki, K.; Okuma, Y.; Uchiyama, T.; Miyamoto, M.; Sakakibara, R.; Shimo, Y.; Hattori, N.; Kuwabara, S.; Yamamoto, T.; Kaji, Y.; et al. Impact of sleep-related symptoms on clinical motor subtypes and disability in Parkinson's disease: A multicentre cross-sectional study. *J. Neurol. Neurosurg. Psychiatry* **2017**, *88*, 953–959. [CrossRef] [PubMed]
40. Amara, A.W.; Chahine, L.M.; Caspell-Garcia, C.; Long, J.D.; Coffey, C.; Högl, B.; Videnovic, A.; Iranzo, A.; Mayer, G.; Foldvary-Schaefer, N.; et al. Longitudinal assessment of excessive daytime sleepiness in early Parkinson's disease. *J. Neurol. Neurosurg. Psychiatry* **2017**, *88*, 653–662. [CrossRef] [PubMed]
41. Braak, H.; Del Tredici, K.; Rüb, U.; de Vos, R.A.; Jansen Steur, E.N.; Braak, E. Staging of brain pathology related to sporadic Parkinson's disease. *Neurobiol. Aging* **2003**, *24*, 197–211. [CrossRef] [PubMed]
42. Valko, P.O.; Hauser, S.; Sommerauer, M.; Werth, E.; Baumann, C.R. Observations on sleep-disordered breathing in idiopathic Parkinson's disease. *PLoS ONE* **2014**, *9*, e100828. [CrossRef] [PubMed]
43. Béland, S.G.; Postuma, R.B.; Latreille, V.; Bertrand, J.A.; Panisset, M.; Chouinard, S.; Wolfson, C.; Gagnon, J.F. Observational Study of the Relation between Parkinson's Disease and Sleep Apnea. *J. Park. Dis.* **2015**, *5*, 805–811. [CrossRef]

44. Bahia, C.M.C.S.; Pereira, J.S.; Lopes, A.J. Laryngopharyngeal motor dysfunction and obstructive sleep apnea in Parkinson's disease. *Sleep Breath.* **2019**, *23*, 543–550. [CrossRef]
45. Kapur, V.K.; Auckley, D.H.; Chowdhuri, S.; Kuhlmann, D.C.; Mehra, R.; Ramar, K.; Harrod, C.G. Clinical Practice Guideline for Diagnostic Testing for Adult Obstructive Sleep Apnea: An American Academy of Sleep Medicine Clinical Practice Guideline. *J. Clin. Sleep Med.* **2017**, *13*, 479–504. [CrossRef]
46. Gros, P.; Mery, V.P.; Lafontaine, A.L.; Robinson, A.; Benedetti, A.; Kimoff, R.J.; Kaminska, M. Diagnosis of Obstructive Sleep Apnea in Parkinson's Disease Patients: Is Unattended Portable Monitoring a Suitable Tool? *Park. Dis.* **2015**, *2015*, 258418. [CrossRef]
47. Kay, D.B.; Tanner, J.J.; Bowers, D. Sleep disturbances and depression severity in patients with Parkinson's disease. *Brain Behav.* **2018**, *8*, e00967. [CrossRef]
48. Lauretani, F.; Testa, C.; Salvi, M.; Zucchini, I.; Lorenzi, B.; Tagliaferri, S.; Cattabiani, C.; Maggio, M. Reward System Dysfunction and the Motoric-Cognitive Risk Syndrome in Older Persons. *Biomedicines* **2022**, *10*, 808. [CrossRef] [PubMed]
49. Rietdijk, C.D.; Perez-Pardo, P.; Garssen, J.; van Wezel, R.J.; Kraneveld, A.D. Exploring Braak's Hypothesis of Parkinson's Disease. *Front. Neurol.* **2017**, *8*, 37. [CrossRef] [PubMed]
50. Pitton Rissardo, J.; Fornari Caprara, A.L. Parkinson's disease rating scales: A literature review. *Ann. Mov. Disord.* **2020**, *3*, 3–22. [CrossRef]
51. Seppi, K.; Ray Chaudhuri, K.; Coelho, M.; Fox, S.H.; Katzenschlager, R.; Perez Lloret, S.; Weintraub, D.; Sampaio, C.; The Collaborators of the Parkinson's Disease Update on Non-Motor Symptoms Study Group on behalf of the Movement Disorders Society Evidence-Based Medicine Committee. Update on treatments for nonmotor symptoms of Parkinson's disease-an evidence-based medicine review. *Mov. Disord.* **2019**, *34*, 180–198. [CrossRef]
52. Ma, J.F.; Wan, Q.; Hu, X.Y.; Sun, S.G.; Wang, W.Z.; Zhao, Z.X.; Wang, Y.J.; Liu, C.F.; Li, J.M.; Jiang, Y.P.; et al. Efficacy and safety of pramipexole in chinese patients with restless legs syndrome: Results from a multi-center, randomized, double-blind, placebo-controlled trial. *Sleep Med.* **2012**, *13*, 58–63. [CrossRef] [PubMed]
53. Chung, S.; Bohnen, N.I.; Albin, R.L.; Frey, K.A.; Müller, M.L.; Chervin, R.D. Insomnia and sleepiness in Parkinson disease: Associations with symptoms and comorbidities. *J. Clin. Sleep Med.* **2013**, *9*, 1131–1137. [CrossRef] [PubMed]
54. Oertel, W.H.; Benes, H.; Garcia-Borreguero, D.; Högl, B.; Poewe, W.; Montagna, P.; Ferini-Strambi, L.; Sixel-Döring, F.; Trenkwalder, C.; Partinen, M.; et al. Rotigotine transdermal patch in moderate to severe idiopathic restless legs syndrome: A randomized, placebo-controlled polysomnographic study. *Sleep Med.* **2010**, *11*, 848–856. [CrossRef]
55. Walters, A.S.; Ondo, W.G.; Dreykluft, T.; Grunstein, R.; Lee, D.; Sethi, K.; TREAT RLS 2 (Therapy with Ropinirole: Efficacy and Tolerability in RLS 2) Study Group. Ropinirole is effective in the treatment of restless legs syndrome. TREAT RLS 2: A 12-week, double-blind, randomized, parallel-group, placebo-controlled study. *Mov. Disord.* **2004**, *19*, 1414–1423. [CrossRef]
56. Garcia-Borreguero, D.; Silber, M.H.; Winkelman, J.W.; Högl, B.; Bainbridge, J.; Buchfuhrer, M.; Hadjigeorgiou, G.; Inoue, Y.; Manconi, M.; Oertel, W.; et al. Guidelines for the first-line treatment of restless legs syndrome/Willis-Ekbom disease, prevention and treatment of dopaminergic augmentation: A combined task force of the IRLSSG, EURLSSG, and the RLS-foundation. *Sleep Med.* **2016**, *21*, 1–11. [CrossRef]
57. Winkelman, J.W.; Armstrong, M.J.; Allen, R.P.; Chaudhuri, K.R.; Ondo, W.; Trenkwalder, C.; Zee, P.C.; Gronseth, G.S.; Gloss, D.; Zesiewicz, T. Practice guideline summary: Treatment of restless legs syndrome in adults: Report of the Guideline Development, Dissemination, and Implementation Subcommittee of the American Academy of Neurology. *Neurology* **2016**, *87*, 2585–2593. [CrossRef]
58. Walters, A.S.; Ondo, W.G.; Kushida, C.A.; Becker, P.M.; Ellenbogen, A.L.; Canafax, D.M.; Barrett, R.W.; XP045 Study Group. Gabapentin enacarbil in restless legs syndrome: A phase 2b, 2-week, randomized, double-blind, placebo-controlled trial. *Clin. Neuropharmacol.* **2009**, *32*, 311–320. [CrossRef] [PubMed]
59. Allen, R.P.; Chen, C.; Garcia-Borreguero, D.; Polo, O.; DuBrava, S.; Miceli, J.; Knapp, L.; Winkelman, J.W. Comparison of pregabalin with pramipexole for restless legs syndrome. *N. Engl. J. Med.* **2014**, *370*, 621–631. [CrossRef] [PubMed]
60. Kim, Y.; Kim, Y.E.; Park, E.O.; Shin, C.W.; Kim, H.J.; Jeon, B. REM sleep behavior disorder portends poor prognosis in Parkinson's disease: A systematic review. *J. Clin. Neurosci.* **2018**, *47*, 6–13. [CrossRef]
61. St Louis, E.K.; Boeve, B.F. REM Sleep Behavior Disorder: Diagnosis, Clinical Implications, and Future Directions. *Mayo Clin. Proc.* **2017**, *92*, 1723–1736. [CrossRef]
62. Aurora, R.N.; Zak, R.S.; Maganti, R.K.; Auerbach, S.H.; Casey, K.R.; Chowdhuri, S.; Karippot, A.; Ramar, K.; Kristo, D.A.; Morgenthaler, T.I.; et al. Best practice guide for the treatment of REM sleep behavior disorder (RBD). *J. Clin. Sleep Med.* **2010**, *6*, 85–95; Erratum in *J. Clin. Sleep Med.* **2010**, *6*, table of contents. [PubMed]
63. McCarter, S.J.; Boswell, C.L.; St Louis, E.K.; Dueffert, L.G.; Slocumb, N.; Boeve, B.F.; Silber, M.H.; Olson, E.J.; Tippmann-Peikert, M. Treatment outcomes in REM sleep behavior disorder. *Sleep Med.* **2013**, *14*, 237–242. [CrossRef] [PubMed]
64. Gros, P.; Mery, V.P.; Lafontaine, A.L.; Robinson, A.; Benedetti, A.; Kimoff, R.J.; Kaminska, M. Obstructive sleep apnea in Parkinson's disease patients: Effect of Sinemet CR taken at bedtime. *Sleep Breath.* **2016**, *20*, 205–212. [CrossRef]
65. Medeiros, C.A.; Carvalhedo de Bruin, P.F.; Lopes, L.A.; Magalhães, M.C.; de Lourdes Seabra, M.; de Bruin, V.M. Effect of exogenous melatonin on sleep and motor dysfunction in Parkinson's disease. A randomized, double blind, placebo-controlled study. *J. Neurol.* **2007**, *254*, 459–464. [CrossRef] [PubMed]
66. Dowling, G.A.; Mastick, J.; Colling, E.; Carter, J.H.; Singer, C.M.; Aminoff, M.J. Melatonin for sleep disturbances in Parkinson's disease. *Sleep Med.* **2005**, *6*, 459–466. [CrossRef]

67. Batla, A.; Simeoni, S.; Uchiyama, T.; deMin, L.; Baldwin, J.; Melbourne, C.; Islam, S.; Bhatia, K.P.; Pakzad, M.; Eriksson, S.; et al. Exploratory pilot study of exogenous sustained-release melatonin on nocturia in Parkinson's disease. *Eur. J. Neurol.* **2021**, *28*, 1884–1892. [CrossRef]
68. De Berardis, D.; Fornaro, M.; Serroni, N.; Olivieri, L.; Marini, S.; Moschetta, F.S.; Srinivasan, V.; Assetta, M.; Valchera, A.; Salone, A.; et al. Agomelatine treatment of major depressive disorder in Parkinson's disease: A case series. *J. Neuropsychiatry Clin. Neurosci.* **2013**, *25*, 343–345. [CrossRef]
69. Ahn, J.H.; Kim, M.; Park, S.; Jang, W.; Park, J.; Oh, E.; Cho, J.W.; Kim, J.S.; Youn, J. Prolonged-release melatonin in Parkinson's disease patients with a poor sleep quality: A randomized trial. *Park. Relat. Disord.* **2020**, *75*, 50–54. [CrossRef]
70. Kashihara, K.; Nomura, T.; Maeda, T.; Tsuboi, Y.; Mishima, T.; Takigawa, H.; Nakashima, K. Beneficial Effects of Ramelteon on Rapid Eye Movement Sleep Behavior Disorder Associated with Parkinson's Disease—Results of a Multicenter Open Trial. *Intern. Med.* **2016**, *55*, 231–236. [CrossRef]
71. Huang, K.H.; Tai, C.J.; Kuan, Y.H.; Chang, Y.C.; Tsai, T.H.; Lee, C.Y. Pneumonia Risk Associated with the Use of Individual Benzodiazepines and Benzodiazepine Related Drugs among the Elderly with Parkinson's Disease. *Int. J. Environ. Res. Public Health* **2021**, *18*, 9410. [CrossRef]
72. De Almeida, C.M.O.; Pachito, D.V.; Sobreira-Neto, M.A.; Tumas, V.; Eckeli, A.L. Pharmacological treatment for REM sleep behavior disorder in Parkinson disease and related conditions: A scoping review. *J. Neurol. Sci.* **2018**, *393*, 63–68. [CrossRef] [PubMed]
73. Gilat, M.; Marshall, N.S.; Testelmans, D.; Buyse, B.; Lewis, S.J.G. A critical review of the pharmacological treatment of REM sleep behavior disorder in adults: Time for more and larger randomized placebo-controlled trials. *J. Neurol.* **2022**, *269*, 125–148. [CrossRef] [PubMed]
74. Shin, C.; Park, H.; Lee, W.W.; Kim, H.J.; Kim, H.J.; Jeon, B. Clonazepam for probable REM sleep behavior disorder in Parkinson's disease: A randomized placebo-controlled trial. *J. Neurol. Sci.* **2019**, *401*, 81–86. [CrossRef]
75. Werneck, A.L.; Rosso, A.L.; Vincent, M.B. The use of an antagonist 5-HT2a/c for depression and motor function in Parkinson' disease. *Arq. Neuropsiquiatr.* **2009**, *67*, 407–412. [CrossRef] [PubMed]
76. Hadi, F.; Agah, E.; Tavanbakhsh, S.; Mirsepassi, Z.; Mousavi, S.V.; Talachi, N.; Tafakhori, A.; Aghamollaii, V. Safety and efficacy of melatonin, clonazepam, and trazodone in patients with Parkinson's disease and sleep disorders: A randomized, double-blind trial. *Neurol. Sci.* **2022**, *43*, 6141–6148. [CrossRef] [PubMed]
77. Lebrun, C.; Gély-Nargeot, M.C.; Rossignol, A.; Geny, C.; Bayard, S. Efficacy of cognitive behavioral therapy for insomnia comorbid to Parkinson's disease: A focus on psychological and daytime functioning with a single-case design with multiple baselines. *J. Clin. Psychol.* **2020**, *76*, 356–376. [CrossRef]
78. Menza, M.; Dobkin, R.D.; Marin, H.; Gara, M.; Bienfait, K.; Dicke, A.; Comella, C.L.; Cantor, C.; Hyer, L. Treatment of insomnia in Parkinson's disease: A controlled trial of eszopiclone and placebo. *Mov. Disord.* **2010**, *25*, 1708–1714. [CrossRef]
79. Cochen De Cock, V. Therapies for Restless Legs in Parkinson's Disease. *Curr. Treat. Options Neurol.* **2019**, *21*, 56. [CrossRef]
80. Silber, M.H.; Becker, P.M.; Earley, C.; Garcia-Borreguero, D.; Ondo, W.G.; Medical Advisory Board of the Willis-Ekbom Disease Foundation. Willis-Ekbom Disease Foundation revised consensus statement on the management of restless legs syndrome. *Mayo Clin. Proc.* **2013**, *88*, 977–986. [CrossRef]
81. Trenkwalder, C.; Allen, R.; Högl, B.; Clemens, S.; Patton, S.; Schormair, B.; Winkelmann, J. Comorbidities, treatment, and pathophysiology in restless legs syndrome. *Lancet Neurol.* **2018**, *17*, 994–1005. [CrossRef]
82. Anderson, S.L.; Vande Griend, J.P. Quetiapine for insomnia: A review of the literature. *Am. J. Health Syst. Pharm.* **2014**, *71*, 394–402. [CrossRef] [PubMed]
83. Juri, C.; Chaná, P.; Tapia, J.; Kunstmann, C.; Parrao, T. Quetiapine for insomnia in Parkinson disease: Results from an open-label trial. *Clin. Neuropharmacol.* **2005**, *28*, 185–187. [CrossRef]
84. Fernandez, H.H.; Okun, M.S.; Rodriguez, R.L.; Malaty, I.A.; Romrell, J.; Sun, A.; Wu, S.S.; Pillarisetty, S.; Nyathappa, A.; Eisenschenk, S. Quetiapine improves visual hallucinations in Parkinson disease but not through normalization of sleep architecture: Results from a double-blind clinical-polysomnography study. *Int. J. Neurosci.* **2009**, *119*, 2196–2205. [CrossRef] [PubMed]
85. Hinze-Selch, D.; Mullington, J.; Orth, A.; Lauer, C.J.; Pollmächer, T. Effects of clozapine on sleep: A longitudinal study. *Biol. Psychiatry* **1997**, *42*, 260–266. [CrossRef]
86. Neufeld, M.Y.; Rabey, J.M.; Orlov, E.; Korczyn, A.D. Electroencephalographic findings with low-dose clozapine treatment in psychotic Parkinsonian patients. *Clin. Neuropharmacol.* **1996**, *19*, 81–86. [CrossRef]
87. Pham Nguyen, T.P.; Abraham, D.S.; Thibault, D.; Weintraub, D.; Willis, A.W. Low continuation of antipsychotic therapy in Parkinson disease—Intolerance, ineffectiveness, or inertia? *BMC Neurol.* **2021**, *21*, 240. [CrossRef]
88. Patel, R.S.; Bhela, J.; Tahir, M.; Pisati, S.R.; Hossain, S. Pimavanserin in Parkinson's Disease-induced Psychosis: A Literature Review. *Cureus* **2019**, *11*, e5257. [CrossRef]
89. Ancoli-Israel, S.; Vanover, K.E.; Weiner, D.M.; Davis, R.E.; van Kammen, D.P. Pimavanserin tartrate, a 5-HT(2A) receptor inverse agonist, increases slow wave sleep as measured by polysomnography in healthy adult volunteers. *Sleep Med.* **2011**, *12*, 134–141. [CrossRef]

90. Jha, M.K.; Fava, M.; Freeman, M.P.; Thase, M.E.; Papakostas, G.I.; Shelton, R.C.; Trivedi, M.H.; Dirks, B.; Liu, K.; Stankovic, S. Effect of Adjunctive Pimavanserin on Sleep/Wakefulness in Patients with Major Depressive Disorder: Secondary Analysis from CLARITY. *J. Clin. Psychiatry* **2020**, *82*, 20m13425. [CrossRef]
91. Patel, N.; LeWitt, P.; Neikrug, A.B.; Kesslak, P.; Coate, B.; Ancoli-Israel, S. Nighttime Sleep and Daytime Sleepiness Improved With Pimavanserin during Treatment of Parkinson's Disease Psychosis. *Clin. Neuropharmacol.* **2018**, *41*, 210–215. [CrossRef]
92. Rios Romenets, S.; Creti, L.; Fichten, C.; Bailes, S.; Libman, E.; Pelletier, A.; Postuma, R.B. Doxepin and cognitive behavioural therapy for insomnia in patients with Parkinson's disease—A randomized study. *Park. Relat. Disord.* **2013**, *19*, 670–675. [CrossRef] [PubMed]
93. Xu, S.; Cui, Y.; Shen, J.; Wang, P. Suvorexant for the prevention of delirium: A meta-analysis. *Medicine* **2020**, *99*, e21043. [CrossRef]
94. Prange, S.; Klinger, H.; Laurencin, C.; Danaila, T.; Thobois, S. Depression in Patients with Parkinson's Disease: Current Understanding of its Neurobiology and Implications for Treatment. *Drugs Aging* **2022**, *39*, 417–439. [CrossRef] [PubMed]
95. Agüera-Ortiz, L.; García-Ramos, R.; Grandas Pérez, F.J.; López-Álvarez, J.; Montes Rodríguez, J.M.; Olazarán Rodríguez, F.J.; Olivera Pueyo, J.; Pelegrín Valero, C.; Porta-Etessam, J. Focus on Depression in Parkinson's Disease: A Delphi Consensus of Experts in Psychiatry, Neurology, and Geriatrics. *Park. Dis.* **2021**, *2021*, 6621991. [CrossRef] [PubMed]
96. Antonini, A.; Poewe, W.; Chaudhuri, K.R.; Jech, R.; Pickut, B.; Pirtošek, Z.; Szasz, J.; Valldeoriola, F.; Winkler, C.; Bergmann, L.; et al. Levodopa-carbidopa intestinal gel in advanced Parkinson's: Final results of the GLORIA registry. *Park. Relat. Disord.* **2017**, *45*, 13–20. [CrossRef]
97. Giladi, N.; Fichtner, A.; Poewe, W.; Boroojerdi, B. Rotigotine transdermal system for control of early morning motor impairment and sleep disturbances in patients with Parkinson's disease. *J. Neural Transm.* **2010**, *117*, 1395–1399. [CrossRef]
98. Xiang, W.; Sun, Y.Q.; Teoh, H.C. Comparison of nocturnal symptoms in advanced Parkinson's disease patients with sleep disturbances: Pramipexole sustained release versus immediate release formulations. *Drug Des. Dev. Ther.* **2018**, *12*, 2017–2024. [CrossRef]
99. Mizuno, Y.; Nomoto, M.; Hasegawa, K.; Hattori, N.; Kondo, T.; Murata, M.; Takeuchi, M.; Takahashi, M.; Tomida, T.; Rotigotine Trial Group. Rotigotine vs ropinirole in advanced stage Parkinson's disease: A double-blind study. *Park. Relat. Disord.* **2014**, *20*, 1388–1393. [CrossRef]
100. Pahwa, R.; Stacy, M.A.; Factor, S.A.; Lyons, K.E.; Stocchi, F.; Hersh, B.P.; Elmer, L.W.; Truong, D.D.; Earl, N.L.; EASE-PD Adjunct Study Investigators. Ropinirole 24-hour prolonged release: Randomized, controlled study in advanced Parkinson disease. *Neurology* **2007**, *68*, 1108–1115. [CrossRef] [PubMed]
101. Romigi, A.; Stanzione, P.; Marciani, M.G.; Izzi, F.; Placidi, F.; Cervellino, A.; Giacomini, P.; Brusa, L.; Grossi, K.; Pierantozzi, M. Effect of cabergoline added to levodopa treatment on sleep-wake cycle in idiopathic Parkinson's disease: An open label 24-hour polysomnographic study. *J. Neural Transm.* **2006**, *113*, 1909–1913. [CrossRef]
102. Trenkwalder, C.; Benes, H.; Grote, L.; Happe, S.; Högl, B.; Mathis, J.; Saletu-Zyhlarz, G.M.; Kohnen, R.; CALDIR Study Group. Cabergoline compared to levodopa in the treatment of patients with severe restless legs syndrome: Results from a multi-center, randomized, active controlled trial. *Mov. Disord.* **2007**, *22*, 696–703. [CrossRef] [PubMed]
103. Wilson, S.M.; Wurst, M.G.; Whatley, M.F.; Daniels, R.N. Classics in Chemical Neuroscience: Pramipexole. *ACS Chem. Neurosci.* **2020**, *11*, 2506–2512. [CrossRef]
104. Kakar, R.S.; Kushida, C.A. Ropinirole in the treatment of restless legs syndrome. *Expert Rev. Neurother.* **2005**, *5*, 35–42. [CrossRef]
105. Kesayan, T.; Shaw, J.D.; Jones, T.M.; Staffetti, J.S.; Zesiewicz, T.A. Critical appraisal of rotigotine transdermal system in management of Parkinson's disease and restless legs syndrome—Patient considerations. *Degener. Neurol. Neuromuscul. Dis.* **2015**, *5*, 63–72, Erratum in: *Degener. Neurol. Neuromuscul. Dis.* **2016**, *6*, 13–15.
106. Dusek, P.; Busková, J.; Růžicka, E.; Majerová, V.; Srp, A.; Jech, R.; Roth, J.; Sonka, K. Effects of ropinirole prolonged-release on sleep disturbances and daytime sleepiness in Parkinson disease. *Clin. Neuropharmacol.* **2010**, *33*, 186–190. [CrossRef] [PubMed]
107. Hoel, R.W.; Giddings Connolly, R.M.; Takahashi, P.Y. Polypharmacy Management in Older Patients. *Mayo Clin. Proc.* **2021**, *96*, 242–256. [CrossRef]
108. Gilat, M.; Coeytaux Jackson, A.; Marshall, N.S.; Hammond, D.; Mullins, A.E.; Hall, J.M.; Fang, B.A.M.; Yee, B.J.; Wong, K.K.H.; Grunstein, R.R.; et al. Melatonin for rapid eye movement sleep behavior disorder in Parkinson's disease: A randomised controlled trial. *Mov. Disord.* **2020**, *35*, 344–349. [CrossRef]
109. Amara, A.W.; Wood, K.H.; Joop, A.; Memon, R.A.; Pilkington, J.; Tuggle, S.C.; Reams, J.; Barrett, M.J.; Edwards, D.A.; Weltman, A.L.; et al. Randomized, Controlled Trial of Exercise on Objective and Subjective Sleep in Parkinson's Disease. *Mov. Disord.* **2020**, *35*, 947–958. [CrossRef]
110. Meloni, M.; Figorilli, M.; Carta, M.; Tamburrino, L.; Cannas, A.; Sanna, F.; Defazio, G.; Puligheddu, M. Preliminary finding of a randomized, double-blind, placebo-controlled, crossover study to evaluate the safety and efficacy of 5-hydroxytryptophan on REM sleep behavior disorder in Parkinson's disease. *Sleep Breath.* **2022**, *26*, 1023–1031. [CrossRef]
111. Peball, M.; Krismer, F.; Knaus, H.G.; Djamshidian, A.; Werkmann, M.; Carbone, F.; Ellmerer, P.; Heim, B.; Marini, K.; Valent, D.; et al. Non-Motor Symptoms in Parkinson's Disease are Reduced by Nabilone. *Ann. Neurol.* **2020**, *88*, 712–722. [CrossRef]
112. Stefani, A.; Santamaria, J.; Iranzo, A.; Hackner, H.; Schenck, C.H.; Högl, B. Nelotanserin as symptomatic treatment for rapid eye movement sleep behavior disorder: A double-blind randomized study using video analysis in patients with dementia with Lewy bodies or Parkinson's disease dementia. *Sleep Med.* **2021**, *81*, 180–187. [CrossRef]

113. Garcia-Borreguero, D.; Garcia-Malo, C.; Granizo, J.J.; Ferré, S. A Randomized, Placebo-Controlled Crossover Study with Dipyridamole for Restless Legs Syndrome. *Mov. Disord.* **2021**, *36*, 2387–2392. [CrossRef]
114. Pierantozzi, M.; Placidi, F.; Liguori, C.; Albanese, M.; Imbriani, P.; Marciani, M.G.; Mercuri, N.B.; Stanzione, P.; Stefani, A. Rotigotine may improve sleep architecture in Parkinson's disease: A double-blind, randomized, placebo-controlled polysomnographic study. *Sleep Med.* **2016**, *21*, 140–144. [CrossRef]
115. Schrempf, W.; Fauser, M.; Wienecke, M.; Brown, S.; Maaß, A.; Ossig, C.; Otto, K.; Brandt, M.D.; Löhle, M.; Schwanebeck, U.; et al. Rasagiline improves polysomnographic sleep parameters in patients with Parkinson's disease: A double-blind, baseline-controlled trial. *Eur. J. Neurol.* **2018**, *25*, 672–679. [CrossRef] [PubMed]
116. Trenkwalder, C.; Kies, B.; Rudzinska, M.; Fine, J.; Nikl, J.; Honczarenko, K.; Dioszeghy, P.; Hill, D.; Anderson, T.; Myllyla, V.; et al. Rotigotine effects on early morning motor function and sleep in Parkinson's disease: A double-blind, randomized, placebo-controlled study (RECOVER). *Mov. Disord.* **2011**, *26*, 90–99. [CrossRef]
117. Silva-Batista, C.; de Brito, L.C.; Corcos, D.M.; Roschel, H.; de Mello, M.T.; Piemonte, M.E.P.; Tricoli, V.; Ugrinowitsch, C. Resistance Training Improves Sleep Quality in Subjects with Moderate Parkinson's Disease. *J. Strength Cond. Res.* **2017**, *31*, 2270–2277. [CrossRef] [PubMed]
118. Larsson, V.; Aarsland, D.; Ballard, C.; Minthon, L.; Londos, E. The effect of memantine on sleep behaviour in dementia with Lewy bodies and Parkinson's disease dementia. *Int. J. Geriatr. Psychiatry* **2010**, *25*, 1030–1038. [CrossRef] [PubMed]
119. Di Giacopo, R.; Fasano, A.; Quaranta, D.; Della Marca, G.; Bove, F.; Bentivoglio, A.R. Rivastigmine as alternative treatment for refractory REM behavior disorder in Parkinson's disease. *Mov. Disord.* **2012**, *27*, 559–561. [CrossRef] [PubMed]
120. Büchele, F.; Hackius, M.; Schreglmann, S.R.; Omlor, W.; Werth, E.; Maric, A.; Imbach, L.L.; Hägele-Link, S.; Waldvogel, D.; Baumann, C.R. Sodium Oxybate for Excessive Daytime Sleepiness and Sleep Disturbance in Parkinson Disease: A Randomized Clinical Trial. *JAMA Neurol.* **2018**, *75*, 114–118. [CrossRef]
121. Ray Chaudhuri, K.; Martinez-Martin, P.; Rolfe, K.A.; Cooper, J.; Rockett, C.B.; Giorgi, L.; Ondo, W.G. Improvements in nocturnal symptoms with ropinirole prolonged release in patients with advanced Parkinson's disease. *Eur. J. Neurol.* **2012**, *19*, 105–113. [CrossRef]
122. Adler, C.H.; Hauser, R.A.; Sethi, K.; Caviness, J.N.; Marlor, L.; Anderson, W.M.; Hentz, J.G. Ropinirole for restless legs syndrome: A placebo-controlled crossover trial. *Neurology* **2004**, *62*, 1405–1407. [CrossRef] [PubMed]
123. Adler, C.H.; Caviness, J.N.; Hentz, J.G.; Lind, M.; Tiede, J. Randomized trial of modafinil for treating subjective daytime sleepiness in patients with Parkinson's disease. *Mov. Disord.* **2003**, *18*, 287–293. [CrossRef]
124. De Almeida, C.M.O.; Brito, M.M.C.; Bosaipo, N.B.; Pimentel, A.V.; Tumas, V.; Zuardi, A.W.; Crippa, J.A.S.; Hallak, J.E.C.; Eckeli, A.L. Cannabidiol for Rapid Eye Movement Sleep Behavior Disorder. *Mov. Disord.* **2021**, *36*, 1711–1715. [CrossRef] [PubMed]
125. Plastino, M.; Gorgone, G.; Fava, A.; Ettore, M.; Iannacchero, R.; Scarfone, R.; Vaccaro, A.; De Bartolo, M.; Bosco, D. Effects of safinamide on REM sleep behavior disorder in Parkinson disease: A randomized, longitudinal, cross-over pilot study. *J. Clin. Neurosci.* **2021**, *91*, 306–312. [CrossRef]
126. De Cock, V.C.; Dodet, P.; Leu-Semenescu, S.; Aerts, C.; Castelnovo, G.; Abril, B.; Drapier, S.; Olivet, H.; Corbillé, A.G.; Leclair-Visonneau, L.; et al. Safety and efficacy of subcutaneous night-time only apomorphine infusion to treat insomnia in patients with Parkinson's disease (APOMORPHEE): A multicentre, randomised, controlled, double-blind crossover study. *Lancet Neurol.* **2022**, *21*, 428–437. [CrossRef]
127. Wailke, S.; Herzog, J.; Witt, K.; Deuschl, G.; Volkmann, J. Effect of controlled-release levodopa on the microstructure of sleep in Parkinson's disease. *Eur. J. Neurol.* **2011**, *18*, 590–596. [CrossRef] [PubMed]
128. Bagautdinova, J.; Mayeli, A.; Wilson, J.D.; Donati, F.L.; Colacot, R.M.; Meyer, N.; Fusar-Poli, P.; Ferrarelli, F. Sleep Abnormalities in Different Clinical Stages of Psychosis: A Systematic Review and Meta-analysis. *JAMA Psychiatry* **2023**, *80*, 202–210. [CrossRef]
129. Weintraub, D.; Aarsland, D.; Chaudhuri, K.R.; Dobkin, R.D.; Leentjens, A.F.; Rodriguez-Violante, M.; Schrag, A. The neuropsychiatry of Parkinson's disease: Advances and challenges. *Lancet Neurol.* **2022**, *21*, 89–102. [CrossRef]
130. Jankovic, J.; Tan, E.K. Parkinson's disease: Etiopathogenesis and treatment. *J. Neurol. Neurosurg. Psychiatry* **2020**, *91*, 795–808. [CrossRef]
131. Bloem, B.R.; Okun, M.S.; Klein, C. Parkinson's disease. *Lancet* **2021**, *397*, 2284–2303. [CrossRef]
132. Aarsland, D.; Batzu, L.; Halliday, G.M.; Geurtsen, G.J.; Ballard, C.; Ray Chaudhuri, K.; Weintraub, D. Parkinson disease-associated cognitive impairment. *Nat. Rev. Dis. Primers* **2021**, *7*, 47. [CrossRef] [PubMed]

Disclaimer/Publisher's Note: The statements, opinions and data contained in all publications are solely those of the individual author(s) and contributor(s) and not of MDPI and/or the editor(s). MDPI and/or the editor(s) disclaim responsibility for any injury to people or property resulting from any ideas, methods, instructions or products referred to in the content.

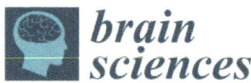 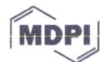

Systematic Review

Treatment of Vascular Parkinsonism: A Systematic Review

Cristina del Toro-Pérez [1], Eva Guevara-Sánchez [1] and Patricia Martínez-Sánchez [1,2,*]

1. Stroke Centre, Department of Neurology, Torrecárdenas University Hospital, University of Almería, 04009 Almería, Spain
2. Faculty of Health Sciences, CEINSA (Center of Health Research), University of Almería, 04120 Almería, Spain
* Correspondence: patrinda@ual.es

Abstract: Background and aims: Although the distinction between vascular parkinsonism (VP) and idiopathic Parkinson's disease (IPD) is widely described, it is not uncommon to find parkinsonisms with overlapping clinical and neuroimaging features even in response to levodopa treatment. In addition, several treatments have been described as possible adjuvants in VP. This study aims to update and analyze the different treatments and their efficacy in VP. Methods: A literature search was performed in PubMed, Scopus and Web of Science for studies published in the last 15 years until April 2022. A systematic review was performed. No meta-analysis was performed as no new studies on response to levodopa in VP were found since the last systematic review and meta-analysis in 2017, and insufficient studies on other treatments were located to conduct it in another treatment subgroup. Results: Databases and other sources yielded 59 publications after eliminating duplicates, and a total of 12 original studies were finally included in the systematic review. The treatments evaluated included levodopa, vitamin D, repetitive transcranial magnetic stimulation (rTMS) and intracerebral transcatheter laser photobiomodulation therapy (PBMT). The response to levodopa was lower in patients with VP with respect to IPD. Despite this, there has been described a subgroup of patients with good response, it being possible to identify them by means of neuroimaging techniques and the olfactory identification test. Other therapies showed encouraging results in studies with some risk of bias. Conclusions: The response of VP to different therapeutic strategies is modest. However, there is evidence that a subgroup of patients can be identified as more responsive to L-dopa based on clinical and neuroimaging criteria. This subgroup should be treated with L-dopa at appropriate doses. New therapies such as vitamin D, rTMS and PBMT warrant further studies to demonstrate their efficacy.

Keywords: vascular parkinsonism; treatment; therapy; systematic review; levodopa; vitamin D; repetitive transcranial magnetic stimulation; intracerebral transcatheter laser photobiomodulation

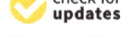

Citation: del Toro-Pérez, C.; Guevara-Sánchez, E.; Martínez-Sánchez, P. Treatment of Vascular Parkinsonism: A Systematic Review. *Brain Sci.* 2023, 13, 489. https://doi.org/10.3390/brainsci13030489

Academic Editor: Abdelaziz M. Hussein

Received: 20 February 2023
Revised: 9 March 2023
Accepted: 13 March 2023
Published: 14 March 2023

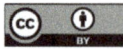

Copyright: © 2023 by the authors. Licensee MDPI, Basel, Switzerland. This article is an open access article distributed under the terms and conditions of the Creative Commons Attribution (CC BY) license (https://creativecommons.org/licenses/by/4.0/).

1. Introduction

The term vascular parkinsonism (VP) is one of the most controversial in neurology since its introduction in the early 20th century given the heterogeneity of the clinical picture that defines it, the topography of the ischemic lesions that cause it and the response to treatment among patients [1]. This parkinsonism is accompanied by ischemic brain lesions of different characteristics demonstrated by neuroimaging, without findings suggestions of other causes of parkinsonism. Winikates and Jankovic first proposed clinical criteria for vascular parkinsonism (VP) in 1999 [2]. New, stricter criteria based on a clinicopathological study were defined in 2004 [3], although a definitive diagnosis can only be reached by autopsy [4].

Currently, VP encompasses a heterogeneous set of clinical pictures in which the predominant syndrome is similar to parkinsonism but without meeting the necessary diagnostic criteria, which can present in various forms. VP has also been termed "lower body parkinsonism" because it can manifest as predominant parkinsonism of the lower extremities, with difficulty walking, absence of tremors and minimal or no response to levodopa treatment, especially in hypertensive patients. However, cases with clinical features difficult to distinguish from idiopathic Parkinson's disease (IPD) have also been described, with a response to levodopa, even without evidence of Lewy bodies in post-mortem studies [4].

Classically, it has been considered that VP did not show a good response to levodopa treatment. However, a study published in 2004 showed that a subgroup of patients with vascular lesions in or near the nigrostriatal pathway could be responders to levodopa regardless of VP characteristics [5]. Following this, several studies have tried to identify clinical or radiological features that might explain or anticipate a good treatment efficacy, with different response rates described, and therapies other than levodopa or dopaminergic agonists have also been tested. Given the limitations of VP treatment and the emergence of new therapeutic strategies since the last meta-analysis [6], the present systematic review has been performed.

2. Materials and Methods

2.1. Search Strategy

This paper follows the guidelines according to the preferred reporting items for systematic reviews and meta-analysis protocol (PRISMA-P) [7]. It was registered in the PROSPERO international database of prospectively registered systematic reviews (CRD 42021250195). Pubmed, Scopus and Web of Science electronic databases were searched for articles in English or Spanish, published in the last 15 years until April 2022 and with the following criteria: randomized clinical trials, cross-sectional, case-control and cohort observational studies including patients with VP and treatment of VP, analyzing differences between given therapies and their efficacy. Case reports and animal-model studies were excluded. The search query was: ("Parkinson Disease, Secondary" OR "Parkinsonism, Symptomatic" OR "Symptomatic Parkinson Disease" OR "Symptomatic Parkinsonism" OR "Secondary Parkinsonism" OR "Parkinson Disease, Symptomatic" OR "Parkinsonism, Secondary" OR "Parkinson Disease, Secondary Vascular" OR "Secondary Vascular Parkinson Disease" OR "Atherosclerotic Parkinsonism" OR "Parkinsonism, Atherosclerotic" OR "Parkinson's disease" OR "PD" OR "Lower Body Parkinsonism" OR "Pseudo-parkinsonism" OR "acute parkinsonism" or "vascular parkinsonism") AND ("vascular" OR "stroke" OR "brain ischemia") AND ("treatment" OR "disease management" OR "Therapeutic" OR "Therapy" OR "Therapies" OR "Treatments"). In addition to the database search, a manual revision of the reference lists of all relevant articles was performed to identify additional studies of interest.

2.2. Selection of Studies

Two researchers (CT and EG) separately reviewed the titles and abstracts of the retrieved articles to determine the presence of the abovementioned criteria. Disagreements were solved by the consensus of a third author (PM). Two investigators (CT and EG) separately reviewed the titles and abstracts of the retrieved articles to determine the presence of the abovementioned criteria. Disagreements were resolved by consensus of a third author (PM). These results were transferred to Rayyan (https://www.rayyan.ai/), accessed on 25 April 2022.

For systematic, independent screening for exclusion or inclusion by two reviewers (CT and EG). Duplicate entries, studies on diseases other than vascular parkinsonism or studies evaluating another aspect of vascular parkinsonism other than its treatment, papers not written in English or Spanish, publications that were not research studies, and any other articles that did not fit the scope of the review were excluded.

2.3. Data Extraction

After manuscript selection, the following information was extracted: the number of participants and socio-demographic characteristics, the assessed scales and the evaluation protocol or diagnostic strategies, the type of vascular lesion, response to evaluated treatment and the major findings reported. We expected to find a limited number of studies that could eventually be included in the review.

2.4. Quality Assessment

To improve the quality of detection of the risk of bias in non-randomized studies, these will be assessed using the Newcastle–Ottawa scale, with a subsequent comparison with the STROBE scale used in the last systematic review of 2017. The Cochrane risk-of-bias tool for randomized trials (RoB 2) will be used for randomized studies [6,8–10].

3. Results

The Databases search yielded 4738 results. Overall, 4687 publications involving different pathologies were excluded. After removing duplicates, 59 publications were screened for eligibility. Of them, 8 studies were identified through the references of the principal records. A total of 46 studies were excluded for the following reasons: publications that evaluated different pathologies, no evaluation of response to treatment, systematic reviews, studies in languages other than Spanish or English, experimental studies with animals or studies prior to the last 15 years.

A PRISMA flow diagram is shown in Figure 1. After reading the articles and removing duplicates, a total of 12 original studies were finally included in the systematic review and are summarized in Tables 1 and 2. Table 3 shows the studies performed using neuroimaging studies. Finally, a meta-analysis was not performed as we have not found studies on the response to levodopa in VP since the last systematic review and meta-analysis of 2017 and there are insufficient studies on other treatments to perform it on another treatment subgroup.

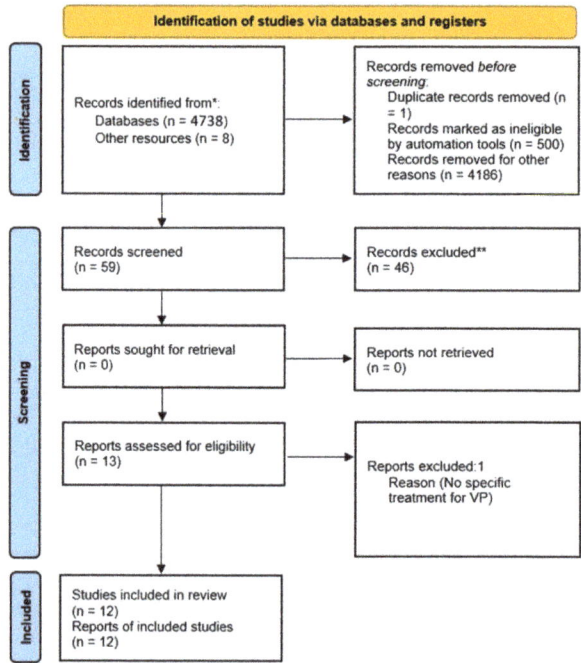

Figure 1. PRISMA Flow Diagram. * Pubmed, Scopus and Web of Science electronic databases. ** Studies excluded for the following reasons: publications that evaluated different pathologies, no evaluation of response to treatment, systematic reviews, studies in languages other than Spanish or English, experimental studies with animals.

Table 1. Studies methodology and clinical-demographic characteristics.

Study	Design	Mean Age (n)	Main Symptoms	Comparative Group (vs. VP)	Follow-Up	Blinded	Diagnostic Criteria for VP
Zijlmans, J. et al., 2007 [ ]	Case-control	Group I (VP): 74.1 years ± 11.5 (13) Group II (IPD): 66.0 ± 14.5 (14) Group III (controls): 66.3 ± 18 (14)	Gait disorder, acute contralateral bradykinetic rigid syndrome, cognitive dysfunction	VP/IPD	No	Nuclear Medicine specialists	Zijlmans et al.
Antonini, A. et al., 2012 [ ]	Case-control	Group I (SPECT no pathological): 72.8 ± 4.8 (59–80) (28) Group II (SPECT pathological): 72.6 ± 5.7 (48)	Lower body parkinsonism	VP/IPD	No	Radiologists and Nuclear Medicine specialists	Zijlmans et al.
Sato, Y., et al. 2013 [ ]	Case-control	Group I (VP): 73.9 ± 6.2 (94) Group II (IPD): 73.6 ± 5.9 (92)	Bradykinetic rigid syndrome, rest tremor	VP/IPD	2 years	A therapist that evaluated muscle strength	Zijlmans et al.
Vale, T.C. et al., 2013 [ ]	Case series	Group I (VP): 75.8 ± 10.1 (17)	Lower body parkinsonism, pyramidal signs, urinary incontinence	Their selves	No	No	Zijlmans et al.
Benítez-Rivero, S. et al., 2013 [ ]	Case series to correlate image to VP clinic. Case control to find clinical and image differences between PD and VP	Group I (VP): 72.6 ± 6.8 (106) Group II (IPD): 55.3 ± 12.6 (280)	Gait disorder, postural tremor, mixed tremor, rest tremor, falls, postural instability, dysphagia, urinary incontinence, cognitive dysfunction, emotional lability	VP/IPD	5 years	Nuclear Medicine specialists	Zijlmans et al.
Yip, C.W. et al., 2013 [ ]	Case series	Group I (VP): 64.2 (5)	Bradykinetic rigid syndrome, tremor, postural instability	No	6 months	No	Winikates et al.
Gago, M.F. et al., 2014 [ ]	Case-control	Group I (VP): 77 (5) Group II (IPD): 73 (10)	Worse MoCA and UPDRS III scores, gait impairment, difficulty getting up from the chair and low global spontaneity of movement	VP/IPD	No	No	Zijlmans et al.

Table 1. *Cont.*

Study	Design	Mean Age (n)	Main Symptoms	Comparative Group (vs. VP)	Follow-Up	Blinded	Diagnostic Criteria for VP
Navarro-Otano, J. et al., 2014 [ ]	Case-control	Group I (VP): 68.11 ± 8.2 (15) Group II (IPD): 66.2 ± 9.5 (15) Group III (controls): 66.2 ± 8.2 (9)	Gait disorder, postural tremor, falls, postural instability	VP/IPD/controls	No	Nuclear medicine specialists	Zijlmans et al.
Vale, T.C. et al., 2015 [ ]	Case-control	Group I: (VP) 75.7 ± 10.4 (15) Group II: (IPD) 67.3 ± 7.5 (30)	Lower body parkinsonism, pyramidal signs, instability urinary incontinence	VP/IPD	No	No	Zijlmans et al.
Lee, M.J. et al., 2015 [ ]	Case-control	Group I: (no pathological) 75.77 ± 6.16 (22) Group II: (pathological) 75.15 ± 6.75. (20)	Gait disorder, postural tremor, resting tremor, falls, postural instability, urinary incontinence supranuclear palsy, dysphagia, emotional lability	NDD+/NDD−	No	No	Zijlmans et al.
Maksimovich, I.V. et al., 2019 [ ]	Case-control	Group I (VP): 52–80 (37) Group II (control group): (25)	Cognitive dysfunction	VP/ Binswanger Disease/ controls	8 years	No	Does not specify
Fernandes, C. et al., 2021 [ ]	Case-control	Group I (VP): 80.53 ± 4.63 (14) Group II (IPD): 76.60 ± 4.29 (15) Group III (controls): 52.76 ± 22.91 (34)	Gait disorder	VP/IPD/controls	No	No	Zijlmans et al.

Table 2. Study methodology (continuation) and main results.

Study	Used Scales Image Testing	Type of Vascular Lesion Specified	Primary Endpoint	VP Treatment as Primary Endpoint	Definition of Treatment Response	Response to Treatment
Zijlmans, J. et al., 2007 [ ]	UPDRS III [123I] FP-CIT SPECT	In or near areas that can increase the basal ganglia motor output or decrease the thalamocortical drive directly (substantia nigra in one, globus pallidum/putamen area in the others). Extensive subcortical white matter lesions	To compare pre-synaptic dopaminergic function VP vs IPD; VPa vs VPi and if severity and response to levodopa can be related to pre-synaptic dopaminergic function	Yes	Based on the mean % reduction in motor UPDRS	(L-dopa) Mean reduction in motor UPDRS in Group I (VP patients): 14% "Good" response: 0.07%
Antonini, A. et al., 2012 [ ]	UPDRS III, UPDRS II, Y&H, DAT SCAN	Periventricular hyperintensities, lesions in hemispheric white matter, basal ganglia, infra-tentorial foci	Clinical and neuroimage profile	No	≥30% changes in total UPDRS motor scores from the baseline	(L-dopa) Negative response: Group I (VP patients): 68.4% Group II (IPD patients): 40%
Sato, Y. et al., 2013 [ ]	Barthel index, SSS arm score, SSS leg score	Cerebral infarction/Cerebral hemorrhage	Clinical profile	Yes	The number of falls per person and incidence of hip fractures	(Vitamin D supplementation) VP patients: 59% reduction in falls IPD patients: 0% reduction in falls Increase of strength in both groups (does not provide details)
Vale, T.C. et al., 2013 [ ]	DSM-UPDRS, HY, MMSE, FAB, EIS, Pfeffer, Katz, NINDS-AIREN	Substance nigra, White matter disease, Multiple lacunar infarcts	Clinic and radiological profile	No	Based on the percentage of reduction in Part III of DSM-UPDRS and Hoehn-Yahr	(L-dopa) Improvement in part III DSM-UPDRS: 5.8 ± 4.4 (Efficacy is based on mean scale score reduction, no control group)
Benítez-Rivero, S. et al., 2013 [ ]	UPDRS, HY, Stchelten's scale DAT SCAN,	Supratentorial lesions: Subcortical basal gabglia>thalamus>internal capsule Infratentorial	(A) To find clinical and image (SPECT) differences between IPD and VP. (B) Among VP patients, to study possible clinical features related to SPECT or structural image (CT or MRI)	No	Does not specify criteria for responsiveness	(L-Dopa) Group I (VP patients): 47.9% Group II (IPD patients): 100%

Table 2. Cont.

Study	Used Scales Image Testing	Type of Vascular Lesion Specified	Primary Endpoint	VP Treatment as Primary Endpoint	Definition of Treatment Response	Response to Treatment
Yip, C.W. et al., 2013 [16]	UPDRS rTMS	Multiple lacunar infarcts, lentiform nuclei, caudate, Multiple subcortical lesions	Gait improvement	Yes	Mean timing measured in seconds of 10 m walk and the improvement of UPDRS score	(rTMS) At 4 weeks post-rTMS:11.9%, At 2 weeks post-rTMS: 6.8%, Not statistically significant by 6 weeks For the UPDRS post-rTMS over time: 11.8%
Gago, M.F. et al., 2014 [17]	MDS-UPDRS III, MoCA	Subcortical or basal ganglia lesions	Clinical improvement on postural stability	Yes	Percentage of the difference between "off" and "on" states	(L-dopa) Group I (VP patients): 19% Group II (IPD patients): 57.5%
Navarro-Otano, J. et al., 2014 [8]	UPDRS, HY 123I-MIBG cardiac gammagraphy, UPSIT, DaT-SPECT	Decreased uptake with a pattern typical for IPD (symmetric or asymmetric levodopa uptake reduction or absent uptake) or decreased uptake pattern non-typical of PD (as a local or patchy defect where cerebral MR imaging showed an ischemic lesion)	To ascertain the clinical value of 123I-MIBG cardiac gammagraphy, UPSIT and DaT-SPECT to diagnosis	No	Levodopa response was codified as good, partial and absent, does not specify criteria for responsiveness	(L-dopa) Group I (VP patients with normal H/M ratio): 0% Group II (VP patients with low H/M ratio): 28.6% In total good response: 14.3% Group III (IPD patients): 100%
Vale, T.C. et al., 2015 [19]	MDS-UPDRS, MMSE, FAB, EXIT25, Hachinski scale, Katz index, Pfeffer, FOG-Q, HY	Extensive white matter disease, Multiple lacunar infarcts	Clinic and radiological profile	No	Based on the percentage of reduction in Part III of MDS-UPDRS	(L-dopa) Yes Not percentages
Lee, M.J. et al., 2015 [18]	MMSE, UPDRS III [18F] FP-CIT PET, MRI	Moderate or severe white matter lesions in the lobar subcortical or periventricular regions Deep subcortical lesions in frontal, temporal, parietal and occipital regions	Clinical and MRI findings that indicate NDD	No	≥30% changes in total UPDRS motor scores from the baseline	(L-dopa) Group I (Normal uptake): 4.5% Group II (reduced uptake): 40% In total good response: 44,5%

Table 2. Cont.

Study	Used Scales Image Testing	Type of Vascular Lesion Specified	Primary Endpoint	VP Treatment as Primary Endpoint	Definition of Treatment Response	Response to Treatment
Maksimovich, I.V. et al., 2019 [ ]	Clinical Dementia Rating scale, MMSE, BI MRI, CT, SG, REG, MUGA.	Signs of brain involutional changes, Subarachnoid space expansion, Nonocclusive hydrocephalus signs, Local focal subcortical demyelization, Leukoaraiosis signs	Clinical and image improvement	Yes	Mental and motor functions, an improvement in blood flow measured through SG and REG and a narrowing of the subarachnoid space	(PBMT) Group I (case group VP with PBMT):94.60% Group II (control group VP without PBMT): 56.00% Group III (case group BD with PBMT): 53.85%
Fernandes, C. et al., 2021 [ ]	CDR, Hoehn-Yahr CNNs	Does not specify	Clinical improvement	Yes	Based on gait time series with and without the influence of levodopa medication	(L-dopa) Group I (VP patients): 79.33% Group II (IPD patients): 82.33% Group III (controls): 86%

(123I)-MIBG cardiac gamma-graphy: (123)I-metaiodobenzylguanidine on cardiac gammagraphy; (123I) FP-CIT SPECT: Single Photon Emission Tomography with 123Ioflupane; 18F-FDG-PET: Fluorodeoxyglucose labeled with 18F Positron Emission Tomography; CDR: Clinical Dementia Rating; CNNs: Calibrated Neuropsychological Normative System; CT: Computerized Tomography; DaT: Dopamine Transporter; DSM/MDS: Diagnostic and Statistical Manual of Mental Disorders; EIS: Executive Interview Scale; EXIT-25: The Executive Interview; FAB: Frontal Assessment Battery; FOG-Q: Freezing of Gait Questionnaire; HY: Hoehn & Yahr; BD: Binswanger's Disease; BI: Bartels Index; IPD: Idiopathic Parkinson's Disease; MMSE: Mini Mental State Examination; MoCA: Montreal; Cognitive Assessment test; MRI: Magnetic Resonance Imaging; MUGA: Multigated Angiography; NDD: Nigrostriatal Dopaminergic Denervation; NINDS-AIREN: Association International pour la Recherche et l'Enseignement in Neurosciences and Hachinski Scores; PBMT: Intracerebral Transcatheter Laser Photobiomodulation Therapy; rTMS: repetitive Transcranial Magnetic Stimulation; REG: rheoencephalography; SG: Scintigraphy, reg: rheoencephalography; SPECT: Single Photon Emission Computed Tomography; SSS: Scandinavian Stroke Scale; UPDRS: Unified Parkinson's Disease Rating Scales; UPSIT: Smell Identification Test; VP: Vascular Parkinsonism.

Table 3. Studies results based on imaging techniques.

Study	Image Testing	Response to Treatment (Levodopa) Depending on Image	Comments
Navarro-Otano, J. et a, 2014 [18]	123I-MIBG cardiac image	VP patients with normal H/M ratio (non-suggesting IPD): 0% (0/7) VP patients with low H/M ratio: 28.6% (2/8)	A normal H/M ratio (not suggestive of IPD) predicted a poor response to treatment.
Lee, M.J. et al. 2015 [20]	[18F] FP-CIT PET	Group I: 4.5 (1/22) Group II: 40.0% (8/20)	Patients with a pathological PET study showed significantly better response to levodopa. Good response based on ≥30% changes in UPDRS.
Benítez-Rivero, S. et al., 2012 [15]	123 I-FP-CIT SPECT	Does not compare the response to treatment according to an image.	SPECT results were only associated with the presence of falls.
Zijlmans, J. et al., 2007 [11]	[123I] FP-SPECT Based on BP%	Two L-dopa responders with a BG BP% similar to the 11 non-responders (mean 29.5 (28.4–30.5) vs mean 26.0 (6.9–56.5))	[123I] FP-SPECT uptake not correlated to levodopa response based on reduction in UPDRS III scale.
Antonini, A. et al., 2012 [12]	FP-CIT SPECT	SPECT (no pathological) l: 93% (26/28) SPECT (pathological): 48% (23/48)	They confirm that a normal FP-CIT SPECT is associated with a poor levodopa effect.

(123I)-MIBG cardiac gamma-graphy: (123)I-metaiodobenzylguanidine on cardiac gammagraphy; (123I) FP-CIT SPECT: Single Photon Emission Tomography with 123Ioflupane; 18F-FDG-PET: Fluorodeoxyglucose labeled with 18F Positron Emission Tomography; BP: radiotracer pickup.

As no randomized studies were found in the search, the Cochrane Collaboration tool for assessing risk of bias was not used. The risk of bias in the included studies was assessed using the Newcastle–Ottawa Scale. This can be seen in Figure 2 together with a comparison of the results of this scale with the STROBE scale used in the previous systematic review.

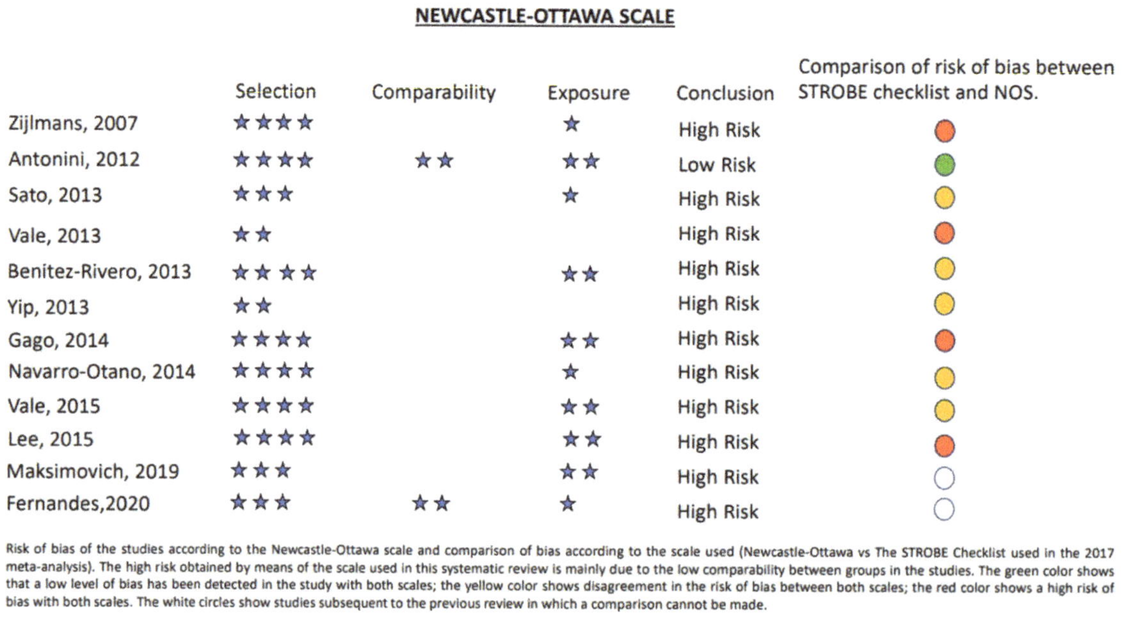

NEWCASTLE-OTTAWA SCALE

Study	Selection	Comparability	Exposure	Conclusion	Comparison of risk of bias between STROBE checklist and NOS.
Zijlmans, 2007	★★★★		★	High Risk	🟠
Antonini, 2012	★★★★	★★	★★	Low Risk	🟢
Sato, 2013	★★★		★	High Risk	🟡
Vale, 2013	★★			High Risk	🟠
Benítez-Rivero, 2013	★★★★		★★	High Risk	🟡
Yip, 2013	★★			High Risk	🟡
Gago, 2014	★★★★		★★	High Risk	🟠
Navarro-Otano, 2014	★★★★		★	High Risk	🟡
Vale, 2015	★★★★		★★	High Risk	🟡
Lee, 2015	★★★★		★★	High Risk	🟠
Maksimovich, 2019	★★★		★★	High Risk	⚪
Fernandes, 2020	★★★	★★	★	High Risk	⚪

Risk of bias of the studies according to the Newcastle-Ottawa scale and comparison of bias according to the scale used (Newcastle-Ottawa vs The STROBE Checklist used in the 2017 meta-analysis). The high risk obtained by means of the scale used in this systematic review is mainly due to the low comparability between groups in the studies. The green color shows that a low level of bias has been detected in the study with both scales; the yellow color shows disagreement in the risk of bias between both scales; the red color shows a high risk of bias with both scales. The white circles show studies subsequent to the previous review in which a comparison cannot be made.

Figure 2. Newcastle–Ottawa scale and comparison of bias with STROBE scale [11–22].

4. Treatments

4.1. Levodopa

A cross-sectional study assessed the characteristics and response to levodopa in 17 patients with a diagnosis of VP [14]. VP was divided into four types based on Fenelon and Houéto classification [23]: (1) VP identical to IPD, (2) Unilateral after a contralateral vascular lesion, (3) Atypical parkinsonism and (4) Parkinsonian gait disorder. They added three categories depending on the course: (1) Rapidly progressive (worse before a year from its onset), (2) stable and (3) slowly progressive (worsening after a year from its onset). Response to levodopa was based on the percentage of reduction on Part III of MDS-UPDRS and the Hoehn and Yahr stage (HY), evaluated in an "off" state (12 h after interruption of levodopa) and an "on" state (1 h after levodopa). The patients had been treated with levodopa at a mean dose of 530.9 ± 218.2 mg/day for a mean period of 2.9 years. There was a mean of 5.8 ± 4.4 point reduction in UPDRS Part III after levodopa, with no change in the HY stage. Most patients had a poor response to the drug and no complications of levodopa were seen, such as dyskinesia or fluctuation. Two years later, the same first author designed a case-control study to further study VP, comparing baseline, imaging and response characteristics to levodopa compared to IPD patients. He observed that 33.3% of IPD patients with freezing of gait "off" (50%) responded to levodopa, whereas no patients with VP responded. The percentage of patients responding to levodopa was lower in the VP group, although the mean MDS-UPDRS part III score did decrease [19].

Two studies have relied on gait to assess VP response to levodopa. The first of them [24] is a non-blinded, non-randomized, case-control study adding levodopa response to increase the accuracy of the differential diagnosis between IPD and VP according to gait characteristics and response to treatment, based on a previous study that succeeded in discriminating between IPD, VP and healthy controls by gait assessment thanks to machine learning strategies (accuracy for distinguish IPD and VP was 50–63.3%) [22,24,25]. 14 VP and 15 IPD were included, excluding patients with resting tremors, dementia CDR > 2, musculoskeletal disease and an HY stage. Similar to previous studies, 36 controls were added for the normalization process of gait data. Patients were evaluated after 12 h in the "off" state and after 60 min after taking >50% over their usual dose of levodopa ("on" state). Speed, stride length and foot clearance were the independent variables included to predict differences between patients with and without IPD, based on previous studies [26–28]. The results showed increased discrimination due to levodopa comparing "on" and "off" status, achieving IPD diagnostic accuracies of $86\% \pm 7.12$, the sensitivity of $80\% \pm 16.33$ and $90\% \pm 20$, as well as a VP diagnostic accuracy of 72.8% without levodopa testing. These results show that the inferior response to levodopa treatment in VP is also reflected in gait. In the second one, Gago M.F. et al. evaluated the effect of levodopa on postural stability [17]. Two groups (VP and IPD) with normal retropulsion tests were included. The included IPD patients were of the akinetic-rigid type. Both groups were age-matched since gait is altered by age. Wearable sensor-based gait was compared when patients were in their best "on" state with gait "off". The best dopaminergic therapy to reach their best "on" state was assessed over the three months prior to the start of the study. Five VP and 10 PD were included. The IPD group had better MoCA scores, gait, lower UPDRS III scores, easier getting out of a chair and global spontaneity of movement after levodopa treatment, with a motor benefit of 19% of VP patients vs. 57.5% of IPD patients.

On the other hand, several studies have added imaging studies for the study of the response to levodopa in VP (Table 3). In the study by J. Navarro-Otano. et al. the aim was to add diagnostic accuracy to the difference between VP and IPD using the University of Pennsylvania smell identification test (UPSIT) to cardiac imaging by 123I-MIBG [18]. Patients were diagnosed with VP using the criteria of Ziljmans 2004, and patients with IPD using the criteria based on Huges, 1992. The discrimination ability between IPD and VP of the tests as well as the response to treatment were studied. A greater response to levodopa was observed in patients with IPD compared to VP (100% vs. 14.3%). However, the response rates to levodopa were different within the group of VP patients according to the results of the tests performed. No VP patient with a normal H/M ratio in the 123I-MIBG test (not suggestive of IPD) responded to levodopa, whereas 28.6% of VP with a low ratio presented a good response ($p = 0.0462$). Of note, 123 I-MIBG SPECT can be positive in diabetic patients.

It has been seen that VP patients with nigrostriatal dysfunction assessed by PET study showed significantly better response to levodopa, although VP patients with vascular lesions in the basal ganglia were excluded [20]. Greater than or equal to 30% improvement in UPDRS motor score was observed in 40% of patients with pathological PET vs. 4.5% of patients with normal PET. Also, a partial response (improvement between 10–30% UPDRS motor scale improvement) was observed in 20% vs. 13.6%. Finally, poor response to levodopa was observed in 40% of patients with pathologic PET versus 81.8% with normal PET (change of less than 10%. $p = 0.036$). Clinical differences between patients in whom nigrostriatal dysfunction was observed and between those without this dysfunction did not predict response to levodopa. MRI imaging also failed to predict response to levodopa, with no differences in the degree and regional distribution of white matter lesions between responders and non-responders.

On the contrary, in the study by Benítez-Rivero et al. when clinical characteristics and levodopa response were analyzed with the results of normal or pathological 123 I-FP-CIT SPECT in patients with VP (pathological in 67.5% vs. 100% of patients with IPD), pathological SPECT was only associated with the presence of falls and not with levodopa response [15]. In patients with VP, 47.9% of patients who received levodopa treatment had an improvement vs. 100% of patients with PD.

Zijlmans J. et al. performed a case-control study that aimed to compare by [123I] FP-SPECT uptake: (1) pre-synaptic dopaminergic function VP vs. EPI; (2) acute-onset VP vs. insidious-onset VP; (3) severity of parkinsonism and (4) response to levodopa [11]. It included 13 VP (6 with acute onset, 7 with progressive onset), 14 controls and 14 IPD. It included 13 VP (6 with acute onset, 7 with progressive onset), 14 controls and 14 IPD. Withdrawal of dopaminergic therapy was performed 12 h before the levodopa challenge test. There was a good response in one patient, transient in two, poor in three and uncertain in five. No patients with VP had an excellent response to levodopa, with no difference between acute-onset VP and insidious-onset VP. 123I] FP-SPECT uptake does not correlate with response to levodopa based on UPDRS III scale reduction.

Finally, in the Antonini et al. study [12], a greater negative response to levodopa was observed in VP concerning IPD. A total of 47.8% of VP patients responded to treatment, being their negative response associated with symmetrical symptom onset ($p < 0.001$), HY status (negative 2.43 ± 0.8 vs. positive 2.16 ± 7; $p = 0.007$), absence of dyskinesia ($p = 0.04$) and hypertension and diabetes ($p = 0.04$ and $p = 0.04$). Higher HY status was associated with hypertension and smoking ($p = 0.005$; $p = 0.05$). The strongest predictor variables for a negative response to levodopa (failure to achieve > 30% improvement on the UPDRSIII scale with levodopa 500 mg/day for more than 3 months) were hypertension (systolic blood pressure > 140 mmHg and/or diastolic blood pressure > 90 mmHg) ($p = 0.022$), basal ganglia lesions ($p = 0.045$) and normal FP-CIT SPECT uptake ($p < 0.001$). More of these and other vascular risk factors (family history, hyperlipidemia, heart disease and hypotension) predicted a negative response to chronic levodopa. In patients with pathological uptake on FP-CIT SPECT, vascular lesions in the basal ganglia predicted a negative response to levodopa, and hypertension and vascular lesions in infratentorial areas were associated with worsening disease ($p = 0.007$; $p = 0.045$). VP patients with normal FP-CIT SPECT showed no effect with levodopa. However, in IPD patients with normal FP-CIT SPECT, although they had a worse response to levodopa than those with pathological uptake (48% vs. 93%, $p < 0.001$), we did find a percentage with response to levodopa that was not found in those VP with normal FP-CIT SPECT. Cerebral vascular disease is found to be associated with increased severity of parkinsonism and poor response to levodopa, especially in patients with non-pathological FP-CIT SPECT.

4.2. Vitamin D

Sato et al. designed a 2-year case-control study [13]. The objective was to reduce falls in patients with VP and IPD by vitamin D supplementation of 1200 IU ergocalciferol in vitamin D-deficient patients (mean vitamin D at baseline 22 nmol/L, low compared to the reference range of the normal Japanese population). It is speculated that the protective effect of vitamin D is due not only to its benefits on bone mineral density but also to the enhancement of atrophy of type II muscle fibers, which prevents falls [29,30]. In addition, one study showed that deterioration of muscle function can be observed before signs of bone density loss [31].

Between 92 IPD and 94 VP patients participated. No changes in diet, physical activity or medication that could alter bone or calcium were introduced. Sunlight exposure and muscle strength were assessed and fall schedules and medication adherence were recorded. No differences in baseline clinical characteristics were found. After 12 and 24 months, no differences were found in PD patients, while the percentage of falls was reduced from 34% to 16% in the VP group ($p < 0.001$). A significant increase in muscle strength was observed in both groups. This study adds evidence to the fact that falls have a different etiology in VP and PD, with a possibly greater role of muscle weakness in VP than in PD.

4.3. Repetitive Transcranial Magnetic Stimulation (rTMS)

rTMS has shown beneficial outcomes in bradykinesia and UPDRS scales in IPD [16]. The study of Jang et al. aims to improve gait in VP, based on the mean timing measured in seconds of 10 metres walk and the improvement of UPDRS scores. This study was unblinded and non-randomised. The leg region was identified for each patient by motor-evoked potential. Five patients were included, with 4/5 presenting a headache response to simple analgesics as adverse events. Improvement was observed after 4 weeks of treatment that did not persist in week 6. UPDRS score reduction was observed at weeks number 2, 4 and 6 after rTMS. Also, two 7-point scales were performed based on the Patient's Global Impression of Change and Clinicians' Global Impression of Change, with a significant increase in both of them after rTMS.

4.4. Intracerebral Transcatheter Lase Photobiomodulation Therapy (PBMT)

Cerebral small vessel disease progresses causing leukoaraiosis. Cerebral hypoperfusion and hypoxia stimulate angiogenesis with the development of collateral capillary supplementation [32], facilitating angiogenesis neurogenesis [33]. Intracerebral transcatheter PBMT has shown good results in the treatment of stroke, neurodegenerative diseases, trauma and depression [34–36].

The study by Maksimovich et al. aims to evaluate intracerebral transcatheter PBMT as a treatment for Binswanger's disease and VP, using a case-control study [21]. Sixty-two subjects with VP and 27 with BD were enrolled. After PBMT the VP patients continued dopaminergic therapy (levodopa 250 mg three-four times daily + Amantadinum 100–200 mg daily). The control group of the VP arm was prescribed the same dopaminergic therapy. In the first 6 months after therapy, 94.6% of the VP case group vs. 56% of the controls had significant improvement in mental and motor functions. 100% of cases vs. 52% of controls in the VP group had improvement in blood flow measured by scintigraphy (SG) and rheoencephalography (REG) as well as narrowing of the subarachnoid space assessed by CT and MRI vs. 0% of controls. After 8 years, the restoration of mental and motor functions remained at the same percentage in the case group, while the patients who improved in the control group suffered a clinical worsening at 12–24 months. Improvement in OS and REG was maintained in 94.6% of patients versus 52% in the control group. CT and MRI showed a decrease in involutional changes in 91.89% and a narrowing of the sylvian fissure in 86.5%, while 100% of the control group had greater involutional changes.

5. Discussion

Classically, VP has been considered a homogeneous entity with poor response to levodopa treatment. However, the reviewed studies suggest that VP is a heterogeneous entity that should be properly subclassified to identify those patients with a response to levodopa. Several treatments have been added in recent years as possible adjuvants and even as effective treatments, but further studies are needed to confirm their efficacy.

Levodopa resistance has been considered a useful feature to distinguish between PD and VP. However, despite not showing excellent response to levodopa in a high percentage of patients, a decrease in part III of the UPDRS scale has been observed in this review. Moreover, some patients with VP have been shown to have clinical benefits from levodopa treatment for several months [5,37], and even an excellent positive response to levodopa has been described in pathologically confirmed VP [5]. Furthermore, the fact that the clinic cannot reliably distinguish patients with nigrostriatal dopaminergic denervation (NDD) a Lee et al. study provides additional evidence that in case of non-response to levodopa in patients with VP, levodopa should be increased to the maximum tolerable dose (up to 1 g L-dopa daily for 3 months) [11].

S Benítez-Rivero, et al. together with Ziljmans et al. [15,38], reported dopaminergic deficits in patients with VP, sometimes as marked as in patients with IPD. Other studies did not find this dopaminergic deficit [39]. Also, neuropathology studies have shown a heterogeneous clinical presentation of VP, sometimes with an overlap between VP and IPD that increases in VP patients with a response to levodopa [3,5]. Therefore, although the distinction between both entities by clinical features is widely described, it is not uncommon to find parkinsonisms with overlapping clinical and neuroimaging features and even in the response to levodopa treatment. Although structural imaging based on magnetic resonance imaging (MRI) or computed tomography (CT) shows vascular lesions in all VP, these are also prevalent in IPD patients in up to 25%, their contribution to the clinical features is unknown [12,15]. Levodopa has shown very variable response rates in VP patients in different studies, but almost always much lower than the response rates in patients with IPD. It has been described that a presynaptic dopaminergic deficit evidenced by SPECT and corresponding to ischemic lesions in MRI, simulating the pathological mechanism of IPD, could have a response to levodopa administration. That is why several studies try to delve into their clinical and imaging features to facilitate the differential diagnosis and especially to identify those patients who may benefit from treatment.

In a cross-sectional study of 15 patients with VP, 15 patients with EPD and 9 healthy subjects, the usefulness of olfactory function assessment measured with the University of Pennsylvania Smell Identification Test (UPSIT), cardiac SPECT with 123 I-meta-iodobenzylguanidine (123 I-MIBG) and SPECT with I-FP-CIT assessed by a blinded nuclear medicine specialist was studied [18]. The heart-to-mediastinum ratio was higher in VP versus IPD, with discrimination between VP and IPD under the ROC curve of 0.85. UPSIT scores were similar between VP and IPD. However, patients with normal H/M radius were more likely to have higher UPSIT scores. No VP H/M normal ratio patients (non-suggesting IPD) responded to levodopa, whereas 28.6% of VP with a low ratio presented a good response with statistical significance. As previously mentioned, it is worth noticing that 123 I-MIBG SPECT can be positive in diabetic patients. Other studies did find higher UPSIT scores in patients with VP vs. IPD [40], but the response to levodopa as a function of UPSIT scores was not studied.

Other studies show that a higher burden of cerebral vascular disease is associated with more severe parkinsonism and a negative effect of levodopa, especially in patients with non-pathological FP-CIT SPECT [12]. The location of vascular lesions has also been shown to be related to different clinical features of patients with VP and their response to treatment; Antonini et al. showed that the lesion most strongly predicting a negative effect of levodopa is in the basal ganglia [12], and Benítez-Rivero found that territorial infarction was related to lower response to treatment [15]. The study of Benítez-Rivero et al. found no association between pathological SPECT imaging in VP patients and their response to levodopa and no association between CT/MRI and SPECT findings [15]. On the contrary, the VADO study found several differences in terms of structural imaging with CT or MRI according to the SPECT result [12]. IPD patients with normal FP-CIT SPECT had a worse response to levodopa, a higher HY scale score and greater periventricular leukoaraiosis, while pathological FP-CIT SPECT was associated with vascular lesions in basal ganglia and infratentorial regions. Classic VP clinic (symmetrical onset, higher disease severity based on HY stage, negative response to levodopa) was associated with higher vascular scores [4,12,41]. Interestingly, despite vascular burden, IPD patients with abnormal MRI and pathological SPECT FP-CIT showed a good response to levodopa. These findings are consistent with a worse response to levodopa in patients with non-classical IPD clinic, as well as opening the possibility that those IPD patients with higher vascular lesion burden get a worse response given the irruption of striatal pathways [12]. Other studies have also added evidence that abnormal uptake on FP-SPECT [123I] correlates with disease duration and severity of parkinsonism [4,41]. Nevertheless, some studies show that a chronic response to levodopa can be seen in 50% even in those patients with a normal SPECT FP-CIT [11,12,15,18]. A negative response to levodopa was associated with the symmetrical onset of symptoms characteristic of VP, as well as an absence of dyskinesia (and thus the response to levodopa), hypertension and diabetes [12].

The [123I] FP-SPECT study performed by Zijlmans J. et al. [11] showed a lower uptake in both acute-onset and progressive-onset VP patients versus controls, as well as a higher caudate/putamen ratio. However, interhemispheric asymmetry did not differ between VP and controls nor between both VP groups. This is further evidence alongside the study by Lee et al. [20] that VP patients have a significant presynaptic dopaminergic deficit. Postmortem studies in which nigral cell loss and substantia nigra gliosis in VP occur in a similar pattern to IPD support these findings, with greater involvement of the rostral parts of the striatum compared to the lateral striatum [20,41]. In this study [123I] FP-SPECT uptake did not correlate with response to levodopa based on UPDRS III scale reduction. Lee et al. suggested that leukoaraiosis in VP may cause NDD detectable by [(18)F] FP-CIT PET. Clinical differences between VP NND+ and NND− did not predict levodopa response but the presence of NDD did predict a better response to levodopa treatment [20]. These findings are consistent with those of the study by Antonini et al. in which patients with VP with abnormal MRI and normal FP-CIT SPECT had a poor response to levodopa. In this study, 90% of patients (including IPD and VP) with normal FP-CIT SPECT showed no effect with levodopa [12].

The research designed by Fernandes et al. also shows lower response to levodopa treatment in the VP group in terms of gait disorders. It also adds a useful tool for the differential diagnosis between both entities through the effect of treatment on various gait characteristics assessed by machine learning [22]. The study by Gago M.F. et al. also showed the validity of the gait study of patients with IPD and VP to differentiate both entities, especially in the "on" state. It also evidenced the better response to levodopa treatment in terms of gait disturbances in patients with IPD versus VP. However, it should be noted that some patients with VP did benefit in this respect with treatment, albeit to a lesser extent [22].

Regarding vitamin D treatment, Sato et al. showed a significant difference in the bivariate analysis between VP and IPD in the number of falls per subject over the 2 years after treatment with 1200 IU of ergocalciferol per day, with an increase in muscle strength in the lower extremities that was also observed in both groups. Therefore, this study suggests that vitamin D decreases falls and hip fractures in VP by increasing muscle strength and should be confirmed with further studies that include an analysis adjusted for confounding variables.

Treatment by repetitive transcranial magnetic stimulation (rTMS) at 5 Hz on 5 consecutive days showed improvement in a timed 10-m walk (T10MW), motor portion of the Unified PD Rating Scale (UPDRS-III), global impression of medical change (CGIC), and global impression of patient change (PGIC), up to 6 weeks after rTMS. The treatment was well tolerated, and all patients completed the study. This work demonstrated for the first time that 5 sessions of rTMS could measurably improve gait for up to 6 weeks without significant side effects, so it could be a potentially useful adjunct in the rehabilitation of VP patients and warrants further investigation as these results need to be validated with other studies with a control group and multivariate analysis.

More recently, treatment with intracerebral transcatheter laser photobiomodulation therapy (PBMT) has been successfully studied for VP. After 8 years the restoration of mental and motor functions was maintained with the same percentage in the testing group whereas the control group suffered a clinical worsening. Improvement in blood flow persisted in virtually all patients with VP, twice as many as in control patients. Likewise, a decrease in the signs of brain involution was observed, while 100% of the control group presented greater involutionary changes during the observation period. Despite obtaining encouraging results, this study does not specify the definition of VP and lacks control of the treatment effect through a blinded study and a confounder-adjusted analysis.

It is important to highlight that the articles included in this systematic review show a high risk of bias according to the Newcastle–Ottawa scale. This bias has been compared with that described in the previous systematic review which used the STROBE checklist with a lower bias rate. Despite this, most of the studies also showed a high risk of bias even when using this other scale. This bias clearly increases when performed in response to levodopa, which was not the primary endpoint in several of the articles. Few articles make a good case-control comparison using a statistical study adjusted for confounding variables probably due to the low number of patients in some of them and some articles have no control group, as can be seen in the comparability part of Table 1. Neither have they been performed in a blind manner for the patient or physician providing the medication. Only one of them did not mention the diagnostic criterion of VP. Both systematic reviews show that there is a lack of high-quality evidence regarding the treatment of VP.

6. Conclusions

The response of VP to different therapeutic strategies is modest. However, there is evidence that a subgroup of patients can be identified as more responsive to L-dopa based on clinical and neuroimaging criteria. This subgroup should be treated with L-dopa at appropriate doses. New therapies such as vitamin D, rTMS and PBMT deserve further studies to demonstrate their efficacy.

Author Contributions: C.d.T.-P., E.G.-S. and P.M.-S. conceived and designed the methodology of the systematic review. C.d.T.-P. and E.G.-S. extracted and collected the relevant information and drafted the manuscript. P.M.-S. supervised the article selection and reviewed and edited the manuscript. All authors have read and agreed to the published version of the manuscript.

Funding: This study is part of the Spanish Health Outcomes-Oriented Cooperative Research Networks (RICORS-ICTUS), Instituto de Salud Carlos III (Carlos III Health Institute), Ministerio de Ciencia e Innovación (Ministry of Science and Innovation), RD21/0006/0010.

Institutional Review Board Statement: Not applicable.

Informed Consent Statement: Not applicable.

Data Availability Statement: The data presented in this study are available upon request from the corresponding author.

Conflicts of Interest: The authors declare no conflict of interest.

References

1. Critchley, M. Arteriosclerotic parkinsonism. *Brain* **1929**, *52*, 23–83. [CrossRef]
2. Winikates, J.; Jankovic, J. Clinical Correlates of Vascular Parkinsonism. *Arch. Neurol.* **1999**, *56*, 98–102. [CrossRef] [PubMed]
3. Zijlmans, J.C.M.; Daniel, S.E.; Hughes, A.J.; Révész, T.; Lees, A.J. Clinicopathological investigation of vascular parkinsonism, including clinical criteria for diagnosis. *Mov. Disord.* **2004**, *19*, 630–640. [CrossRef]
4. Benamer, H.T.S.; Grosset, D.G. Vascular Parkinsonism: A Clinical Review. *Eur. Neurol.* **2009**, *61*, 11–15. [CrossRef]

5. Zijlmans, J.C.M.; Katzenschlager, R.; Daniel, S.E.; Lees, A.J.L. The L-dopa response in vascular parkinsonism. *J. Neurol. Neurosurg. Psychiatry* **2004**, *75*, 545–547. [CrossRef]
6. Miguel-Puga, A.; Villafuerte, G.; Salas-Pacheco, J.; Arias-Carrión, O. Therapeutic Interventions for Vascular Parkinsonism: A Systematic Review and Meta-analysis. *Front. Neurol.* **2017**, *22*, 8. [CrossRef] [PubMed]
7. Moher, D.; Shamseer, L.; Clarke, M.; Ghersi, D.; Liberati, A.; Petticrew, M.; Shekelle, P.; Stewart, L.A. Preferred Reporting Items for Systematic Review and meta-analysis Protocols (PRISMA-P) 2015 Statement. *Syst. Rev.* **2015**, *4*, 1. [CrossRef]
8. Vandenbroucke, J.P.; von Elm, E.; Altman, D.G.; Gøtzsche, P.C.; Mulrow, C.D.; Pocock, S.J.; Poole, C.; Schlesselman, J.J.; Egger, M.; Strobe Initiative. Strengthening the Reporting of Observational Studies in Epidemiology (STROBE): Explanation and Elaboration. *PLoS Med.* **2007**, *4*, e297. [CrossRef]
9. Wells, G.; Wells, G.; Shea, B.; Shea, B.; O'Connell, D.; Peterson, J.; Welch, V.; Losos, M. The Newcastle-Ottawa Scale (NOS) for Assessing the Quality of Nonrandomised Studies in Meta-Analyses. *Appl. Eng. Agric.* **2014**, *18*, 727–734.
10. Higgins, J.P.T.; Altman, D.G.; Gotzsche, P.C.; Juni, P.; Moher, D.; Oxman, A.D.; Savović, J.; Schulz, K.F.; Weeks, L.; Sterne, J.A.C.; et al. The Cochrane Collaboration's tool for assessing risk of bias in randomised trials. *BMJ* **2011**, *343*, d5928. [CrossRef]
11. Zijlmans, J.; Evans, A.; Fontes, F.; Katzenschlager, R.; Gacinovic, S.; Lees, A.J.; Costa, D. [123I] FP-CIT spect study in vascular parkinsonism and Parkinson's disease. *Mov. Disord.* **2007**, *22*, 1278–1285. [CrossRef]
12. Benítez-Rivero, S.; Marín-Oyaga, V.A.; García-Solís, D.; Huertas-Fernández, I.; García-Gomez, F.J.; Jesus, S.; Cáceres, M.T.; Carrillo, F.; Ortiz, A.M.; Carballo, M.; et al. Clinical features and 123I-FP-CIT SPECT imaging in vascular parkinsonism and Parkinson's disease. *J. Neurol. Neurosurg. Psychiatry* **2013**, *84*, 122–129. [CrossRef] [PubMed]
13. Sato, Y.; Iwamoto, J.; Honda, Y.; Amano, N. Vitamin D reduces falls and hip fractures in vascular Parkinsonism but not in Parkinson's disease. *Clin. Risk Manag.* **2013**, *9*, 171–176. [CrossRef]
14. Vale, T.C.; Caramelli, P.; Cardoso, F. Vascular parkinsonism: A case series of 17 patients. *Arq. Neuropsiquiatr.* **2013**, *71*, 757–762. [CrossRef]
15. Alcock, L.; Galna, B.; Perkins, R.; Lord, S.; Rochester, L. Step length determines minimum toe clearance in older adults and people with Parkinson's disease. *J. Biomech.* **2018**, *71*, 30–36. [CrossRef]
16. Stern, L.Z. Diphenylhydantoin for steroid-induced muscle weakness. *JAMA* **1973**, *223*, 1287–1288. [CrossRef]
17. Gago, M.F.; Fernandes, V.; Ferreira, J.; Silva, H.; Rodrigues, M.L.; Rocha, L.; Bicho, E.; Sousa, N. The effect of levodopa on postural stability evaluated by wearable inertial measurement units for idiopathic and vascular Parkinson's disease. *Gait Posture* **2014**, *41*, 459–464. [CrossRef]
18. Navarro-Otano, J.; Gaig, C.; Muxi, A.; Lomeña, F.; Compta, Y.; Buongiorno, M.T.; Martí, M.J.; Tolosa, E.; Valldeoriola, F. 123I-MIBG cardiac uptake, smell identification and 123I-FP-CIT SPECT inthe differential diagnosis between vascular parkinsonism and Parkinson's disease. *Park. Relat Disord.* **2014**, *20*, 192–197. [CrossRef]
19. Vale, T.C.; Caramelli, P.; Cardoso, F. Clinicoradiological comparison between vascular parkinsonism and Parkinson's disease. *J. Neurol. Neurosurg. Psychiatry* **2015**, *86*, 547–553. [CrossRef]
20. Lee, M.J.; Kim, S.L.; Kim, H.I.; Oh, Y.J.; Lee, S.H.; Kim, H.K.; Lyoo, C.; Ryu, Y. [18F] FP-CIT PET study in parkinsonian patients with leukoaraiosis. *Park. Relat Disord.* **2015**, *21*, 704–708. [CrossRef]
21. Maksimovich, I.V. Intracerebral Transcatheter Laser Photobiomodulation Therapy in the Treatment of Binswanger's Disease and Vascular Parkinsonism: Research and Clinical Experience. *Photobiomodul. Photomed. Laser Surg.* **2019**, *37*, 606–614. [CrossRef]
22. Fernandes, C.; Ferreira, F.; Lopes, R.L.; Bicho, E.; Erlhagen, W.; Sousa, N.; Gago, M.F. Discrimination of idiopathic Parkinson's disease and vascular parkinsonism based on gait time series and the levodopa effect. *J. Biomech.* **2021**, *125*, 110214. [CrossRef]
23. Fénelon, G.; Houéto, J.L. Vascular Parkinson syndromes: A controversial concept. *Rev. Neurol.* **1998**, *154*, 291–302. [PubMed]
24. Manap, H.H.; Tahir, N.; Yassin, A. Statistical analysis of parkinson disease gait classification using Artificial Neural Network. In Proceedings of the 2011 IEEE International Symposium on Signal Processing and Information Technology (ISSPIT), Bilbao, Spain, 14–17 December 2011.
25. Tahir, N.; Manap, H.H. Parkinson Disease Gait Classification based on Machine Learning Approach. *J. Appl. Sci.* **2012**, *12*, 180–185. [CrossRef]
26. Bejek, Z.; Paróczai, R.; Illyés, Á.; Kiss, R.M. The influence of walking speed on gait parameters in healthy people and in patients with osteoarthritis. *Knee Surg. Sport. Traumatol. Arthrosc.* **2006**, *14*, 612–622. [CrossRef] [PubMed]
27. Zeni, J.A.; Richards, J.G.; Higginson, J.S. Two simple methods for determining gait events during treadmill and overground walking using kinematic data. *Gait Posture* **2008**, *27*, 710–714. [CrossRef]
28. Antonini, A.; Vitale, C.; Barone, P.; Cilia, R.; Righini, A.; Bonuccelli, U.; Abbruzzese, G.; Ramat, S.; Petrone, A.; Quatrale, R.; et al. The relationship between cerebral vascular disease and parkinsonism: The VADO study. *Park. Relat Disord.* **2012**, *18*, 775–780. [CrossRef]
29. Dawson-Hughes, B.; Harris, S.S.; Krall, E.A.; Dallal, G.E. Effect of Calcium and Vitamin D Supplementation on Bone Density in Men and Women 65 Years of Age or Older. *N. Engl. J. Med.* **1997**, *337*, 670–676. [CrossRef]
30. Sato, Y.; Iwamoto, J.; Kanoko, T.; Satoh, K. Low-dose vitamin D prevents muscular atrophy and reduces falls and hip fractures in women after stroke: A randomized controlled trial. *Cerebrovasc. Dis.* **2005**, *20*, 187–192. [CrossRef] [PubMed]

31. Yip, C.W.; Cheong, P.W.; Green, A.; Prakash, P.K.; Fook-Cheong, S.K.; Tan, E.K.; Lo, Y.L. A prospective pilot study of repetitive transcranial magnetic stimulation for gait dysfunction in vascular parkinsonism. *Clin. Neurol. Neurosurg.* **2013**, *115*, 887–891. [CrossRef]
32. Prins, N.D.; van Dijk, E.J.; den Heijer, T.; Vermeer, S.E.; Jolles, J.; Koudstaal, P.J.; Hofman, A.; Breteler, M.M.B. Cerebral small-vessel disease and decline in information processing speed, executive function and memory. *Brain* **2005**, *128*, 2034–2041. [CrossRef]
33. Jin, K.; Wang, X.; Xie, L.; Mao, X.O.; Zhu, W.; Wang, Y.; Shen, J.; Mao, Y.; Banwait, S.; Greenberg, D.A. Evidence for stroke-induced neurogenesis in the human brain. *Proc. Natl. Acad. Sci. USA* **2006**, *103*, 13198–13202. [CrossRef]
34. Oron, A.; Oron, U.; Chen, J.; Eilam, A.; Zhang, C.; Sadeh, M.; Lampl, Y.; Streeter, J.; De Taboada, L.; Chopp, M. Low-level laser therapy applied transcranially to rats after induction of stroke significantly reduces long-term neurological deficits. *Stroke* **2006**, *37*, 2620–2624. [CrossRef] [PubMed]
35. Hamblin, M.R. Mechanisms and Mitochondrial Redox Signaling in Photobiomodulation. *Photochem. Photobiol.* **2018**, *94*, 199–212. [CrossRef] [PubMed]
36. Cassano, P.; Petrie, S.R.; Mischoulon, D.; Cusin, C.; Katnani, H.; Yeung, A.; De Taboada, L.; Archibald, A.; Bui, E.; Baer, L.; et al. Transcranial Photobiomodulation for the Treatment of Major Depressive Disorder. the ELATED-2 Pilot Trial. *Photomed. Laser Surg.* **2018**, *36*, 634–646. [CrossRef] [PubMed]
37. Glass, P.G.; Lees, A.J.; Bacellar, A.; Zijlmans, J.; Katzenschlager, R.; Silveira-Moriyama, L. The clinical features of pathologically confirmed vascular parkinsonism. *J. Neurol. Neurosurg. Psychiatry* **2012**, *83*, 1027–1029. [CrossRef] [PubMed]
38. Zijlmans, J.C.M. The Role of Imaging in the Diagnosis of Vascular Parkinsonism. *Neuroimaging Clin. N. Am.* **2010**, *20*, 69–76. [CrossRef] [PubMed]
39. Gerschlager, W.; Bencsits, G.; Pirker, W.; Bloem, B.R.; Asenbaum, S.; Prayer, D.; Zijlmans, J.C.M.; Hoffmann, M.; Brücke, T. [123I]β-CIT SPECT distinguishes vascular parkinsonism from Parkinson's disease. *Mov. Disord.* **2002**, *17*, 518–523. [CrossRef]
40. Katzenshlager, R.; Evans, A.; Manson, A.; Palsalos, P.N.; Ratnaraj, N.; Watt, H.; Timmermann, L.; Van Der Giessen, R.; Lees, A.J. Mucuna pruriens in Parkinson's disease: A double blind clinical and pharmacological study. *J. Neurol. Neurosurg. Psychiatry* **2004**, *75*, 1672–1677. [CrossRef]
41. Fearnley, J.M.; Lees, A.J. Ageing and Parkinson's Disease: Substantia Nigra Regional Selectivity. *Brain* **1991**, *114*, 2283–2301. [CrossRef]

Disclaimer/Publisher's Note: The statements, opinions and data contained in all publications are solely those of the individual author(s) and contributor(s) and not of MDPI and/or the editor(s). MDPI and/or the editor(s) disclaim responsibility for any injury to people or property resulting from any ideas, methods, instructions or products referred to in the content.

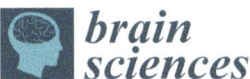

Review

Apathy in Parkinson's Disease: Defining the Park Apathy Subtype

Ségolène De Waele [1,2,*], Patrick Cras [1,2] and David Crosiers [1,2]

[1] Translational Neurosciences, Born-Bunge Institute, Faculty of Medicine and Health Sciences, University of Antwerp, 2650 Edegem, Belgium; patrick.cras@uza.be (P.C.); david.crosiers@uza.be (D.C.)
[2] Department of Neurology, Antwerp University Hospital, 2650 Edegem, Belgium
* Correspondence: segolene.dewaele@uantwerpen.be

Abstract: Apathy is a neurobehavioural symptom affecting Parkinson's disease patients of all disease stages. Apathy seems to be associated with a specific underlying non-motor disease subtype and reflects dysfunction of separate neural networks with distinct neurotransmitter systems. Due to the complicated neuropsychiatric aetiology of apathy, clinical assessment of this invalidating non-motor symptom remains challenging. We aim to summarize the current findings on apathy in Parkinson's disease and highlight knowledge gaps. We will discuss the prevalence rates across the different disease stages and suggest screening tools for clinically relevant apathetic symptoms. We will approach the fundamental knowledge on the neural networks implicated in apathy in a practical manner and formulate recommendations on patient-tailored treatment. We will discuss the Park apathy phenotype in detail, shedding light on different clinical manifestations and implications for prognosis. With this review, we strive to distil the vast available theoretical knowledge into a clinical and patient-oriented perspective.

Keywords: Parkinson's disease; apathy; neuropsychiatry; non-motor subtyping

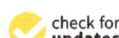

Citation: De Waele, S.; Cras, P.; Crosiers, D. Apathy in Parkinson's Disease: Defining the Park Apathy Subtype. *Brain Sci.* **2022**, *12*, 923. https://doi.org/10.3390/brainsci12070923

Academic Editors: Patricia Martinez-Sanchez and Francisco Nieto-Escamez

Received: 27 June 2022
Accepted: 12 July 2022
Published: 14 July 2022

Publisher's Note: MDPI stays neutral with regard to jurisdictional claims in published maps and institutional affiliations.

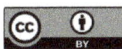

Copyright: © 2022 by the authors. Licensee MDPI, Basel, Switzerland. This article is an open access article distributed under the terms and conditions of the Creative Commons Attribution (CC BY) license (https://creativecommons.org/licenses/by/4.0/).

1. Introduction

Non-motor subtyping in Parkinson's disease (PD) has garnered increasing interest in the past few years. While useful, motor subtyping does not adequately portray PD's highly heterogeneous clinical presentations, as motor symptoms change during the disease course. Non-motor subtyping may prove a valid and more precise alternative, allowing for a patient-tailored approach and treatment [1,2]. Current findings point towards apathy as a distinct marker of a non-motor disease subtype: the Park Apathy subtype [3,4]. The manifestation of apathy within the non-motor spectrum of PD was first described in 1982 by Dr. Rabin. In his case series of 13 patients, he described that 'apathy is also common [. . .] this can be the most debilitating symptom' [5]. In the past, it was considered a late-stage symptom occurring predominantly in elderly patients [6]. Research has shown however that apathy manifests itself in all disease stages, and may serve as a prodromal symptom in some [6–9]. Presence of apathy in PD patients has been linked to increased motor burden, reduced quality of life (QoL) and has been identified as a risk factor for motor complications and cognitive decline [10–14]. Despite the profound implications, screening for apathy is generally not included in daily clinical practice. Patients and their loved ones may struggle to pinpoint the underlying problem, attributing the symptoms to fatigue or unwillingness on the patient's part [15,16]. Medical professionals as well struggle to identify it during routine follow-up and often apathetic patients are thought to suffer from depression or cognitive decline [16]. Trials have been undertaken to identify treatment options but successful results are sparse [17]. This is in part due to the one-dimensional approach undertaken in most trials. Apathy is usually described as a neuropsychiatric symptom, but it is more accurate to consider apathy as a behavioural state: the quantitative reduction of self-generated voluntary and purposeful behaviours [...] [18]. This altered behavioural state can arise from dysfunction in different neural networks, regulated by specific neurotransmitters, manifesting itself clinically into separate syndromes [18]. These symptoms may present themselves separately or in combination, requiring a customized approach.

This review aims to summarize the current knowledge about apathy in PD in the different disease stages. Subsequently, we will approach the underlying psychological and neural concepts and the pathophysiology practically, including possible helpful imaging biomarkers. Lastly, we detail the phenotype of the Park Apathy subtype and discuss potential treatment options.

2. Materials and Methods

We collected articles published between 1 January 2014 and 1 December 2021 by searching the following databases: Pubmed, Web of Science, and Google Scholar. We used the following search terms: 'apathy', 'neuropsychiatric symptoms', 'motivation', 'Parkinson', 'Parkinson's disease', 'imaging', 'pathophysiology', 'prodromal', 'prevalence', and 'treatment', or a combination thereof. The abstracts of the resulting articles were scanned and only those relevant to the scope of this review article were included. References of the included articles were browsed and pertinent papers were included after analysing their respective abstracts.

3. Prevalence of Apathy during the Disease Course

Epidemiological studies show a wide range of prevalence rates of apathy in PD (see Table 1) [4,11,14,19–41]. These discrepancies can be attributed to several factors.

First, methodologies to determine apathy vary significantly across the studies. Several scales are available to the clinician to evaluate apathy. Symptoms can be rated by the patients, their caregivers, or the clinician. The assessment tools range from quoting one item on an non-motor symptoms (NMS) scale to apathy-specific scales, which are quoted numerically or through a Likert scale [42]. Despite wide and frequent use, many scales have poor sensitivity or are less appropriate to evaluate apathy in specific disease populations. The Movement Disorders Society Unified Parkinson's Disease Rating Scale (MDS-UPDRS) part I is a frequently used scale to assess NMS. Yet, it performs poorly compared to apathy-specific scales such as the Apathy Scale (AS) or the Lille Apathy Rating Scale (LARS). Compared to the LARS, the UPDRS apathy item has a sensitivity of only 33% [31,43]. The Geriatric Depression Scale-15 (GDS-15) is used in the Parkinson's Progression Markers Initiative (PPMI) cohort (ClinicalTrials.gov Identifier: NCT01141023). Some studies have used a subscore of the GDS-15 to identify apathy [44,45]. However, this subscore is unsuited for use in de novo PD patients [46]. The MDS Task Force on rating scales for PD recommends the use of the UPDRS item 1.5, AS or LARS [47,48]. The UPDRS item 1.5 must be considered a screening tool, due to its apparent limitations [48]. The LARS scale was not granted the classification 'recommended' by the Task Force in 2008, but now fulfils the necessary criteria for recommendation following further research [47]. The LARS has an additional benefit, allowing for differentiation of subtypes of apathy, which we discuss further below [49].

Second, apathy can reflect an underlying mood disorder, a confounding factor that is not consistently excluded. Current apathy scales may not be sufficiently refined to detect these subtleties, and a separate evaluation of concurrent depression is recommended [47]. Third, apathy is common in the elderly without underlying neurological or psychiatric conditions. Apathy in community-dwelling adults is estimated to be about 11–29.4%, and the prevalence increases with age and functional decline [50,51]. Lastly, apathy in a patient can fluctuate during disease progression, which could either be attributed to the introduction of medication or the symptom's natural course [14,36,52]. Few studies have undertaken longitudinal follow-up of apathy or have monitored the evolution of this symptom at the individual patient level [14,19]. Martin and colleagues mapped the development of apathy scores per patient for two years, yet no clear pattern emerged [52].

Considering these confounding factors, current data suggest that apathy in PD is present in all disease stages. It can even manifest in the prodromal phase, e.g., PD patients start traveling less almost 8 years before diagnosis, in the absence of overt functional decline, mood disorders or motor deficits at that time [53]. In retrospective studies, 14.3–31% of PD patients reported decreased initiative 2–9 years predating their diagnosis [2,54,55]. Recall bias is, however, inherent to retrospective studies; therefore, evaluating individuals at high risk of developing PD may offer a more objective insight into the prodromal stage. Patients suffering from REM sleep behaviour disorder (RBD) have a 34–73% chance of converting to a clinically manifest synucleinopathy within five to ten years [56–58]. Apathy is common in these patients, affecting around 46% [43]. Following conversion to manifest PD, apathy remains more prevalent in patients with RBD than those without RBD [59,60]. An additional common prodromal PD sign is hyposmia; idiopathic anosmia has a lower PD conversion rate than RBD, with reports of 10% at ten years [61]. Apathy may be more prevalent in hyposmic PD patients, possibly associated with a higher odour threshold and decreased discrimination and identification of odours [8,62–64]. It was not related to subjective changes in smell [4].

The decline in the prevalence of apathy in the first few years after PD diagnosis has been attributed to the introduction of dopaminergic medication [19,30,36], which was corroborated by several studies [19,30,36]. Prevalence rates during the disease course vary (see Table 1). In de novo, treatment-naive PD patients, reported rates vary from 15% to 40.8% [4,11,20,30,37–39,41]. Patient cohorts around 1–1.5 year disease duration show similar prevalence rates: 18.6 to 48.3% [21–23,39]. At 2–4 years after diagnosis, the proportion of apathetic patients drops to 20.2–28%, possibly reflecting an increased dosage of dopaminergic replacement treatment (DRT) [20,23,65]. Further progression of the disease accompanies a further increase in the number of apathetic patients. [23] Reported prevalence rates vary from 14.7–72% in patients with 5–10 years of disease duration, [24–29,31] to 13.9–63% after more than 10 years of disease [14,32,34,35]. Longitudinal follow-up studies with sensitive apathy-specific scales can shed more light on this complex matter.

Table 1. Prevalence rates of apathy during the disease course. * Marks studies in which underlying depression was excluded.

Author (Year)	Rate of Apathy (%)	Disease Stage (Mean ± SD (Years))	Measuring Tool
Prodromal stage			
Pont-Sunyer et al. (2015) [2]	50%	−10–2 years	Patient perception
Gaenslen et al. (2011) [54]	23.7%	−8.8 years	Patient perception
Darweesh et al. (2017) [53]	NA (case-control)	−7.7 years	IADL–traveling subscore
Durcan et al. (2019) [55]	14.3%	−2.1–0.7 years	NMSQuest
High-risk populations			
Barber et al. (2018) [43]	46%	RBD	LARS
De novo, untreated			
De La Riva et al. (2014) [39]	16.7%	±0.5	UPDRS
Hinkle et al. (2021) [11]	16.9%	0.5 ± 0.5	UPDRS
Liu et al. (2017) [37]	17.29% *	1.26 ± 1.25	LARS
Dujardin et al. (2014) [4]	13.7% *	1.3 ± 0.9	LARS
Oh et al. (2021) [41]	30.1%	1.6 ± 1.9	NPI
Santangelo et al. (2015) [30]	33.3%	<2	Diagnostic criteria [66]
Cho et al. (2018) [38]	58.8%	2.1 ± 1.97	NMSS
Leiknes et al. (2010) [20]	29.1%	2.3 [0.4–10]	NPI

Table 1. Cont.

Author (Year)	Rate of Apathy (%)	Disease Stage (Mean ± SD (Years))	Measuring Tool
Early disease stage			
Benito-León et al. (2012) [21]	21.7% *	1.3 ± 0.6	LARS
Cubo et al. (2012) [22]	33.4%	1.3 ± 0.6	LARS
Ou et al. (2021) [23]	18.6%	1.5	LARS
De La Riva (2014) [39]	30.2%	±3	UPDRS
Mild disease			
Isella et al. (2002) [25]	43.3%	4.9 ± 4.4	AES-S
Eglit et al. (2021) [29]	71.7%	5.5 ± 5.2	AS
Kulisevsky et al. (2008) [26]	48.3%	5.65 ± 4.94	NPI
Lieberman et al. (2006) [28]	44% *	6.2 ± 5.9	NPI
Oguru et al. (2010) [27]	17% *	6.3 ± 4.4	AS
Kirsch-Darrow et al. (2006) [24]	28.8% *	6.4 ± 5.7	AES
Butterfield et al. (2010) [33]	14.7% *	7.07 ± 4.96	AES-S
Kirsch-Darrow et al. (2009) [31]	31.4% *	8.1 ± 5.9	AS
Advanced disease			
Aarsland et al. (1999) [34]	16.5% / 4.3% *	12.6 ± 5.1	NPI
Stella et al. (2009) [32]	38%	12.7 ± 6.2	NPI
Pedersen et al. (2009) [14]	13.9%	13.0 ± 4.7	NPI

Abbreviations: SD: standard deviation; NA: not applicable; IADL Lawton Instrumental Activities of Daily Living; NMSQuest: Non-Motor Symptom Questionnaire; RBD: REM sleep behaviour disorder; LARS: Lille Apathy Rating Scale; NPI: Neuropsychiatric Inventory; NMSS: Non-Motor Symptom Scale; UPDRS: Unified Parkinson's Disease Rating Scale; AES-S: Apathy Evaluation Scale–Self-rated; AS: Apathy Scale.

4. Pathophysiology

4.1. Psychological Model

To understand the pathophysiology of apathy it is necessary to evaluate how apathy arises as a behavioural concept. Apathy is essentially the reduction of voluntary, goal-directed behaviour (GDB) [18]. The neuro-cognitive formulation of how GDB arises is convoluted, so we provide an abbreviated model based on Brown and Pluck's theory (Figure 1) [67]. The process of GDB emerges from an interaction of internal and external drives, intention, planning, motivation, and emotional state. Theoretically, interference in any of these processes can lead to apathy [18,67].

Stuss and coworkers described three distinct subtypes of apathy. First, difficulties with self-activating thoughts or initiating the necessary motor functions for GDB are the predominant feature in the first type. We summarized this as a reduction of 'internal drive'. This reduced internal drive and response starkly contrast the preserved reaction to external drives and stimuli [18,68]. In an everyday setting, these patients do little unless instructed [69,70]. Daily productivity is low and there is no variation in activities in daily life [49], resulting in severe inertia that can be reversed successfully with external stimuli [18]. This subtype of apathy is sometimes referred to as 'behavioural apathy'; however since all forms of apathy lead to a reduction in GDB, we suggest an alternative terminology [71]. Aphrenic apathy, derived from the Greek word for 'inability to think', is a more apt description of this subtype.

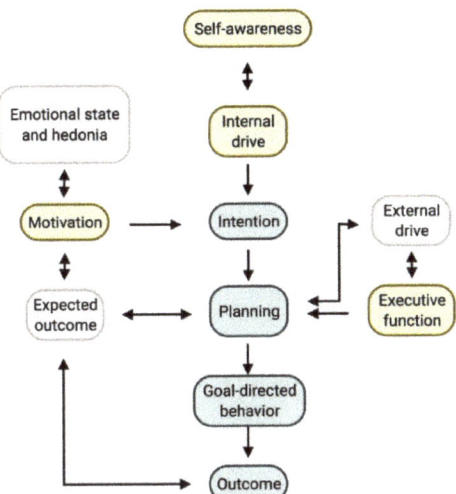

Figure 1. Proposed model for goal-directed behaviour. The three accepted subtypes and where they plug into the model are shown in yellow. Self-awareness, which is currently not yet considered a subtype, could interact with the internal drive and planning. Note on the left the importance of the hedonic state, which can affect those suffering from depression. Created with https://biorender.com/ (accessed on 27 June 2022).

A disruption in the planning aspect of GDB leads to 'cognitive' apathy or cognitive inertia. Faulty executive processing lies at the basis here, rendering difficulties with planning, working memory, rule-finding, and set-shifting [18]. The underlying executive dysfunction makes it difficult to plan the actions needed to perform GDB [18,67,68]. Executive dysfunction does not always reflect underlying dementia but may herald it [72]. This clinically manifests as a decreased interest, or more accurately, a decreased (intellectual) curiosity [69]. These patients spend little or no time on leisure activities and have few interests. Often, they do not wish to pursue (new) hobbies or social engagements. They quickly give up on a task when facing difficulties, reflecting their executive dysfunction [49,69].

A final subtype of apathy is an underlying reward deficiency syndrome, in which a patient cannot relate the GDB to the (pleasurable) outcome or reward. This is the result of emotional blunting or reduced emotional resonance [18,68,69]. This third subtype is often referred to as 'motivational' apathy [18,68]. It results in a reduced emotional response, for instance when the patient is confronted with upsetting news or watching something humorous. Patients can also display a decreased concern for their families and often no longer inquire after their health and well-being spontaneously [18,49].

It is necessary to differentiate this apathy subtype from the symptoms of an underlying depression or mood disorder. Apathy can also be related to anhedonia, resulting in decreased GDB [67,73]. Apathy in patients suffering from a depressive episode can improve with adequate treatment of their mood disorder [74].

Aside from these three widely accepted apathy subtypes, a fourth dimension called 'self-awareness' was initially proposed by Stuss and coworkers [68]. These authors described self-awareness as a critical component of GDB. They defined it as '[. . .] a metacognitive ability, necessary to mediate information from a personal, social past and current history with projections to the future [. . .]' [68]. The LARS was developed with this fourth dimension in mind, reflected by a fourth and independent cluster in their data analysis, separate from depression [49]. The question remains whether reduced self-awareness can be considered an underlying mechanism of apathy or a different construct altogether [69]. Self-awareness in essence organizes an individual's understanding of a social environment and the function of this individual within it [75]. Clinically, impaired self-awareness can manifest as anosognosia, or reduced insight into one's own physical limitations due to an illness. Reduced self-awareness has often been described in PD patients and is associated with cognitive decline [76–78]. Clinically, this may manifest itself in social interactions, where the patient might be quite headstrong in an argument, unwilling to concede to another's point of view. This results from a decrease in self-reflection, making it difficult to assess one's own faults accurately [49].

4.2. Neural Networks

It is often assumed that apathy results from a pure hypodopaminergic state, as it often can arise following dopamine withdrawal for Deep Brain Stimulation (DBS) surgery. Dopaminergic treatment has shown improvement in some patients, but a more complex model is required to explain the implicated neurotransmitter systems [19]. Despite adequate dopaminergic treatment, apathy occurs in PD patients, and the severity of apathy is independent of medication dosage [39,79]. Apathy can co-occur in PD patients suffering from impulse control disorders related to a hyperdopaminergic state [80,81]. Co-occurrence of apathy and impulse disorders was also reported in other neurological disorders [82]. Lastly, animal models and imaging studies in patients have shown the involvement of other neurotransmitter systems [83–85]. To further study the complex underlying physiology of apathy, the definition of the neuroanatomical correlates is an important starting point. Generally, the occurrence of apathy can be reduced to a dysfunctional circuitry between the frontal lobes and the basal ganglia. Within this circuitry, separate networks can be identified (see Figure 2) [68,86,87].

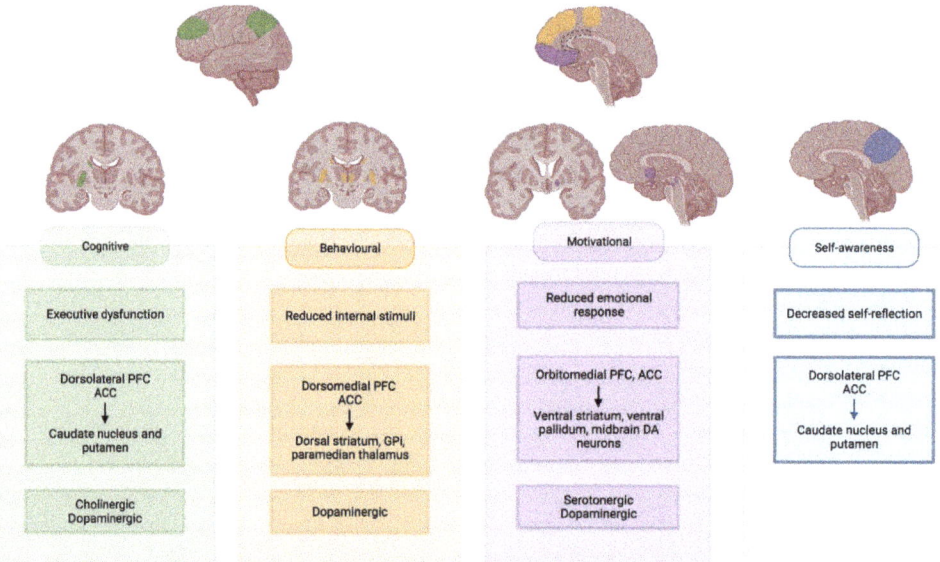

Figure 2. Neural networks underlying apathy subtypes. Involved cortical regions and basal ganglia regions are highlighted for each subtype. Created with https://biorender.com/ (accessed on 27 June 2022). Abbreviations: PFC: prefrontal cortex; ACC: anterior cingulate cortex; Gpi: internal globus pallidus; DA: dopaminergic.

'Behavioural' or 'aphrenic' apathy is often equated to a lack of initiation or internal drive to perform the GDB [18,68]. It is often referred to as an auto-activation deficit, with a reduced response to internal stimuli [18]. This type of apathy is often considered the most severe form. It has been described in bilateral dysfunction of the pathway between the dorsomedial prefrontal cortex (dmPFC) and anterior cingulate cortex (ACC) with the dorsal striatum, paramedian thalamus and the internal part of the globus pallidus (GPi) [88–96]. Similar syndromes have been described in uni- or bilateral lesions of the supplementary motor area (SMA) [70]. These are regions of interest in the 'lateral orbitofrontal cortex' circuit as described by Garrett and colleagues, which also receives input from temporal gryi and projects to the substantia nigra pars reticulata [87]. This circuit is partially dopamine-mediated, as evidenced by reduced dopaminergic binding and response to DRT [88,89,92,97].

Executive dysfunction leads to 'cognitive' apathy, where planning difficulties interfere with GDB. The dorsolateral PFC, cooperating with the ACC, is vital to executive processing, resulting in apathetic behaviour when lesioned [18,87,98,99]. This region has projections to the lateral parts of the dorsal striatum [87,92,100–102]. The lateral dorsal striatum also receives input from the posterior parietal cortex [87]. Cognitive apathy has been linked to decreased functional connectivity (FC) between the orbitofrontal cortex (OFC) and the right putamen [103]. We assume that the 'dorsolateral PFC' circuit is largely acetylcholine-mediated due to its implication in executive dysfunction [104]. In Alzheimer's disease patients with predominant cognitive apathy, there was reduced response to dextroamphetamine administration, suggesting some possible dopaminergic involvement as well [105].

'Motivational' apathy is mediated by the mesocorticolimbic pathway or the reward system [18,68,106]. Involved regions are the orbitomedial PFC, the ACC, the ventral striatum, the ventral pallidum and the dopaminergic midbrain neurons [18,107]. This system is mediated by the amygdala, hippocampus, thalamus, lateral habenular nucleus, the dorsal PFC, as well as the pedunculopontine nucleus and raphe nucleus in the brainstem [107,108]. Patients with 'motivational' apathy according to the LARS showed altered FC between the left inferior frontal gyrus and the left pallidum. There was an increased FC between the left inferior frontal gyrus and the right caudate [103]. Apathetic PD patients showed selective impairment of reward processing, reducing their ability to differentiate between favourable and unfavourable outcomes [109]. Dopamine plays an important role in this circuit, yet its relation to manifest apathy is complex [110]. Administration of dopamine agonists blunts reward sensitivity in healthy adults, while use in apathetic patients shows promise as a potential therapy [111,112]. Yet, some studies found no difference in dopaminergic uptake between apathetic and non-apathetic patients [84]. Serotonin could act as a modulator, with reduced uptake found in critical parts of the mesocorticolimbic pathway in apathetic PD patients [84,85]. The uptake reduction was proportional to apathy's severity [84]. Reduced serotonergic uptake in the raphe nucleus was also associated with the presence and severity of apathy in possible prodromal PD patients [113].

In our abbreviated and modified model in Figure 1, we propose a new role for self-awareness in developing GDB. Recent imaging findings have identified common underlying brain regions and networks in patients with reduced self-awareness and apathy. The precuneus is part of the default-mode network and plays an important role in self-awareness [114–116]. Studies found that isolated apathy in PD was associated with atrophy and hypometabolism of the precuneus compared to healthy controls [117,118]. Other regions of interest in self-awareness are the ACC, the posterior cingulate cortex (PCC), the temporoparietal junction, the ventromedial and dorsolateral prefrontal cortex and the insula [119–121].

It is unlikely that a different type of apathy develops in each patient. Patients with typical auto-activation deficit lesions were also shown to have reduced reward sensitivity [97,122]. One study found that apathy profiles differed, depending on disease stage. In stable PD patients, defined by the authors as well-controlled motor symptoms without fluctuations and absence of dementia, there was a trend towards decreased intellectual curiosity or 'cognitive' apathy. In PD patients with motor fluctuations without dementia, mostly intellectual curiosity and action initiation were inhibited. In PDD, both domains as well as self-awareness were decreased. Interestingly, in all groups, motivational apathy, as measured by the emotion subscore of the LARS, did not differ significantly from healthy controls [13]. Another study found a predominant decrease in intellectual curiosity in early-stage PD patients [4]. These findings suggest that apathy subtypes might have a distinct temporal profile.

4.3. Imaging Biomarkers

Aside from neurotransmitter changes in different networks, additional imaging biomarkers of apathy have been investigated. Changes have been reported in grey-matter volume (GMV), white and grey matter integrity, FC and network analysis, regional homogeneity (ReHo), glucose metabolism, and resting activity pattern.

Decrease in GMV in the subgenual AAC, left superior temporal, left precuneus, inferior parietal, right superior frontal, and the dorsolateral part of the caput of the left caudate nucleus is related to the presence of apathy. Severity of apathy was related to morphological abnormalities in the superior cerebellar peduncle decussation, bilateral posterior cerebellum and vermis, left superior frontal gyrus, and left nucleus accumbens [84,117,123]. GMV increases were noted in the left superior frontal gyrus and cerebellar vermis [117]. Other imaging studies, however, could not confirm these changes [86,124,125]. The connectivity between the parietal cortex and frontal lobes might explain part of these findings, as frontal lesions lead to parietal hyperactivity [116]. Input of temporal gyri has also been described in the 'lateral orbitofrontal cortex' circuit of the basal ganglia, implicated in 'behavioural' apathy [87].

Fractional anisotropy (FA) was significantly decreased in the genu and body of the corpus callosum, bilaterally in the anterior corona radiata and the left superior part of the corona radiata and left cingulum in apathetic PD patients. The grade of integrity was related to apathy severity [126]. Another study found reduced FA in the anterior thalamic fibres, the cingulate bundle, and the corpus callosum's interhemispheric connections and projection fibres. FA was also decreased bilaterally in the medial thalamus [84].

FC was reduced between the left ventral striatum and left frontal lobe in apathetic PD patients. Reduced FC between ventral and dorsal striatum and left frontal lobe, between the limbic region of the left frontal lobe and left striatum, between the caudal and rostral frontal lobe and right striatum and in between subdivisions of the left frontal lobe was related to increased severity of apathy [86] A regional network analysis could not find differences in connectivity between apathetic and non-apathetic PD patients [124].

Analysis of low-frequency function (ALFF), which evaluates the resting state of the entire brain, showed decreased ALFF signal in the left supplementary motor region, left inferior parietal love, left fusiform gyrus, and bilaterally in the cerebellum [127].

ReHo measures synchronization of local neural activity. In apathetic PD patients, ReHo was decreased in right caudate and dorsal ACC [128]. Some studies found reduced glucose metabolism in the precuneus bilaterally and right lingual gyrus and increased metabolism in the middle frontal gyrus in apathetic patients [117]. Additionally, the severity of white matter hyperintensities on FLAIR sequence also showed a link to apathy in PD, independent of depression [129]. These findings suggest top-down control from other cortical regions and support the involvement of the parietal cortex in certain subtypes [87,116].

5. Park Apathy

The Park apathy subtype has been associated with more severe motor symptoms, confirmed in observational studies [3]. Apathetic patients score higher on the UPDRS motor scale than their non-apathetic peers, excluding confounding factors such as disease duration or age [8,9,22,130,131]. This difference is already manifest at diagnosis, before the introduction of DRT [4,7,8,22,37]. As discussed above, apathy may fluctuate during the disease course [14,19]. Persisting apathy was linked to a more significant increase in motor symptoms during a four-year follow-up period compared to those with incidental apathy [14]. Severity may also play a role, as the grade of motor disability and apathy go hand-in-hand in specific cohorts [4,7,23,37]. Despite extensive research, not all research groups found increased motor severity in this group [13]. The discrepancy may be explained by the effect of persistent and incidental apathy [14].

Specific motor symptoms in apathetic patients differ as well. They have increased body sway in a quiet stance compared to non-apathetic patients, reflecting a more pronounced underlying postural instability [132]. Even in early PD, axial symptoms are more frequent and pronounced in this group [8,22,37,133]. Freezing of gait in ON state is linked to a higher grade of apathy and was less responsive to medication in this group [134]. They are at increased risk of developing motor complications such as fluctuations and dyskinesias earlier in the disease course [11]. However, the relation of apathy to motor fluctuations may be more complex, as dyskinesias at baseline were a predictive factor of worsening apathy [36]. Apathy is possibly more common in patients with right-sided PD onset, and patients with left-sided onset had decreased odds of developing apathetic behaviour [22,135].

Apathetic patients also suffer from more NMS, evidenced by higher scores on non-motor scales at disease initiation [37]. Symptoms such as anhedonia, sleeping difficulties and fatigue occur more often [4]. Increased fatigue has quite consistently been linked to apathy [4,64,136,137]. Especially 'motivational' apathy is a predictor of worsening fatigue in early PD [138]. On fatigue-specific scales, apathetic patients primarily report mental fatigue related to decreased intellectual curiosity [136].

The relationship between apathy and depression is complex. Apathy can arise as a symptom of an underlying depression but can also manifest as a distinct symptom altogether. In most cohorts, apathetic patients score higher on depression scales in early and advanced PD [7,8,13,14,23,130], whereas in another sample depressive symptoms were not noted [139]. Possibly higher depression scores are a risk factor for developing apathy [14,36]. There is a possible overlap between the assessment scales for depression and apathy, and a separate evaluation of both is still recommended [49].

Early on, apathetic patients generally perform normally on basic cognitive screening tests [4,8,140]. Executive dysfunction and memory deficits, however, do become apparent when an extensive neuropsychological battery is performed. These patients display mild executive dysfunction, evidenced by lower scores on the interference task of the Stroop test, the Benton Judgment of Line Orientation Test, and the Letter Fluency test [30,125,140]. These impairments become more conspicuous over the years [9,14,141]. In more advanced stages, persistent apathy was linked to greater global cognitive decline [14]. Dujardin and coworkers found preserved cognitive efficiency in advanced apathetic PD patients without dementia. Attention, working memory, executive functions, language, and visuospatial skills were significantly decreased nonetheless [142]. Others report similar declines in executive function and visuospatial abilities in the absence of dementia [33,139,141,143].

Apathy is a possible risk factor for the development of dementia. Prevalence of PD with minimal cognitive impairment (PD-MCI) increases with disease progression, but conversion to either normal cognition or PD dementia (PDD) is possible [144]. Combined with the fluctuating nature of apathy, this may impede forming robust conclusions [19]. It is generally assumed that apathy is more frequent in both PD-MCI and PDD [77,145]. In a longitudinal analysis, self-rated apathy scores were linked to current and future cognitive scores, but were not predictive of conversion to PDD [52]. A longitudinal study found that those with both incident and persistent apathy had a more significant decrease in cognitive functions after four years, with a more pronounced change in those with persistent apathy. The rate of dementia in the persistent apathy group did not significantly differ from the baseline [14]. In another sample, the conversion rate to dementia was higher in apathetic patients. They also noted decreased cognitive scores at baseline, but a much more pronounced reduction in scores at follow-up in the apathetic group [9].

The above suggests that apathy is a marker of a more severe disease phenotype, with a higher motor and non-motor burden. Subtyping based on the presence of apathy has yet to be applied in large cohorts, but current evidence shows promise [146]. Evidence suggests that persistent apathy may be a more significant risk factor than purely incidental apathy [14].

6. Treatment

Despite quality research on the topic, effective treatment for apathy in PD is lacking [17]. This is partly due to the variety of screening methods and follow-up duration as discussed above. The one-size-fits-all approach complicates matters further. Patients may suffer from different subtypes or combinations thereof, requiring customized treatment. Screening for and identifying the dominant subtype(s) per patient might be helpful in future research, allowing for a more patient-oriented approach. We highlight the most promising strategies below. For a more extensive overview, we would like to direct the reader to a review article that delves deeper into the subject [17].

6.1. Pharmacological

As discussed above, many neurotransmitters are involved in the underlying process of apathy. Evidence has been found of dopaminergic, serotonergic, and cholinergic involvement [79,83,88,89,92,97].

Use of DRT has shown promising results, and administration of dopamine agonists is often most successful. A recent meta-analysis concluded that using rotigotine improved apathy scores, which was not confirmed in a more recent placebo-controlled study [147,148]. Other dopamine agonists such as pramipexole or apomorphine might also be beneficial, as patients score better on the items 'intellectual curiosity' and 'self-awareness' after administration [112,149]. Global apathy scores improved in those receiving apomorphine when combined with rotigotine [149,150]. Rotigotine and pramipexol were effective in reversing an auto-activation deficit in a case series [151].

DRT is assumed to improve apathy in the long term, as evidenced by the decreasing prevalence after the introduction of medication [23]. Apathy scores do not differ significantly in ON or OFF stages, showing no significant response to DRT in the acute phase [152]. No studies comparing different DRT strategies in these patients are available.

Results on serotonergic treatment are scarce. Selective serotonin receptor inhibitors are known to induce flat affect and apathy, both in healthy individuals and PD patients [153]. A cross-over study in 25 PD subjects with 5-hydroxytryptophan, a precursor of serotonin, had no significant impact on apathy scores [154]. Use of both selective serotonin and serotonin noradrenaline reuptake inhibitors (SSRI and SNRI respectively) did not significantly alter apathy scores compared to baselines [155].

In those already receiving optimized dopaminergic treatment without PDD, add-on of rivastigmine improved apathy scores [79]. Although rivastigmine was reported to improve apathy in PDD in a few case reports, a more extensive patient series showed no improvement in this group [104,156]. Use of rivastigmine decreased caregiver distress associated with apathy [157]. Galantamine might be effective in apathetic PDD patients [158].

Other strategies include the use of stimulants. Administration of dextroamphetamine in a PD sample with cognitive decline improved apathy scores in nearly a third of patients. Most of these patients were already receiving cholinesterase inhibitors [159]. Singular positive reports have been published on the use of methylphenidate, istradefylline, MAO inhibitors, yokukansan, and exenatide [160–165]. Bupropion and choline alphoscerate, a cholinergic precursor, was shown to be effective in treating apathy in other neurodegenerative diseases [166–168]. A case report of a patient suffering from an auto-activation deficit reported spectacular improvement of symptoms following administration of tricyclic antidepressants [169].

6.2. Non-Pharmacological

Non-pharmacological treatment options have garnered increasing interest. Exercise especially is beneficial in the treatment of both motor and NMS [170,171]. For the treatment of apathy, exercise and physical activity may also prove useful. A longitudinal study found that patients with baseline higher activity levels had improved apathy scores at follow-up. Apathy scores at baseline were not related to activity level [172]. Others however found very little difference between those following an intensive exercise schedule with sessions thrice a week and those without intervention. Only those following individual therapy showed slight improvement [173]. Apathy scores did improve in patients following biweekly Nordic walking sessions over 12 weeks, compared to control patients [174]. Though there is some evidence for a positive effect of dance, a recent meta-analysis concluded it was not superior to self-directed exercise or the best medical treatment [175,176]. There is need for structured research into the matter, wherein different physical activities and interventions are systematically researched and compared. As current evidence does not support one type of physical activity above another, it is advised to tailor the type of physical exercise to the patients' needs and preferences [177].

A small body of evidence exists for using repetitive transcranial magnetic stimulation (rTMS). A cross-over study found that rTMS over the supplementary motor area improved apathy scores compared to placebo [178]. Stimulation of the M1 area in the precentral gyrus showed similar improvement [179]. Benefit was also found after targeting the dorsolateral PFC, after which both apathy and emotional processing improved [180]. Cognitive rehabilitation is beneficial in treating apathy in the healthy elderly, but no such benefits were observed in PD patients [181–183]. A pilot project showed slight benefits in the short term, but longitudinal data is not available [184].

7. Conclusions

Apathy is a marker of a distinct PD phenotype. It manifests itself during all stages of the disease, both in the prodromal stage and in advanced PD patients. Presence of apathy may fluctuate in individual patients, making assessment challenging. It is associated with earlier onset of axial symptoms, gait difficulties, motor complications, fatigue, and cognitive impairment. Patients with persistent apathy during follow-up may be at greater risk of developing these complications than those with incidental apathy. Whether severity of apathy plays a role is currently unclear. The underlying pathophysiology of apathy is complex, with different underlying neural networks resulting in separate apathy dimensions. These dimensions can be assessed through use of the LARS questionnaire. The LARS may prove a useful tool for tailoring therapy, as each dimension is associated with distinct neurotransmitter deficits. Additional studies are needed to elucidate how these different apathy dimensions present themselves in PD patients, how they evolve and respond to treatment. Thus far, tailored therapy is lacking but adequate DRT is recommended for all patients. Additional exercise interventions might be beneficial.

Future research should focus on follow-up of apathy in individual patients, monitoring evolution of presence, severity, and apathy dimensions during the disease course. Clinical trials focusing on treatment should take heed of apathy's fluctuating nature, providing a long follow-up duration and multiple apathy assessments in time. A one-size-fits-all approach is to be avoided and future endeavours should consider underlying apathy dimensions as a guide of treatment choice and response.

Author Contributions: S.D.W. carried out the literature review, provided the figures and wrote the manuscript with support from D.C., D.C. and P.C. provided proofreading and revision of the manuscript. All authors have read and agreed to the published version of the manuscript.

Funding: This research received no external funding.

Institutional Review Board Statement: Not applicable.

Informed Consent Statement: Not applicable.

Data Availability Statement: Not applicable.

Acknowledgments: The manuscript was read and approved by all named authors. Images for this paper were created using Biorender. Publication and licensing rights were granted for publication in Brain Sciences (Agreement number FU2439NERH and AB2439NGZW). We thank the patient support group 'Move for Parkinson' for their participation in the funding of this study.

Conflicts of Interest: The authors declare that the research was conducted without any commercial or financial relationships that could be construed as a potential conflict of interest.

References

1. Sauerbier, A.; Lenka, A.; Aris, A.; Pal, P.K. Nonmotor Symptoms in Parkinson's Disease: Gender and Ethnic Differences. In *International Review of Neurobiology*; Chaudhuri, K.R., Titova, N., Eds.; Academic Press: Cambridge, MA, USA, 2017; Volume 133, pp. 417–446. ISBN 9780128137086.
2. Pont-Sunyer, C.; Hotter, A.; Gaig, C.; Seppi, K.; Compta, Y.; Katzenschlager, R.; Mas, N.; Hofeneder, D.; Brücke, T.; Bayés, A.; et al. The Onset of Nonmotor Symptoms in Parkinson's Disease (the Onset Pd Study). *Mov. Disord.* **2015**, *30*, 229–237. [CrossRef] [PubMed]
3. Sauerbier, A.; Jenner, P.; Todorova, A.; Chaudhuri, K.R. Non Motor Subtypes and Parkinson's Disease. *Park. Relat. Disord.* **2016**, *22*, S41–S46. [CrossRef] [PubMed]
4. Dujardin, K.; Langlois, C.; Plomhause, L.; Carette, A.S.; Delliaux, M.; Duhamel, A.; Defebvre, L. Apathy in Untreated Early-Stage Parkinson Disease: Relationship with Other Non-Motor Symptoms. *Mov. Disord.* **2014**, *29*, 1796–1801. [CrossRef]
5. Rabins, P.V. Psychopathology of Parkinson's Disease. *Compr. Psychiatry* **1982**, *23*, 421–429. [CrossRef]
6. Aarsland, D.; Brønnick, K.; Ehrt, U.; De Deyn, P.P.; Tekin, S.; Emre, M.; Cummings, J.L. Neuropsychiatric Symptoms in Patients with Parkinson's Disease and Dementia: Frequency, Profile and Associated Care Giver Stress. *J. Neurol. Neurosurg. Psychiatry* **2007**, *78*, 36–42. [CrossRef]
7. Pedersen, K.F.; Alves, G.; Brønnick, K.; Aarsland, D.; Tysnes, O.B.; Larsen, J.P. Apathy in Drug-Naïve Patients with Incident Parkinson's Disease: The Norwegian ParkWest Study. *J. Neurol.* **2010**, *257*, 217–223. [CrossRef]
8. Terashi, H.; Ueta, Y.; Kato, H.; Mitoma, H.; Aizawa, H. Characteristics of Apathy in Treatment-Naïve Patients with Parkinson's Disease. *Int. J. Neurosci.* **2019**, *129*, 16–21. [CrossRef]
9. Dujardin, K.; Sockeel, P.; Delliaux, M.; Destée, A.; Defebvre, L. Apathy May Herald Cognitive Decline and Dementia in Parkinson's Disease. *Mov. Disord.* **2009**, *24*, 2391–2397. [CrossRef]
10. Barone, P.; Antonini, A.; Colosimo, C.; Marconi, R.; Morgante, L.; Avarello, T.P.; Bottacchi, E.; Cannas, A.; Ceravolo, G.; Ceravolo, R.; et al. The PRIAMO Study: A Multicenter Assessment of Nonmotor Symptoms and Their Impact on Quality of Life in Parkinson's Disease. *Mov. Disord.* **2009**, *24*, 1641–1649. [CrossRef]
11. Hinkle, J.T.; Perepezko, K.; Gonzalez, L.L.; Mills, K.A.; Pontone, G.M. Apathy and Anxiety in De Novo Parkinson's Disease Predict the Severity of Motor Complications. *Mov. Disord. Clin. Pract.* **2021**, *8*, 76–84. [CrossRef]
12. Ellmers, T.J.; Maslivec, A.; Young, W.R. Fear of Falling Alters Anticipatory Postural Control during Cued Gait Initiation. *Neuroscience* **2020**, *438*, 41–49. [CrossRef] [PubMed]
13. Dujardin, K.; Sockeel, P.; Devos, D.; Delliaux, M.; Krystkowiak, P.; Destée, A.; Defebvre, L. Characteristics of Apathy in Parkinson's Disease. *Mov. Disord.* **2007**, *22*, 778–784. [CrossRef] [PubMed]
14. Pedersen, K.F.; Alves, G.; Aarsland, D.; Larsen, J.P. Occurrence and Risk Factors for Apathy in Parkinson Disease: A 4-Year Prospective Longitudinal Study. *J. Neurol. Neurosurg. Psychiatry* **2009**, *80*, 1279–1282. [CrossRef]
15. Martinez-Martin, P.; Rodriguez-Blazquez, C.; Forjaz, M.J.; Frades-Payo, B.; Agüera-Ortiz, L.; Weintraub, D.; Riesco, A.; Kurtis, M.M.; Chaudhuri, K.R. Neuropsychiatric Symptoms and Caregiver's Burden in Parkinson's Disease. *Park. Relat. Disord.* **2015**, *21*, 629–634. [CrossRef] [PubMed]
16. Weiss, H.D.; Pontone, G.M. "Pseudo-Syndromes" Associated with Parkinson Disease, Dementia, Apathy, Anxiety, and Depression. *Neurol. Clin. Pract.* **2019**, *9*, 354–359. [CrossRef]
17. Mele, B.; Van, S.; Holroyd-Leduc, J.; Ismail, Z.; Pringsheim, T.; Goodarzi, Z. Diagnosis, Treatment and Management of Apathy in Parkinson's Disease: A Scoping Review. *BMJ Open* **2020**, *10*, e037632. [CrossRef]
18. Levy, R.; Dubois, B. Apathy and the Functional Anatomy of the Prefrontal Cortex-Basal Ganglia Circuits. *Cereb. Cortex* **2006**, *16*, 916–928. [CrossRef]
19. Ou, R.; Hou, Y.; Wei, Q.; Lin, J.; Liu, K.; Zhang, L.; Jiang, Z.; Cao, B.; Zhao, B.; Song, W.; et al. Longitudinal Evolution of Non-Motor Symptoms in Early Parkinson's Disease: A 3-Year Prospective Cohort Study. *NPJ Park. Dis.* **2021**, *7*, 1–6. [CrossRef]
20. Leiknes, I.; Tysnes, O.B.; Aarsland, D.; Larsen, J.P. Caregiver Distress Associated with Neuropsychiatric Problems in Patients with Early Parkinson's Disease: The Norwegian ParkWest Study. *Acta Neurol. Scand.* **2010**, *122*, 418–424. [CrossRef]
21. Benito-León, J.; Cubo, E.; Coronell, C.; Rodríguez-Fernández, R.; Pego-Reigosa, R.; Paz-González, J.M.; Cebrián-Pérez, E.; Suarez-Gil, P.; Marey-López, J.; Corredera-García, E.; et al. Impact of Apathy on Health-Related Quality of Life in Recently Diagnosed Parkinson's Disease: The ANIMO Study. *Mov. Disord.* **2012**, *27*, 211–218. [CrossRef]
22. Cubo, E.; Benito-León, J.; Coronell, C.; Armesto, D. Clinical Correlates of Apathy in Patients Recently Diagnosed with Parkinson's Disease: The ANIMO Study. *Neuroepidemiology* **2012**, *38*, 48–55. [CrossRef]
23. Ou, R.; Lin, J.; Liu, K.; Jiang, Z.; Wei, Q.; Hou, Y.; Zhang, L.; Cao, B.; Zhao, B.; Song, W.; et al. Evolution of Apathy in Early Parkinson's Disease: A 4-Years Prospective Cohort Study. *Front. Aging Neurosci.* **2021**, *12*, 1–9. [CrossRef] [PubMed]
24. Kirsch-Darrow, L.; Fernandez, H.H.; Marsiske, M.; Okun, M.S.; Bowers, D. Dissociating Apathy and Depression in Parkinson Disease. *Neurology* **2006**, *67*, 33–38. [CrossRef] [PubMed]
25. Isella, V.; Melzi, P.; Grimaldi, M.; Iurlaro, S.; Piolti, R.; Ferrarese, C.; Frattola, L.; Appollonio, I. Clinical, Neuropsychological, and Morphometric Correlates of Apathy in Parkinson's Disease. *Mov. Disord.* **2002**, *17*, 366–371. [CrossRef] [PubMed]

26. Kulisevsky, J.; Pagonbarraga, J.; Pascual-Sedano, B.; García-Sánchez, C.; Gironell, A. Prevalence and Correlates of Neuropsychiatric Symptoms in Parkinson's Disease without Dementia. *Mov. Disord.* **2008**, *23*, 1889–1896. [CrossRef]
27. Oguru, M.; Tachibana, H.; Toda, K.; Okuda, B.; Oka, N. Apathy and Depression in Parkinson Disease. *J. Geriatr. Psychiatry Neurol.* **2010**, *23*, 35–41. [CrossRef]
28. Lieberman, A. Are Dementia and Depression in Parkinson's Disease Related? *J. Neurol. Sci.* **2006**, *248*, 138–142. [CrossRef]
29. Eglit, G.M.L.; Lopez, F.; Schiehser, D.M.; Pirogovsky-Turk, E.; Litvan, I.; Lessig, S.; Filoteo, J.V. Delineation of Apathy Subgroups in Parkinson's Disease: Differences in Clinical Presentation, Functional Ability, Health-Related Quality of Life, and Caregiver Burden. *Mov. Disord. Clin. Pract.* **2021**, *8*, 92–99. [CrossRef]
30. Santangelo, G.; Vitale, C.; Trojano, L.; Picillo, M.; Moccia, M.; Pisano, G.; Pezzella, D.; Cuoco, S.; Erro, R.; Longo, K.; et al. Relationship between Apathy and Cognitive Dysfunctions in de Novo Untreated Parkinson's Disease: A Prospective Longitudinal Study. *Eur. J. Neurol.* **2015**, *22*, 253–260. [CrossRef]
31. Kirsch-Darrow, L.; Zahodne, L.B.; Hass, C.; Mikos, A.; Okun, M.S.; Fernandez, H.H.; Bowers, D. How Cautious Should We Be When Assessing Apathy with the Unified Parkinson's Disease Rating Scale? *Mov. Disord.* **2009**, *24*, 684–688. [CrossRef]
32. Stella, F.; Banzato, C.E.M.; Quagliato, E.M.A.B.; Viana, M.A.; Christofoletti, G. Psychopathological Features in Patients with Parkinson's Disease and Related Caregivers' Burden. *Int. J. Geriatr. Psychiatry* **2009**, *24*, 1158–1165. [CrossRef] [PubMed]
33. Butterfield, L.C.; Cimino, C.R.; Oelke, L.E.; Hauser, R.A.; Sanchez-Ramos, J. The Independent Influence of Apathy and Depression on Cognitive Functioning in Parkinson's Disease. *Neuropsychology* **2010**, *24*, 721–730. [CrossRef] [PubMed]
34. Aarsland, D.; Larsen, J.P.; Lim, N.G.; Janvin, C.; Karlsen, K.; Tandberg, E.; Cummings, J.L. Range of Neuropsychiatric Disturbances in Patients with Parkinson's Disease. *J. Neurol. Neurosurg. Psychiatry* **1999**, *67*, 492–496. [CrossRef] [PubMed]
35. Starkstein, S.E.; Mayberg, H.S.; Preziosi, T.J.; Andrezejewski, P.; Leiguarda, R.; Robinson, R.G. Reliability, Validity, and Clinical Correlates of Apathy in Parkinson's Disease. *J. Neuropsychiatry Clin. Neurosci.* **1992**, *4*, 134–139. [CrossRef] [PubMed]
36. Wee, N.; Kandiah, N.; Acharyya, S.; Chander, R.J.; Ng, A.; Au, W.L.; Tan, L.C.S. Baseline Predictors of Worsening Apathy in Parkinson's Disease: A Prospective Longitudinal Study. *Park. Relat. Disord.* **2016**, *23*, 95–98. [CrossRef]
37. Liu, H.; Ou, R.; Wei, Q.; Hou, Y.; Zhang, L.; Cao, B.; Zhao, B.; Song, W.; Shang, H. Apathy in Drug-Naïve Patients with Parkinson's Disease. *Park. Relat. Disord.* **2017**, *44*, 28–32. [CrossRef]
38. Cho, B.H.; Choi, S.M.; Kim, J.T.; Kim, B.C. Association of Coffee Consumption and Non-Motor Symptoms in Drug-Naïve, Early-Stage Parkinson's Disease. *Park. Relat. Disord.* **2018**, *50*, 42–47. [CrossRef]
39. De La Riva, P.; Smith, K.; Xie, S.X.S.X.; Weintraub, D. Course of Psychiatric Symptoms and Global Cognition in Early Parkinson Disease. *Neurology* **2014**, *83*, 1096–1103. [CrossRef]
40. Wang, F.; Pan, Y.; Zhang, M.; Hu, K. Predicting the Onset of Freezing of Gait in de Novo Parkinson's Disease. *medRxiv* **2021**, 2021.03.11.21253192.
41. Oh, Y.S.; Kim, J.H.; Yoo, S.W.; Hwang, E.J.; Lyoo, C.H.; Lee, K.S.; Kim, J.S. Neuropsychiatric Symptoms and Striatal Monoamine Availability in Early Parkinson's Disease without Dementia. *Neurol. Sci.* **2021**, *42*, 711–718. [CrossRef]
42. Radakovic, R.; Harley, C.; Abrahams, S.; Starr, J.M. A Systematic Review of the Validity and Reliability of Apathy Scales in Neurodegenerative Conditions. *Int. Psychogeriatr.* **2015**, *27*, 903–923. [CrossRef]
43. Barber, T.R.; Muhammed, K.; Drew, D.; Lawton, M.; Crabbe, M.; Rolinski, M.; Quinnell, T.; Zaiwalla, Z.; Ben-Shlomo, Y.; Husain, M.; et al. Apathy in Rapid Eye Movement Sleep Behaviour Disorder Is Common and Under-Recognized. *Eur. J. Neurol.* **2018**, *25*, 469-e32. [CrossRef] [PubMed]
44. Weintraub, D.; Xie, S.; Karlawish, J.; Siderowf, A. Differences in Depression Symptoms in Patients with Alzheimer's and Parkinson's Diseases: Evidence from the 15-Item Geriatric Depression Scale (GDS-15). *Int. J. Geriatr. Psychiatry* **2007**, *22*, 1025–1030. [CrossRef] [PubMed]
45. Van Wanrooij, L.L.; Borsboom, D.; Moll Van Charante, E.P.; Richard, E.; Van Gool, W.A. A Network Approach on the Relation between Apathy and Depression Symptoms with Dementia and Functional Disability. *Int. Psychogeriatr.* **2019**, *31*, 1655–1663. [CrossRef] [PubMed]
46. Szymkowicz, S.M.; Ellis, L.J.; May, P.E. The 3-Item "Apathy" Subscale Within the GDS-15 Is Not Supported in De Novo Parkinson's Disease Patients: Analysis of the PPMI Cohort. *J. Geriatr. Psychiatry Neurol.* **2021**. [CrossRef] [PubMed]
47. Martinez-Martin, P.; Rodriguez-Blazquez, C.; Forjaz, M.J.; Kurtis, M.M.; Skorvanek, M. Measurement of Nonmotor Symptoms in Clinical Practice. In *International Review of Neurobiology*; Chaudhuri, K.R., Titova, N., Eds.; Academic Press: Cambridge, MA, USA, 2017; Volume 133, pp. 291–345. ISBN 0074-7742.
48. Leentjens, A.F.G.; Dujardin, K.; Marsh, L.; Martinez-Martin, P.; Richard, I.H.; Starkstein, S.E.; Weintraub, D.; Sampaio, C.; Poewe, W.; Rascol, O.; et al. Apathy and Anhedonia Rating Scales in Parkinson's Disease: Critique and Recommendations. *Mov. Disord.* **2008**, *23*, 2015–2025. [CrossRef] [PubMed]
49. Sockeel, P.; Dujardin, K.; Devos, D.; Denève, C.; Destée, A.; Defebvre, L. The Lille Apathy Rating Scale (LARS), a New Instrument for Detecting and Quantifying Apathy: Validation in Parkinson's Disease. *J. Neurol. Neurosurg. Psychiatry* **2006**, *77*, 579–584. [CrossRef]
50. Groeneweg-Koolhoven, I.; De Waal, M.W.M.; Van Der Weele, G.M.; Gussekloo, J.; Van Der Mast, R.C. Quality of Life in Community-Dwelling Older Persons with Apathy. *Am. J. Geriatr. Psychiatry* **2014**, *22*, 186–194. [CrossRef]
51. Clarke, D.E.; Ko, J.Y.; Lyketsos, C.; Rebok, G.W.; Eaton, W.W. Apathy and Cognitive and Functional Decline in Community-Dwelling Older Adults: Results from the Baltimore ECA Longitudinal Study. *Int. Psychogeriatr.* **2010**, *22*, 819–829. [CrossRef]

52. Martin, G.P.; McDonald, K.R.; Allsop, D.; Diggle, P.J.; Leroi, I. Apathy as a Behavioural Marker of Cognitive Impairment in Parkinson's Disease: A Longitudinal Analysis. *J. Neurol.* **2020**, *267*, 214–227. [CrossRef]
53. Darweesh, S.K.L.; Verlinden, V.J.A.; Stricker, B.H.; Hofman, A.; Koudstaal, P.J.; Ikram, M.A. Trajectories of Prediagnostic Functioning in Parkinson's Disease. *Brain* **2017**, *140*, 429–441. [CrossRef] [PubMed]
54. Gaenslen, A.; Swid, I.; Liepelt-Scarfone, I.; Godau, J.; Berg, D. The Patients' Perception of Prodromal Symptoms before the Initial Diagnosis of Parkinson's Disease. *Mov. Disord.* **2011**, *26*, 653–658. [CrossRef] [PubMed]
55. Durcan, R.; Wiblin, L.; Lawson, R.A.; Khoo, T.K.; Yarnall, A.J.; Duncan, G.W.; Brooks, D.J.; Pavese, N.; Burn, D.J. Prevalence and Duration of Non-Motor Symptoms in Prodromal Parkinson's Disease. *Eur. J. Neurol.* **2019**, *26*, 979–985. [CrossRef] [PubMed]
56. Iranzo, A.; Fernández-Arcos, A.; Tolosa, E.; Serradell, M.; Molinuevo, J.L.; Valldeoriola, F.; Gelpi, E.; Vilaseca, I.; Sánchez-Valle, R.; Lladó, A.; et al. Neurodegenerative Disorder Risk in Idiopathic REM Sleep Behavior Disorder: Study in 174 Patients. *PLoS ONE* **2014**, *9*, e89741. [CrossRef]
57. Barber, T.R.; Lawton, M.; Rolinski, M.; Evetts, S.; Baig, F.; Ruffmann, C.; Gornall, A.; Klein, J.C.; Lo, C.; Dennis, G.; et al. Prodromal Parkinsonism and Neurodegenerative Risk Stratification in REM Sleep Behavior Disorder. *Sleep* **2017**, *40*, 11–13. [CrossRef]
58. Boeve, B.F.; Silber, M.H.; Saper, C.B.; Ferman, T.J.; Dickson, D.W.; Parisi, J.E.; Benarroch, E.E.; Ahlskog, J.E.; Smith, G.E.; Caselli, R.C.; et al. Pathophysiology of REM Sleep Behaviour Disorder and Relevance to Neurodegenerative Disease. *Brain* **2007**, *130*, 2770–2788. [CrossRef]
59. Bargiotas, P.; Ntafouli, M.; Lachenmayer, M.L.; Krack, P.; Schüpbach, W.M.M.; Bassetti, C.L.A. Apathy in Parkinson's Disease with REM Sleep Behavior Disorder. *J. Neurol. Sci.* **2019**, *399*, 194–198. [CrossRef]
60. Iijima, M.; Okuma, Y.; Suzuki, K.; Yoshii, F.; Nogawa, S.; Osada, T.; Hirata, K.; Kitagawa, K.; Hattori, N. Associations between Probable REM Sleep Behavior Disorder, Olfactory Disturbance, and Clinical Symptoms in Parkinson's Disease: A Multicenter Cross-Sectional Study. *PLoS ONE* **2021**, *16*, 0247443. [CrossRef]
61. Haehner, A.; Masala, C.; Walter, S.; Reichmann, H.; Hummel, T. Incidence of Parkinson's Disease in a Large Patient Cohort with Idiopathic Smell and Taste Loss. *J. Neurol.* **2019**, *266*, 339–345. [CrossRef]
62. Morley, J.F.; Weintraub, D.; Mamikonyan, E.; Moberg, P.J.; Siderowf, A.D.; Duda, J.E. Olfactory Dysfunction Is Associated with Neuropsychiatric Manifestations in Parkinson's Disease. *Mov. Disord.* **2011**, *26*, 2051–2057. [CrossRef]
63. Hong, J.Y.; Sunwoo, M.K.; Ham, J.H.; Lee, J.J.; Lee, P.H.; Sohn, Y.H. Apathy and Olfactory Dysfunction in Early Parkinson's Disease. *J. Mov. Disord.* **2015**, *8*, 21–25. [CrossRef] [PubMed]
64. Masala, C.; Solla, P.; Liscia, A.; Defazio, G.; Saba, L.; Cannas, A.; Cavazzana, A.; Hummel, T.; Haehner, A. Correlation among Olfactory Function, Motors' Symptoms, Cognitive Impairment, Apathy, and Fatigue in Patients with Parkinson's Disease. *J. Neurol.* **2018**, *265*, 1764–1771. [CrossRef] [PubMed]
65. Ojagbemi, A.A.; Akinyemi, R.O.; Baiyewu, O. Neuropsychiatric Symptoms in Nigerian Patients with Parkinson's Disease. *Acta Neurol. Scand.* **2013**, *128*, 9–16. [CrossRef]
66. Drijgers, R.L.; Dujardin, K.; Reijnders, J.S.A.M.; Defebvre, L.; Leentjens, A.F.G. Validation of Diagnostic Criteria for Apathy in Parkinson's Disease. *Park. Relat. Disord.* **2010**, *16*, 656–660. [CrossRef] [PubMed]
67. Brown, R.G.; Pluck, G. Negative Symptoms: The "pathology" of Motivation and Goal-Directed Behaviour. *Trends Neurosci.* **2000**, *23*, 412–417. [CrossRef] [PubMed]
68. Stuss, D.T.; Van Reekum, R.; Murphy, K.J. Differentiation of States and Causes of Apathy. In *The Neuropsychology of Emotion*; Borod, J.C., Ed.; Series in Affective Science; Oxford University Press: Oxford, UK, 2000; pp. 340–363. ISBN 0-19-511464-7. (Hardcover).
69. Robert, P.; Onyike, C.U.; Leentjens, A.F.G.; Dujardin, K.; Aalten, P.; Starkstein, S.; Verhey, F.R.J.; Yessavage, J.; Clement, J.P.; Drapier, D.; et al. Proposed Diagnostic Criteria for Apathy in Alzheimer's Disease and Other Neuropsychiatric Disorders. *Eur. Psychiatry* **2009**, *24*, 98–104. [CrossRef]
70. Laplane, D.; Dubois, B. Auto-Activation Deficit: A Basal Ganglia Related Syndrome. *Mov. Disord.* **2001**, *16*, 810–814. [CrossRef]
71. Lazcano-Ocampo, C.; Wan, Y.M.; van Wamelen, D.J.; Batzu, L.; Boura, I.; Titova, N.; Leta, V.; Qamar, M.; Martinez-Martin, P.; Ray Chaudhuri, K. Identifying and Responding to Fatigue and Apathy in Parkinson's Disease: A Review of Current Practice. *Expert Rev. Neurother.* **2020**, *20*, 477–495. [CrossRef]
72. Levy, G.; Jacobs, D.M.; Tang, M.X.; Côté, L.J.; Louis, E.D.; Alfaro, B.; Mejia, H.; Stern, Y.; Marder, K. Memory and Executive Function Impairment Predict Dementia in Parkinson's Disease. *Mov. Disord.* **2002**, *17*, 1221–1226. [CrossRef]
73. Marin, R.S. Apathy: A Neuropsychiatric Syndrome. *J. Neuropsychiatry Clin. Neurosci.* **1991**, *3*, 243–254. [CrossRef]
74. Yuen, G.S.; Gunning, F.M.; Woods, E.; Klimstra, S.A.; Hoptman, M.J.; Alexopoulos, G.S. Neuroanatomical Correlates of Apathy in Late-Life Depression and Antidepressant Treatment Response. *J. Affect. Disord.* **2014**, *166*, 179–186. [CrossRef] [PubMed]
75. Hull, J.G.; Levy, A.S. The Organizational Functions of the Self: An Alternative to the Duval and Wicklund Model of Self-Awareness. *J. Pers. Soc. Psychol.* **1979**, *37*, 756–768. [CrossRef]
76. Leritz, E.; Loftis, C.; Crucian, G.; Friedman, W.; Bowers, D. Self-Awareness of Deficits in Parkinson Disease. *Clin. Neuropsychol.* **2004**, *18*, 352–361. [CrossRef] [PubMed]
77. Orfei, M.D.; Assogna, F.; Pellicano, C.; Pontieri, F.E.; Caltagirone, C.; Pierantozzi, M.; Stefani, A.; Spalletta, G. Anosognosia for Cognitive and Behavioral Symptoms in Parkinson's Disease with Mild Dementia and Mild Cognitive Impairment: Frequency and Neuropsychological/Neuropsychiatric Correlates. *Park. Relat. Disord.* **2018**, *54*, 62–67. [CrossRef]

78. Maier, F.; Prigatano, G.P.; Kalbe, E.; Barbe, M.T.; Eggers, C.; Lewis, C.J.; Burns, R.S.; Morrone-Strupinsky, J.; Moguel-Cobos, G.; Fink, G.R.; et al. Impaired Self-Awareness of Motor Deficits in Parkinson's Disease: Association with Motor Asymmetry and Motor Phenotypes. *Mov. Disord.* **2012**, *27*, 1443–1446. [CrossRef]
79. Devos, D.; Moreau, C.; Maltête, D.; Lefaucheur, R.; Kreisler, A.; Eusebio, A.; Defer, G.; Ouk, T.; Azulay, J.P.; Krystkowiak, P.; et al. Rivastigmine in Apathetic but Dementia and Depression-Free Patients with Parkinson's Disease: A Double-Blind, Placebo-Controlled, Randomised Clinical Trial. *J. Neurol. Neurosurg. Psychiatry* **2014**, *85*, 668–674. [CrossRef]
80. Drew, D.S.; Muhammed, K.; Baig, F.; Kelly, M.; Saleh, Y.; Sarangmat, N.; Okai, D.; Hu, M.; Manohar, S.; Husain, M. Dopamine and Reward Hypersensitivity in Parkinson's Disease with Impulse Control Disorder. *Brain* **2020**, *143*, 2502–2518. [CrossRef]
81. Scott, B.M.; Eisinger, R.S.; Burns, M.R.; Lopes, J.; Okun, M.S.; Gunduz, A.; Bowers, D. Co-Occurrence of Apathy and Impulse Control Disorders in Parkinson Disease. *Neurology* **2020**, *95*, e2769–e2780. [CrossRef]
82. Lansdall, C.J.; Coyle-Gilchrist, I.T.S.; Jones, P.S.; Rodríguez, P.V.; Wilcox, A.; Wehmann, E.; Dick, K.M.; Robbins, T.W.; Rowe, J.B. Apathy and Impulsivity in Frontotemporal Lobar Degeneration Syndromes. *Brain* **2017**, *140*, 1792–1807. [CrossRef]
83. Maillet, A.; Krack, P.; Lhommée, E.; Météreau, E.; Klinger, H.; Favre, E.; Le Bars, D.; Schmitt, E.; Bichon, A.; Pelissier, P.; et al. The Prominent Role of Serotonergic Degeneration in Apathy, Anxiety and Depression in de Novo Parkinson's Disease. *Brain* **2016**, *139*, 2486–2502. [CrossRef]
84. Prange, S.; Metereau, E.; Maillet, A.; Lhommée, E.; Klinger, H.; Pelissier, P.; Ibarrola, D.; Heckemann, R.A.; Castrioto, A.; Tremblay, L.; et al. Early Limbic Microstructural Alterations in Apathy and Depression in de Novo Parkinson's Disease. *Mov. Disord.* **2019**, *34*, 1644–1654. [CrossRef] [PubMed]
85. Maillet, A.; Météreau, E.; Tremblay, L.; Favre, E.; Klinger, H.; Lhommée, E.; Le Bars, D.; Castrioto, A.; Prange, S.; Sgambato, V.; et al. Serotonergic and Dopaminergic Lesions Underlying Parkinsonian Neuropsychiatric Signs. *Mov. Disord.* **2021**, *36*, 2888–2900. [CrossRef] [PubMed]
86. Baggio, H.C.; Segura, B.; Garrido-Millan, J.L.; Marti, M.J.; Compta, Y.; Valldeoriola, F.; Tolosa, E.; Junque, C. Resting-State Frontostriatal Functional Connectivity in Parkinson's Disease-Related Apathy. *Mov. Disord.* **2015**, *30*, 671–679. [CrossRef]
87. Alexander, G.E.; Crutcher, M.D.; Delong, M.R. Basal Ganglia-Thalamocortical Circuits: Parallel Substrates for Motor, Oculomotor, Prefrontal and Limbic Functions. *Prog. Brain Res.* **1990**, *85*, 119–149.
88. Cottencin, O.; Guardia, D.; Warembourg, F.; Gaudry, C.; Goudemand, M. Methadone Overdose, Auto-Activation Deficit, and Catatonia:A Case Study. *Prim. Care Companion J. Clin. Psychiatry* **2009**, *11*, 275–276. [CrossRef] [PubMed]
89. Leroy, A.; Petyt, G.; Pignon, B.; Vaiva, G.; Jardri, R.; Amad, A. Research Letter: Auto-Activation Deficit in Schizophrenia: A Case Report. *Psychol. Med.* **2018**, *48*, 525–527. [CrossRef] [PubMed]
90. Ali-Cherif, A.; Royere, M.L.; Gosset, A.; Poncet, M.; Salamon, G.; Khalil, R. Behavior and mental activity disorders after carbon monoxide poisoning. Bilateral pallidal lesions. *Rev. Neurol.* **1984**, *140*, 401–405.
91. Leu-Semenescu, S.; Uguccioni, G.; Golmard, J.L.; Czernecki, V.; Yelnik, J.; Dubois, B.; Forgeot D'Arc, B.; Grabli, D.; Levy, R.; Arnulf, I. Can We Still Dream When the Mind Is Blank? Sleep and Dream Mentations in Auto-Activation Deficit. *Brain* **2013**, *136*, 3076–3084. [CrossRef]
92. David, R.; Koulibaly, M.; Benoit, M.; Garcia, R.; Caci, H.; Darcourt, J.; Robert, P. Striatal Dopamine Transporter Levels Correlate with Apathy in Neurodegenerative Diseases. A SPECT Study with Partial Volume Effect Correction. *Clin. Neurol. Neurosurg.* **2008**, *110*, 19–24. [CrossRef]
93. Mega, M.S.; Cohenour, R.C. Akinetic Mutism: Disconnection of Frontal-Subcortical Circuits. *Neuropsychiatry. Neuropsychol. Behav. Neurol.* **1997**, *10*, 254–259.
94. Bogousslavsky, J.; Regli, F.; Delaloye, B.; Delaloye-Bischof, A.; Assal, G.; Uske, A. Loss of Psychic Self-Activation with Bithalamic Infarction. *Acta Neurol. Scand.* **1991**, *83*, 309–316. [CrossRef] [PubMed]
95. Laplane, D. La perte d'auto-activation psychique. *Rev. Neurol.* **1990**, *146*, 397–404. [PubMed]
96. Habib, M. Athymhormia and Disorders of Motivation in Basal Ganglia Disease. *J. Neuropsychiatry Clin. Neurosci.* **2004**, *16*, 509–524. [CrossRef] [PubMed]
97. Adam, R.; Leff, A.; Sinha, N.; Turner, C.; Bays, P.; Draganski, B.; Husain, M. Dopamine Reverses Reward Insensitivity in Apathy Following Globus Pallidus Lesions. *Cortex* **2013**, *49*, 1292–1303. [CrossRef]
98. Laine, M.; Tuokkola, T.; Hiltunen, J.; Vorobyev, V.; Bliss, I.; Baddeley, A.; Rinne, J.O. Central Executive Function in Mild Cognitive Impairment: A PET Activation Study: Cognition and Neurosciences. *Scand. J. Psychol.* **2009**, *50*, 33–40. [CrossRef]
99. Kondo, H.; Osaka, N.; Osaka, M. Cooperation of the Anterior Cingulate Cortex and Dorsolateral Prefrontal Cortex for Attention Shifting. *Neuroimage* **2004**, *23*, 670–679. [CrossRef]
100. Baker, S.C.; Rogers, R.D.; Owen, A.M.; Frith, C.D.; Dolan, R.J.; Frackowiak, R.S.J.; Robbins, T.W. Neural Systems Engaged by Planning: A PET Study of the Tower of London Task. *Neuropsychologia* **1996**, *34*, 515–526. [CrossRef]
101. Levy, R.; Friedman, H.R.; Davachi, L.; Goldman-Rakic, P.S. Differential Activation of the Caudate Nucleus in Primates Performing Spatial and Nonspatial Working Memory Tasks. *J. Neurosci.* **1997**, *17*, 3870–3882. [CrossRef]
102. Owen, A.M. Planning and Spatial Working Memory: A Positron Emission Tomography Study in Humans. *Eur. J. Neurosci.* **1996**, *8*, 353–364. [CrossRef]
103. Lucas-Jiménez, O.; Ojeda, N.; Peña, J.; Cabrera-Zubizarreta, A.; Díez-Cirarda, M.; Gómez-Esteban, J.C.; Gómez-Beldarrain, M.Á.; Ibarretxe-Bilbao, N. Apathy and Brain Alterations in Parkinson's Disease: A Multimodal Imaging Study. *Ann. Clin. Transl. Neurol.* **2018**, *5*, 803–814. [CrossRef]

104. Moretti, R.; Caruso, P.; Dal Ben, M. Rivastigmine as a Symptomatic Treatment for Apathy in Parkinson's Dementia Complex: New Aspects for This Riddle. *Parkinsons. Dis.* **2017**, *2017*. [CrossRef] [PubMed]
105. Lanctôt, K.L.; Herrmann, N.; Black, S.E.; Ryan, M.; Rothenburg, L.S.; Liu, B.A.; Busto, U.E. Apathy Associated with Alzheimer Disease: Use of Dextroamphetamine Challenge. *Am. J. Geriatr. Psychiatry* **2008**, *16*, 551–557. [CrossRef]
106. Magnard, R.; Vachez, Y.; Carcenac, C.; Krack, P.; David, O.; Savasta, M.; Boulet, S.; Carnicella, S. What Can Rodent Models Tell Us about Apathy and Associated Neuropsychiatric Symptoms in Parkinson's Disease? *Transl. Psychiatry* **2016**, *6*, e753. [CrossRef] [PubMed]
107. Haber, S.N.; Knutson, B. The Reward Circuit: Linking Primate Anatomy and Human Imaging. *Neuropsychopharmacology* **2010**, *35*, 4–26. [CrossRef]
108. Hong, S.; Hikosaka, O. Pedunculopontine Tegmental Nucleus Neurons Provide Reward, Sensorimotor, and Alerting Signals to Midbrain Dopamine Neurons. *Physiol. Behav.* **2016**, *176*, 139–148. [CrossRef] [PubMed]
109. Martínez-Horta, S.; Riba, J.; Fernández De Bobadilla, R.; Pagonabarraga, J.; Pascual-Sedano, B.; Antonijoan, R.M.; Romero, S.; Ngel Mañanas, M.A.; García-Sanchez, C.; Kulisevsky, J. Apathy in Parkinson's Disease: Neurophysiological Evidence of Impaired Incentive Processing. *J. Neurosci.* **2014**, *17*, 5918–5926. [CrossRef]
110. Schultz, W. Behavioral Dopamine Signals. *Trends Neurosci.* **2007**, *30*, 203–210. [CrossRef]
111. Riba, J.; Krämer, U.M.; Heldmann, M.; Richter, S.; Münte, T.F. Dopamine Agonist Increases Risk Taking but Blunts Reward-Related Brain Activity. *PLoS ONE* **2008**, *3*, e2479. [CrossRef]
112. Leentjens, A.F.G.; Koester, J.; Fruh, B.; Shephard, D.T.S.; Barone, P.; Houben, J.J.G. The Effect of Pramipexole on Mood and Motivational Symptoms in Parkinson's Disease: A Meta-Analysis of Placebo-Controlled Studies. *Clin. Ther.* **2009**, *31*, 89–98. [CrossRef]
113. Barber, T.R.; Griffanti, L.; Muhammed, K.; Drew, D.S.; Bradley, K.M.; McGowan, D.R.; Crabbe, M.; Lo, C.; MacKay, C.E.; Husain, M.; et al. Apathy in Rapid Eye Movement Sleep Behaviour Disorder Is Associated with Serotonin Depletion in the Dorsal Raphe Nucleus. *Brain* **2018**, *141*, 2848–2854. [CrossRef]
114. Cavanna, A.E.; Trimble, M.R. The Precuneus: A Review of Its Functional Anatomy and Behavioural Correlates. *Brain* **2006**, *129*, 564–583. [CrossRef] [PubMed]
115. Shulman, G.L.; Fiez, J.A.; Corbetta, M.; Buckner, R.L.; Miezin, F.M.; Raichle, M.E.; Petersen, S.E. Common Blood Flow Changes across Visual Tasks: II. Decreases in Cerebral Cortex. *J. Cogn. Neurosci.* **1997**, *9*, 648–663. [CrossRef] [PubMed]
116. Mesulam, M.-M. Frontal Cortex and Behavior. *Ann. Neurol.* **1986**, *19*, 320–325. [CrossRef] [PubMed]
117. Shin, J.H.; Shin, S.A.; Lee, J.Y.; Nam, H.; Lim, J.S.; Kim, Y.K. Precuneus Degeneration and Isolated Apathy in Patients with Parkinson's Disease. *Neurosci. Lett.* **2017**, *653*, 250–257. [CrossRef]
118. Reijnders, J.S.A.M.; Scholtissen, B.; Weber, W.E.J.; Aalten, P.; Verhey, F.R.J.; Leentjens, A.F.G. Neuroanatomical Correlates of Apathy in Parkinson's Disease: A Magnetic Resonance Imaging Study Using Voxel-Based Morphometry. *Mov. Disord.* **2010**, *25*, 2318–2325. [CrossRef]
119. Newen, A.; Vogeley, K. Self-Representation: Searching for a Neural Signature of Self-Consciousness. *Conscious. Cogn.* **2003**, *12*, 529–543. [CrossRef]
120. Morin, A. Self-Awareness Part 2: Neuroanatomy and Importance of Inner Speech. *Soc. Personal. Psychol. Compass* **2011**, *5*, 1004–1017. [CrossRef]
121. Robert, G.; Le Jeune, F.; Dondaine, T.; Drapier, S.; Péron, J.; Lozachmeur, C.; Sauleau, P.; Houvenaghel, J.F.; Travers, D.; Millet, B.; et al. Apathy and Impaired Emotional Facial Recognition Networks Overlap in Parkinson's Disease: A PET Study with Conjunction Analyses. *J. Neurol. Neurosurg. Psychiatry* **2014**, *85*, 1153–1158. [CrossRef]
122. Schmidt, L.; D'Arc, B.F.; Lafargue, G.; Galanaud, D.; Czernecki, V.; Grabli, D.; Schüpbach, M.; Hartmann, A.; Lévy, R.; Dubois, B.; et al. Disconnecting Force from Money: Effects of Basal Ganglia Damage on Incentive Motivation. *Brain* **2008**, *131*, 1303–1310. [CrossRef]
123. Carriere, N.; Besson, P.; Dujardin, K.; Duhamel, A.; Defebvre, L.; Delmaire, C.; Devos, D. Apathy in Parkinson's Disease Is Associated with Nucleus Accumbens Atrophy: A Magnetic Resonance Imaging Shape Analysis. *Mov. Disord.* **2014**, *29*, 897–903. [CrossRef]
124. Wen, M.C.; Wen, M.C.; Thiery, A.; Tseng, W.Y.I.; Kok, T.; Xu, Z.; Chua, S.T.; Tan, L.C.S.; Tan, L.C.S.; Tan, L.C.S. Apathy Is Associated with White Matter Network Disruption and Specific Cognitive Deficits in Parkinson's Disease. *Psychol. Med.* **2020**, *52*, 264–273. [CrossRef]
125. Alzahrani, H.; Antonini, A.; Venneri, A. Apathy in Mild Parkinson's Disease: Neuropsychological and Neuroimaging Evidence. *J. Parkinsons. Dis.* **2016**, *6*, 821–832. [CrossRef] [PubMed]
126. Zhang, Y.; Wu, J.; Wu, W.; Liu, R.; Pang, L.; Guan, D.; Xu, Y. Reduction of White Matter Integrity Correlates with Apathy in Parkinson's Disease. *Int. J. Neurosci.* **2018**, *128*, 25–31. [CrossRef]
127. Skidmore, F.M.; Yang, M.; Baxter, L.; von Deneen, K.; Collingwood, J.; He, G.; Tandon, R.; Korenkevych, D.; Savenkov, A.; Heilman, K.M.; et al. Apathy, Depression, and Motor Symptoms Have Distinct and Separable Resting Activity Patterns in Idiopathic Parkinson Disease. *Neuroimage* **2013**, *81*, 484–495. [CrossRef] [PubMed]
128. Sun, H.H.; Pan, P.L.; Hu, J.B.; Chen, J.; Wang, X.Y.; Liu, C.F. Alterations of Regional Homogeneity in Parkinson's Disease with "Pure" Apathy: A Resting-State FMRI Study. *J. Affect. Disord.* **2020**, *274*, 792–798. [CrossRef]

129. Zhang, Y.; Zhang, G.Y.; Zhang, Z.E.; He, A.Q.; Gan, J.; Liu, Z. White Matter Hyperintensities: A Marker for Apathy in Parkinson's Disease without Dementia? *Ann. Clin. Transl. Neurol.* **2020**, *7*, 1692–1701. [CrossRef] [PubMed]
130. Brown, D.S.; Barrett, M.J.; Flanigan, J.L.; Sperling, S.A. Clinical and Demographic Correlates of Apathy in Parkinson's Disease. *J. Neurol.* **2019**, *266*, 507–514. [CrossRef]
131. Álvarez-Avellón, T.; Arias-Carrión, Ó.; Menéndez-González, M. Neuropsychiatric Symptoms and Associated Caregiver Stress in Geriatric Patients with Parkinson's Disease. *Neurol. Neurosci.* **2015**, *201521*, 1–8. [CrossRef]
132. Hassan, A.; Vallabhajosula, S.; Zahodne, L.B.; Bowers, D.; Okun, M.S.; Fernandez, H.H.; Hass, C.J. Correlations of Apathy and Depression with Postural Instability in Parkinson Disease. *J. Neurol. Sci.* **2014**, *338*, 162–165. [CrossRef]
133. Reijnders, J.S.A.M.; Ehrt, U.; Lousberg, R.; Aarsland, D.; Leentjens, A.F.G. The Association between Motor Subtypes and Psychopathology in Parkinson's Disease. *Park. Relat. Disord.* **2009**, *15*, 379–382. [CrossRef]
134. Perez-Lloret, S.; Negre-Pages, L.; Damier, P.; Delval, A.; Derkinderen, P.; Destée, A.; Meissner, W.G.; Schelosky, L.; Tison, F.; Rascol, O. Prevalence, Determinants, and Effect on Quality of Life of Freezing of Gait in Parkinson Disease. *JAMA Neurol.* **2014**, *71*, 884–890. [CrossRef] [PubMed]
135. Harris, E.; McNamara, P.; Durso, R. Apathy in Patients with Parkinson Disease as a Function of Side of Onset. *J. Geriatr. Psychiatry Neurol.* **2013**, *26*, 95–104. [CrossRef] [PubMed]
136. Skorvanek, M.; Gdovinova, Z.; Rosenberger, J.; Ghorbani Saeedian, R.; Nagyova, I.; Groothoff, J.W.; van Dijk, J.P. The Associations between Fatigue, Apathy, and Depression in Parkinson's Disease. *Acta Neurol. Scand.* **2015**, *131*, 80–87. [CrossRef]
137. Sáez-Francàs, N.; Hernández-Vara, J.; Roso, M.C.; Martín, J.A.; Brugué, M.C. The Association of Apathy with Central Fatigue Perception in Patients with Parkinson's Disease. *Behav. Neurosci.* **2013**, *127*, 237–244. [CrossRef] [PubMed]
138. Siciliano, M.; Trojano, L.; De Micco, R.; Giordano, A.; Russo, A.; Tedeschi, G.; Chiorri, C.; Tessitore, A. Predictors of Fatigue Severity in Early, de Novo Parkinson Disease Patients: A 1-Year Longitudinal Study. *Park. Relat. Disord.* **2020**, *79*, 3–8. [CrossRef] [PubMed]
139. Meyer, A.; Zimmermann, R.; Gschwandtner, U.; Hatz, F.; Bousleiman, H.; Schwarz, N.; Fuhr, P. Apathy in Parkinson's Disease Is Related to Executive Function, Gender and Age but Not to Depression. *Front. Aging Neurosci.* **2015**, *7*, 1–6. [CrossRef] [PubMed]
140. Santangelo, G.; D'Iorio, A.; Maggi, G.; Cuoco, S.; Pellecchia, M.T.; Amboni, M.; Barone, P.; Vitale, C. Cognitive Correlates of "Pure Apathy" in Parkinson's Disease. *Park. Relat. Disord.* **2018**, *53*, 101–104. [CrossRef] [PubMed]
141. D'Iorio, A.; Maggi, G.; Vitale, C.; Trojano, L.; Santangelo, G. "Pure Apathy" and Cognitive Dysfunctions in Parkinson's Disease: A Meta-Analytic Study. *Neurosci. Biobehav. Rev.* **2018**, *94*, 1–10. [CrossRef]
142. Dujardin, K.; Moonen, A.J.H.; Behal, H.; Defebvre, L.; Duhamel, A.; Duits, A.A.; Plomhause, L.; Tard, C.; Leentjens, A.F.G. Cognitive Disorders in Parkinson's Disease: Confirmation of a Spectrum of Severity. *Park. Relat. Disord.* **2015**, *21*, 1299–1305. [CrossRef]
143. Costa, A.; Peppe, A.; Zabberoni, S.; Scalici, F.; Caltagirone, C.; Carlesimo, G.A. Apathy in Individuals with Parkinson's Disease Associated with Mild Cognitive Impairment. A Neuropsychological Investigation. *Neuropsychologia* **2018**, *118*, 4–11. [CrossRef]
144. Goldman, J.G.; Holden, S.K.; Litvan, I.; McKeith, I.; Stebbins, G.T.; Taylor, J.P. Evolution of Diagnostic Criteria and Assessments for Parkinson's Disease Mild Cognitive Impairment. *Mov. Disord.* **2018**, *33*, 503–510. [CrossRef]
145. Baiano, C.; Barone, P.; Trojano, L.; Santangelo, G. Prevalence and Clinical Aspects of Mild Cognitive Impairment in Parkinson's Disease: A Meta-Analysis. *Mov. Disord.* **2020**, *35*, 45–54. [CrossRef] [PubMed]
146. Campbell, M.C.; Myers, P.S.; Weigand, A.J.; Foster, E.R.; Cairns, N.J.; Jackson, J.J.; Lessov-Schlaggar, C.N.; Perlmutter, J.S. Parkinson Disease Clinical Subtypes: Key Features & Clinical Milestones. *Ann. Clin. Transl. Neurol.* **2020**, *7*, 1–12. [CrossRef]
147. Wang, H.T.; Wang, L.; He, Y.; Yu, G. Rotigotine Transdermal Patch for the Treatment of Neuropsychiatric Symptoms in Parkinson's Disease: A Meta-Analysis of Randomized Placebo-Controlled Trials. *J. Neurol. Sci.* **2018**, *393*, 31–38. [CrossRef] [PubMed]
148. Castrioto, A.; Thobois, S.; Anheim, M.; Quesada, J.L.; Lhommée, E.; Klinger, H.; Bichon, A.; Schmitt, E.; Durif, F.; Azulay, J.P.; et al. A Randomized Controlled Double-Blind Study of Rotigotine on Neuropsychiatric Symptoms in de Novo PD. *NPJ Park. Dis.* **2020**, *6*, 1–6. [CrossRef]
149. Auffret, M.; Le Jeune, F.; Maurus, A.; Drapier, S.; Houvenaghel, J.F.; Robert, G.H.; Sauleau, P.; Vérin, M. Apomorphine Pump in Advanced Parkinson's Disease: Effects on Motor and Nonmotor Symptoms with Brain Metabolism Correlations. *J. Neurol. Sci.* **2017**, *372*, 279–287. [CrossRef]
150. Todorova, A.; Martinez-Martin, P.; Martin, A.; Rizos, A.; Reddy, P.; Chaudhuri, K.R. Daytime Apomorphine Infusion Combined with Transdermal Rotigotine Patch Therapy Is Tolerated at 2 Years: A 24-h Treatment Option in Parkinson's Disease. *Basal Ganglia* **2013**, *3*, 127–130. [CrossRef]
151. Blundo, C.; Gerace, C. Dopamine Agonists Can Improve Pure Apathy Associated with Lesions of the Prefrontal-Basal Ganglia Functional System. *Neurol. Sci.* **2015**, *36*, 1197–1201. [CrossRef]
152. Ganjavi, H.; Macdonald, P.A. On-off Effects of Dopaminergic Therapy on Psychiatric Symptoms in Parkinson's Disease. *J. Neuropsychiatry Clin. Neurosci.* **2015**, *27*, e134–e139. [CrossRef]
153. Zahodne, L.B.; Bernal-Pacheco, O.; Bowers, D.; Ward, H.; Oyama, G.; Limotai, N.; Velez-Lago, F.; Rodriguez, R.L.; Malaty, I.; McFarland, N.R.; et al. Are Selective Serotonin Reuptake Inhibitors Associated with Greater Apathy in Parkinson's Disease? *J. Neuropsychiatry Clin. Neurosci.* **2012**, *24*, 326–330. [CrossRef]
154. Meloni, M.; Puligheddu, M.; Carta, M.; Cannas, A.; Figorilli, M.; Defazio, G. Efficacy and Safety of 5-Hydroxytryptophan on Depression and Apathy in Parkinson's Disease: A Preliminary Finding. *Eur. J. Neurol.* **2020**, *27*, 779–786. [CrossRef] [PubMed]

155. Takahashi, M.; Tabu, H.; Ozaki, A.; Hamano, T.; Takeshima, T. Antidepressants for Depression, Apathy, and Gait Instability in Parkinson's Disease: A Multicenter Randomized Study. *Intern. Med.* **2019**, *58*, 361–368. [CrossRef] [PubMed]
156. Bullock, R.; Cameron, A. Rivastigmine for the Treatment of Dementia and Visual Hallucinations Associated with Parkinson's Disease: A Case Series. *Curr. Med. Res. Opin.* **2002**, *18*, 258–264. [CrossRef] [PubMed]
157. Oh, Y.-S.; Kim, J.-S.; Lee, P.H. Effect of Rivastigmine on Behavioral and Psychiatric Symptoms of Parkinson's Disease Dementia. *J. Mov. Disord.* **2015**, *8*, 98–102. [CrossRef]
158. Litvinenko, I.V.; Odinak, M.M.; Mogil'naya, V.I.; Emelin, A.Y.U. Efficacy and Safety of Galantamine (Reminyl) for Dementia in Patients with Parkinson's Disease (an Open Controlled Trial). *Neurosci. Behav. Physiol.* **2008**, *38*, 937–945. [CrossRef]
159. Lanctot, K.L.; Chau, S.A.; Herrmann, N.; Drye, L.T.; Rosenberg, P.B.; Scherer, R.W.; Black, S.E.; Vaidya, V.; Bachman, D.L.; Mintzer, J.E. Effect of Methylphenidate on Attention in Apathetic AD Patients in a Randomized, Placebo-Controlled Trial. *Int. Psychogeriatr.* **2014**, *26*, 239–246. [CrossRef]
160. Nagayama, H.; Kano, O.; Murakami, H.; Ono, K.; Hamada, M.; Toda, T.; Sengoku, R.; Shimo, Y.; Hattori, N. Effect of Istradefylline on Mood Disorders in Parkinson's Disease. *J. Neurol. Sci.* **2019**, *396*, 78–83. [CrossRef]
161. Krishna, R.; Ali, M.; Moustafa, A.A. Effects of Combined MAO-B Inhibitors and Levodopa vs Monotherapy in Parkinson's Disease. *Front. Aging Neurosci.* **2014**, *6*, 180. [CrossRef]
162. Hatano, T.; Hattori, N.; Kawanabe, T.; Terayama, Y.; Suzuki, N.; Iwasaki, Y.; Fujioka, T. An Exploratory Study of the Efficacy and Safety of Yokukansan for Neuropsychiatric Symptoms in Patients with Parkinson's Disease. *J. Neural Transm.* **2014**, *121*, 275–281. [CrossRef]
163. Athauda, D.; MacLagan, K.; Budnik, N.; Zampedri, L.; Hibbert, S.; Skene, S.S.; Chowdhury, K.; Aviles-Olmos, I.; Limousin, P.; Foltynie, T. What Effects Might Exenatide Have on Non-Motor Symptoms in Parkinson's Disease: A Post Hoc Analysis. *J. Parkinsons. Dis.* **2018**, *8*, 247–258. [CrossRef]
164. Smith, K.M.; Eyal, E.; Weintraub, D. Combined Rasagiline and Antidepressant Use in Parkinson Disease in the ADAGIO Study: Effects on Nonmotor Symptoms and Tolerability. *JAMA Neurol.* **2015**, *72*, 88–95. [CrossRef] [PubMed]
165. Chatterjee, A.; Fahn, S. Methylphenidate Treats Apathy in Parkinson's Disease. *J. Neuropsychiatry Clin. Neurosci.* **2002**, *14*, 461–462. [CrossRef]
166. Gelderblom, H.; Wüstenberg, T.; McLean, T.; Mütze, L.; Fischer, W.; Saft, C.; Hoffmann, R.; Süssmuth, S.; Schlattmann, P.; Van Duijn, E.; et al. Bupropion for the Treatment of Apathy in Huntington's Disease: A Multicenter, Randomised, Double-Blind, Placebocontrolled, Prospective Crossover Trial. *PLoS ONE* **2017**, *12*, 0173872. [CrossRef] [PubMed]
167. Maier, F.; Spottke, A.; Bach, J.P.; Bartels, C.; Buerger, K.; Dodel, R.; Fellgiebel, A.; Fliessbach, K.; Frölich, L.; Hausner, L.; et al. Bupropion for the Treatment of Apathy in Alzheimer Disease: A Randomized Clinical Trial. *JAMA Netw. Open* **2020**, *3*, e206027. [CrossRef] [PubMed]
168. Rea, R.; Carotenuto, A.; Traini, E.; Fasanaro, A.M.; Manzo, V.; Amenta, F. Apathy Treatment in Alzheimer's Disease: Interim Results of the ASCOMALVA Trial. *J. Alzheimers. Dis.* **2015**, *48*, 377–383. [CrossRef]
169. Laplane, D.; Baulac, M.; Widlocher, D.; Dubois, B. Pure Psychic Akinesia with Bilateral Lesions of Basal Ganglia. *J. Neurol. Neurosurg. Psychiatry* **1984**, *47*, 377–385. [CrossRef]
170. Goodwin, V.A.; Richards, S.H.; Taylor, R.S.; Taylor, A.H.; Campbell, J.L. The Effectiveness of Exercise Interventions for People with Parkinson's Disease: A Systematic Review and Meta-Analysis. *Mov. Disord.* **2008**, *23*, 631–640. [CrossRef]
171. Bloem, B.R.; de Vries, N.M.; Ebersbach, G. Nonpharmacological Treatments for Patients with Parkinson's Disease. *Mov. Disord.* **2015**, *30*, 1504–1520. [CrossRef]
172. Ng, S.Y.-E.; Chia, N.S.-Y.; Abbas, M.M.; Saffari, E.S.; Choi, X.; Heng, D.L.; Xu, Z.; Tay, K.-Y.; Au, W.-L.; Tan, E.-K.; et al. Physical Activity Improves Anxiety and Apathy in Early Parkinson's Disease: A Longitudinal Follow-Up Study. *Front. Neurol.* **2021**, *11*, 625897. [CrossRef]
173. King, L.A.; Wilhelm, J.; Chen, Y.; Blehm, R.; Nutt, J.; Chen, Z.; Serdar, A.; Horak, F.B. Effects of Group, Individual, and Home Exercise in Persons With Parkinson Disease: A Randomized Clinical Trial. *J. Neurol. Phys. Ther.* **2015**, *39*, 204–212. [CrossRef]
174. Cugusi, L.; Solla, P.; Serpe, R.; Carzedda, T.; Piras, L.; Oggianu, M.; Gabba, S.; Di Blasio, A.; Bergamin, M.; Cannas, A.; et al. Effects of a Nordic Walking Program on Motor and Non-Motor Symptoms, Functional Performance and Body Composition in Patients with Parkinson's Disease. *NeuroRehabilitation* **2015**, *37*, 245–254. [CrossRef] [PubMed]
175. Cai, W.; Wang, Y.; Juan, Z.; Cong, Y.; Niu, Y.; Yang, J.; Huang, S. Effects of Dance Therapy on Non-Motor Symptoms in Patients with Parkinson ' s Disease: A Systematic Review and Meta-Analysis. *Aging Clin. Exp. Res.* **2021**, *34*, 1201–1208. [CrossRef]
176. Subramanian, I. Complementary and Alternative Medicine and Exercise in Nonmotor Symptoms of Parkinson's Disease. *Int. Rev. Neurobiol.* **2017**, *134*, 1163–1188. [PubMed]
177. Manera, V.; Abrahams, S.; Agüera-Ortiz, L.; Bremond, F.; David, R.; Fairchild, K.; Gros, A.; Hanon, C.; Husain, M.; König, A.; et al. Recommendations for the Nonpharmacological Treatment of Apathy in Brain Disorders. *Am. J. Geriatr. Psychiatry* **2020**, *28*, 410–420. [CrossRef] [PubMed]
178. Oguro, H.; Nakagawa, T. Randomized Trial of Repetitive Transcranial Magnetic Stimulation for Apathy and Depression in Parkinson's Disease. *J. Neurol. Neurophysiol.* **2014**, *5*, 1–6. [CrossRef]
179. Maruo, T.; Hosomi, K.; Shimokawa, T.; Kishima, H.; Oshino, S.; Morris, S.; Kageyama, Y.; Yokoe, M.; Yoshimine, T.; Saitoh, Y. High-Frequency Repetitive Transcranial Magnetic Stimulation over the Primary Foot Motor Area in Parkinson's Disease. *Brain Stimul.* **2013**, *6*, 884–891. [CrossRef]

180. Wei, W.; Yi, X.; Ruan, J.; Duan, X.; Luo, H. The Efficacy of Repetitive Transcranial Magnetic Stimulation on Emotional Processing in Apathetic Patients with Parkinson's Disease: A Placebo-Controlled ERP Study. *J. Affect. Disord.* **2021**, *282*, 776–785. [CrossRef]
181. Montoya-Murillo, G.; Ibarretxe-Bilbao, N.; Peña, J.; Ojeda, N. Effects of Cognitive Rehabilitation on Cognition, Apathy, Quality of Life, and Subjective Complaints in the Elderly: A Randomized Controlled Trial. *Am. J. Geriatr. Psychiatry* **2020**, *28*, 518–529. [CrossRef]
182. Díez-Cirarda, M.; Ojeda, N.; Peña, J.; Cabrera-Zubizarreta, A.; Lucas-Jiménez, O.; Gómez-Esteban, J.C.; Gómez-Beldarrain, M.; Ibarretxe-Bilbao, N. Long-Term Effects of Cognitive Rehabilitation on Brain, Functional Outcome and Cognition in Parkinson's Disease. *Eur. J. Neurol.* **2018**, *25*, 5–12. [CrossRef]
183. Peña, J.; Ibarretxe-Bilbao, N.; García-Gorostiaga, I.; Gomez-Beldarrain, M.A.; Díez-Cirarda, M.; Ojeda, N. Improving Functional Disability and Cognition in Parkinson Disease Randomized Controlled Trial. *Neurology* **2014**, *83*, 2167–2174. [CrossRef]
184. Butterfield, L.C.; Cimino, C.R.; Salazar, R.; Sanchez-Ramos, J.; Bowers, D.; Okun, M.S. The Parkinson's Active Living (PAL) Program: A Behavioral Intervention Targeting Apathy in Parkinsons Disease. *J. Geriatr. Psychiatry Neurol.* **2017**, *30*, 11–25. [CrossRef] [PubMed]

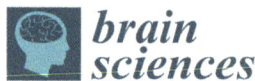 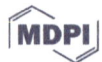

Article

Assessing Anti-Social and Aggressive Behavior in a Zebrafish (*Danio rerio*) Model of Parkinson's Disease Chronically Exposed to Rotenone

Ovidiu-Dumitru Ilie [1], Raluca Duta [1], Roxana Jijie [2,*], Ilinca-Bianca Nita [3], Mircea Nicoara [1,4], Caterina Faggio [5], Romeo Dobrin [6], Ioannis Mavroudis [7], Alin Ciobica [1,*] and Bogdan Doroftei [3]

[1] Department of Biology, Faculty of Biology, "Alexandru Ioan Cuza" University, Carol I Avenue, No 20A, 700505 Iasi, Romania; ovidiuilie90@yahoo.com (O.-D.I.); duta.raluca112@gmail.com (R.D.); mirmag@uaic.ro (M.N.)
[2] Department of Exact and Natural Sciences, Institute of Interdisciplinary Research, "Alexandru Ioan Cuza" University, Carol I Avenue, No 11, 700506 Iasi, Romania
[3] Faculty of Medicine, University of Medicine and Pharmacy "Grigore T. Popa", University Street, No 16, 700115 Iasi, Romania; ilinca.bi@yahoo.com (I.-B.N.); bogdandoroftei@gmail.com (B.D.)
[4] Doctoral School of Geosciences, Faculty of Geography-Geology, "Alexandru Ioan Cuza" University, Carol I Avenue, No 20A, 700505 Iasi, Romania
[5] Department of Chemical, Biological, Pharmaceutical and Environmental Sciences, University of Messina, Viale F. Stagno d'Alcontre 31, 98166 Messina, Italy; caterina.faggio@unime.it
[6] Department of Psychiatry, University of Medicine and Pharmacy "Grigore T. Popa", University Street, No 16, 700115 Iasi, Romania; romeodobrin2002@gmail.com
[7] Department of Neuroscience, Leeds Teaching Hospitals, NHS Trust, Leeds LS2 9JT, UK; i.mavroudis@nhs.net
* Correspondence: roxana.jijie@uaic.ro (R.J.); alin.ciobica@uaic.ro (A.C.)

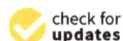

Citation: Ilie, O.-D.; Duta, R.; Jijie, R.; Nita, I.-B.; Nicoara, M.; Faggio, C.; Dobrin, R.; Mavroudis, I.; Ciobica, A.; Doroftei, B. Assessing Anti-Social and Aggressive Behavior in a Zebrafish (*Danio rerio*) Model of Parkinson's Disease Chronically Exposed to Rotenone. *Brain Sci.* **2022**, *12*, 898. https://doi.org/10.3390/brainsci12070898

Academic Editors: Patricia Martinez-Sanchez and Francisco Nieto-Escamez

Received: 4 June 2022
Accepted: 5 July 2022
Published: 8 July 2022

Publisher's Note: MDPI stays neutral with regard to jurisdictional claims in published maps and institutional affiliations.

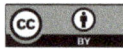

Copyright: © 2022 by the authors. Licensee MDPI, Basel, Switzerland. This article is an open access article distributed under the terms and conditions of the Creative Commons Attribution (CC BY) license (https://creativecommons.org/licenses/by/4.0/).

Abstract: Background: Rotenone (ROT) is currently being used in various research fields, especially neuroscience. Separated from other neurotoxins, ROT induces a Parkinson's disease (PD)-related phenotype that mimics the associated clinical spectrum by directly entering the central nervous system (CNS). It easily crosses through the blood–brain barrier (BBB) and accumulates in mitochondria. Unfortunately, most of the existing data focus on locomotion. This is why the present study aimed to bring novel evidence on how ROT alone or in combination with different potential ant(agonists) might influence the social and aggressive behavior using the counterclockwise rotation as a neurological pointer. Material and Methods: Thus, we exposed zebrafish to ROT—2.5 μg/L, valproic acid (VPA)—0.5 mg/mL, anti-parkinsonian drugs (LEV/CARB)—250 mg + 25 mg, and probiotics (PROBIO)—3 g for 32 days by assessing the anti-social profile and mirror tests and counterclockwise rotation every 4 days to avoid chronic stress. Results: We observed an abnormal pattern in the counterclockwise rotation only in the (a) CONTROL, (c) LEV/CARB, and (d) PROBIO groups, from both the top and side views, this indicating a reaction to medication and supplements administered or a normal intrinsic feature due to high levels of stress/anxiety ($p < 0.05$). Four out of eight studied groups—(b) VPA, (c) LEV/CARB, (e) ROT, and (f) ROT + VPA—displayed an impaired, often antithetical behavior demonstrated by long periods of time on distinct days spent on the right and the central arm ($p < 0.05, 0.005,$ and 0.0005). Interestingly, groups (d) PROBIO, (g) ROT + LEV/CARB, and (h) ROT + PROBIO registered fluctuations but not significant ones in contrast with the above groups ($p > 0.05$). Except for groups (a) CONTROL and (d) PROBIO, where a normalized trend in terms of behavior was noted, the rest of the experimental groups exhibited exacerbated levels of aggression ($p < 0.05, 0.005,$ and 0.001) not only near the mirror but as an overall reaction ($p < 0.05, 0.005,$ and 0.001). Conclusions: The (d) PROBIO group showed a significant improvement compared with (b) VPA, (c) LEV/CARB, and ROT-treated zebrafish (e–h). Independently of the aggressive-like reactions and fluctuations among the testing day(s) and groups, ROT disrupted the social behavior, while VPA promoted a specific typology in contrast with LEV/CARB.

Keywords: anti-social; aggressivity; counterclockwise rotation; zebrafish; *Danio rerio*; Parkinson's disease; rotenone

1. Introduction

The neurotoxic potential of MPTP (1-methyl-4-phenyl-1,2,3,6-tetrahydropyridine), 6-OHDA (6-hydroxydopamine), and paraquat (N, N′-dimethyl-4,4′-bipyridinium dichloride) as viable agents to generate PD-related symptoms is already well documented in the literature. Another compound that has gained increased interest with a toxicological profile and a broad spectrum of utility is ROT [1–3].

This plant-derived isoflavone is one of the oldest natural elements identified in several plants. The leaves, seeds, and stem of Mexican turnip (*Pachyrhizus erosus*), known under the trivial name of Jicama vine plants, and from roots of the *Fabaceae* family belonging to the genera *Derris*, *Lonchocarpus*, *Tephrosia*, and *Mundulea*, are specially processed to obtain ROT [4,5].

The *Lonchocarpus utilis* and *Nolina lindheimeriana*, native to South and North America, and *Lonchocarpus nicou* and *Derris elliptica* are also candidate species for obtaining ROT [4,5]. Due to its nature, the Federal Insecticide Fungicide Rodenticide Act [6] registered ROT in 1947.

ROT in small doses is safe if properly utilized, but it can be toxic to animals, fish, and humans. Compared to incomplete absorption by the gastrointestinal (GI) tract in fish, it is irrespective due to the absence of degrading enzymes in contrast to rodents [5].

Presently, ROT is confirmed to be a dopaminergic antagonistic that crosses the blood–brain barrier (BBB) and directly enters the central nervous system (CNS) and accumulates in cellular organelles, predominantly in the mitochondria, due to its lipophilic structure [1–3].

ROT induces dopamine neuronal toxicity [7], leading to a decline in adenosine triphosphate (ATP) generation and exacerbation in reactive oxygen species (ROS) via the inhibition of the complex I of the mitochondrial electron transport chain (ETC) [8]. Thus, ROT causes microglial activation, reflected by neuroinflammation [9], and aggregation of α-synuclein, known for their involvement in Lewy body pathology [10].

Fortunately, this field of research has received a lot of attention lately. However, little is known about ROT's impacts on zebrafish behavior, particularly sociability and aggression. Based on these considerations, this study aims to evaluate the changes in the social component and level of aggression using the counterclockwise rotation parameter as a neurological pointer in a zebrafish (*Danio rerio*) chronically exposed to ROT for 32 days.

2. Materials and Methods

2.1. Animal Maintenance

We used forty adult (6–8 months), wild-type (WT), AB genetic line zebrafish (*Danio rerio*) purchased from an authorized local breeder from Iasi. The subjects were housed for 14 days in a 90 L dechlorinated water aquarium and for another 7 days in new 10 L tank(s). They were fed twice a day with TetraMin Flakes, while the water was changed daily in each experimental tank. The laboratory temperature was maintained at $26 \pm 2\,°C$, pH 7.5, and 14 h light/10 h night cycle [11].

2.2. Ethical Note

Specimens were maintained and treated under the EU Commission Recommendation (2007), Directive 2010/63/EU of the European Parliament and of the Council of 22 September 2010 norms, referring to the guidelines for accommodation, care and protection of animals used for experimental and other scientific purposes. The implementation of this experiment was approved by the Ethics Committee of the Faculty of Biology, "Alexandru Ioan Cuza" University, Iasi, with the registration number 3936/26/11/2021.

2.3. Ant(Agonists) and Lactic Acid Lacteria Strains

ROT (5 g) was purchased from Toronto Research Chemicals, North York, Canada (# R700580), while VPA (100 g) from Sigma-Aldrich (#SLBC9758V), Saint Louis, MO, USA. LEV (250 mg) + CARB (25 mg) and PROBIO (3 g) that contained six *Lactobacillus* (*casei* W56, *acidophilus* W22, *paracasei* W20, *salivarius* W24, *lactis* W19, and *plantarum* W62) species and three *Bifidobacterium* (*lactis* W51 and W52, and *bifidum* W23) were bought from a local pharmacy. To avoid any conflicts of interest, the brand name of the product was kept under anonymity. ROT (2.5 µg/L) and VPA (0.5 mg/mL) were both dissolved in distilled water, whereas LEV + CARB (250 mg + 25 mg) and PROBIO (3 g) were dissolved and administered before the standard feeding routine for approximately half an hour to ensure the proper ingestion as unique doses using a 100 mL ratted balloon.

Our team [12] and Wang et al. [13] revealed that 2 µg/L over 21–28 days causes mild symptomatology. Thus, we performed some preliminary experiments prior to the actual protocol in which up to 5 zebrafish subjects per tank were exposed to three different doses (from 2 µg/L, 2.5 µg/L, and 5 µg/L) for 24 up to 72 h and concluded that 2.5 µg/L might be optimum, since 5 µg/L led to high mortality (data not shown) despite the existing evidence in the literature indicating a significant locomotor impairment (between 28 and 30 days of exposure) [14–17]. An analogous approach was applied for VPA, where we tested four doses (0.5 mg/mL, 2 mg/mL, 5 mg/mL, and 10 mg/mL). Amounts of 5 mg/mL and 10 mg/mL VPA led to high mortality, while in 2 mg/mL, they exhibited immobility episodes upon touching (data not shown). Based on these considerations, we managed to maintain the survival rate constant among subjects throughout the entire analyzed period.

2.4. Behavioral Testing

After acclimatization for 14 days, zebrafish (n = 5 per group) were randomly divided into eight groups, as follows: Group a was the CONTROL group, while Group b (0.5 mg/mL VPA), Group c (250 mg LEV and 25 mg CARB), Group d (3 g PROBIO), Group e (2.5 µg/L ROT), Group f (2.5 µg/L ROT in combination with 0.5 mg/mL VPA), Group g (2.5 µg/L ROT in combination with 250 mg LEV and 25 mg CARB), and Group h (2.5 µg/L ROT in combination with 3 g PROBIO) were the treated groups. The exposure solution was renewed daily in order to maintain a constant concentration. In addition, during the one-week pre-exposure period, the animals were transferred in vessels similar to the tests performed with the aim to become used to the stress of being caught and transferred as well with the novel configuration for observation. After the experimental accommodation, each experimental group was studied using the 2D and 3D approach over a 4 min period to set the baseline behavior, shown in our study as the initial behavior. No deaths were found in the control and treated groups after chronic exposure to chemicals.

2.4.1. Anti-Social and Aggressivity Behaviors

The anti-social behavior and aggression tests were performed in a multipurpose cross maze closed by a transparent slit of Plexiglas and turned into a T-maze filled with system water (5 cm). We followed the standard protocol by placing the mirror and two social stimuli in the left arm. We focused on the tendency manifested to spend time in the central and right arm concerning the anti-social component and particularly the left arm for aggression. Each subject was left for half a minute for accommodation. The time length of each trial was 4 min per individual. Images were recorded with a professional infrared camera placed above the experimental chamber connected to a computer and analyzed using the software EthoVision XT 11.5, previously calibrated for these tests (Noldus Information Technology, Wageningen, The Netherlands) [12,18].

2.4.2. Cycling Rotation

As already described by members of our group [19] and Kalueff [20], 'tight' cycling rotation but counterclockwise might indicate a high level of anxiety due to abnormal physiological response or selective drugs' action, as in our case. In the counterclockwise rotations, the parameter of interest was analyzed by using the Track3D module of EthoVisionXT 14 video tracking software (Noldus Information Technology, Wageningen, The Netherlands). As above, each subject was left for half a minute to accommodate with the novel tank before starting the trial.

A schematic representation of the present study design can be found below (Figure 1).

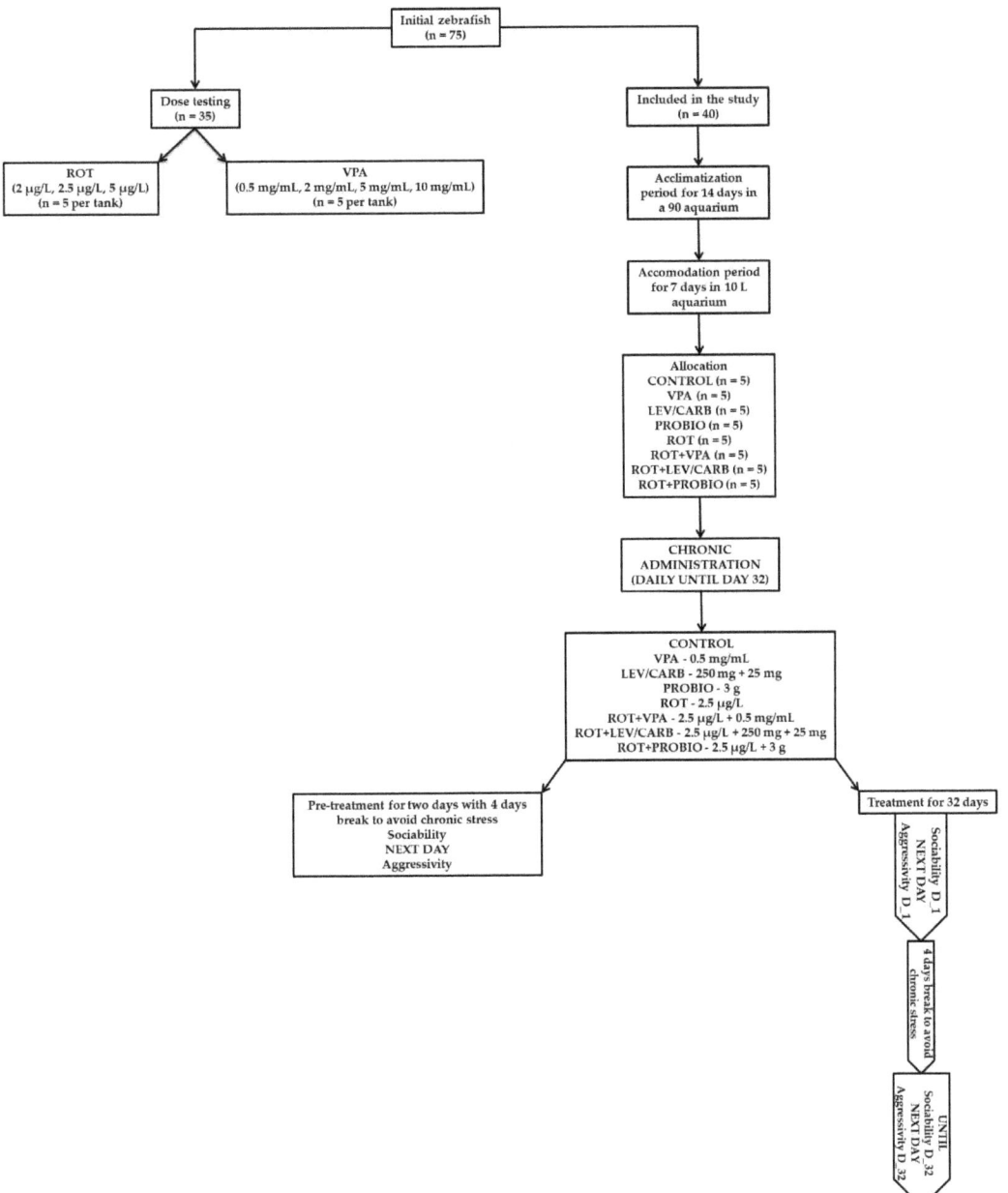

Figure 1. A CONSORT-style flow diagram of the study design.

2.5. Statistical Analyses

The normality and distribution were determined by Shapiro–Wilk test with Graph Pad Prism software (v 9.1.0.221, San Diego, CA, USA). Subsequently, multiple comparisons between the initial behavior and the days of testing within the groups were performed with one-way ANOVA followed by Dunnett's test [21,22]. Trends were generated using OriginPro software (v 9.3-2016, OriginLab Corporation, Northampton, MA, USA).

3. Results

Although fluctuations in behavioral patterns are observable in all eight experimental groups, only in three did we observe a statistically significant difference over 32 days of analysis. We observed an abnormal pattern reflected by their circling tendencies in the (a) CONTROL group (D_24—$p = 0.026$) and (c) LEV/CARB group (D_24—$p = 0.013$) on the same day from a top view. Moreover, a significant difference was observed in the (d) PROBIO group (D_16—$p = 0.022$) from a side view perspective. Additional behavioral impairments in the remaining five groups were not observed ($p > 0.05$). However, in the non-exposed ROT groups (a–d), a constantly increasing pattern of rotation can be observed. In the remaining four groups (e–h) receiving ROT in combination with other agonists, this particular behavior was amplified without a significant difference (Figure 2).

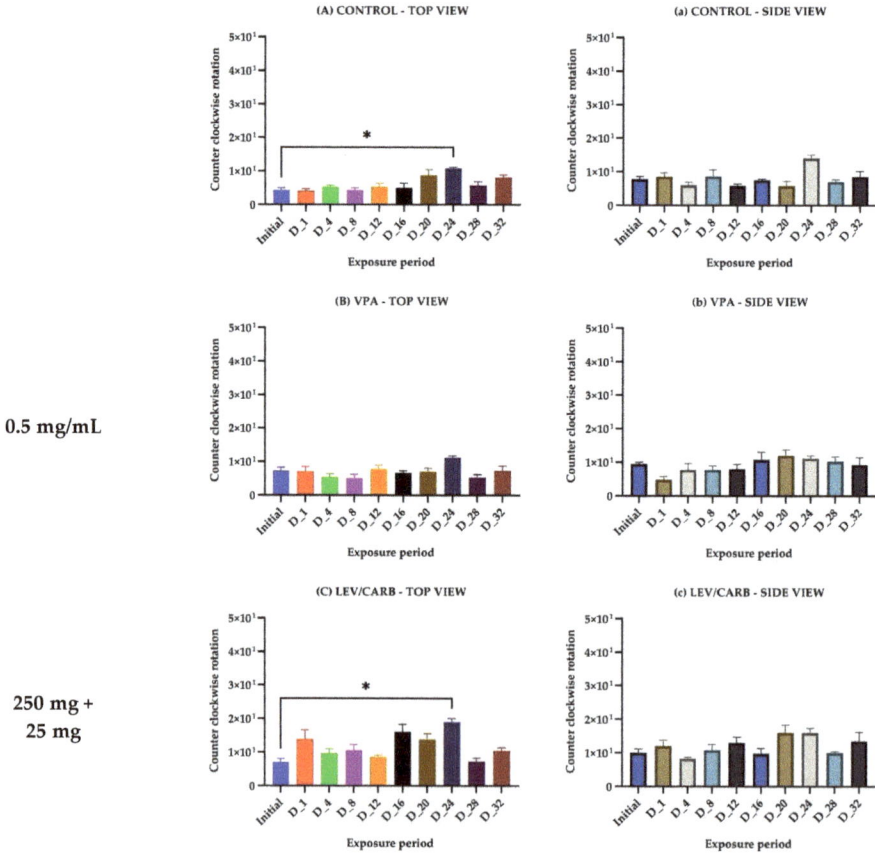

Figure 2. *Cont.*

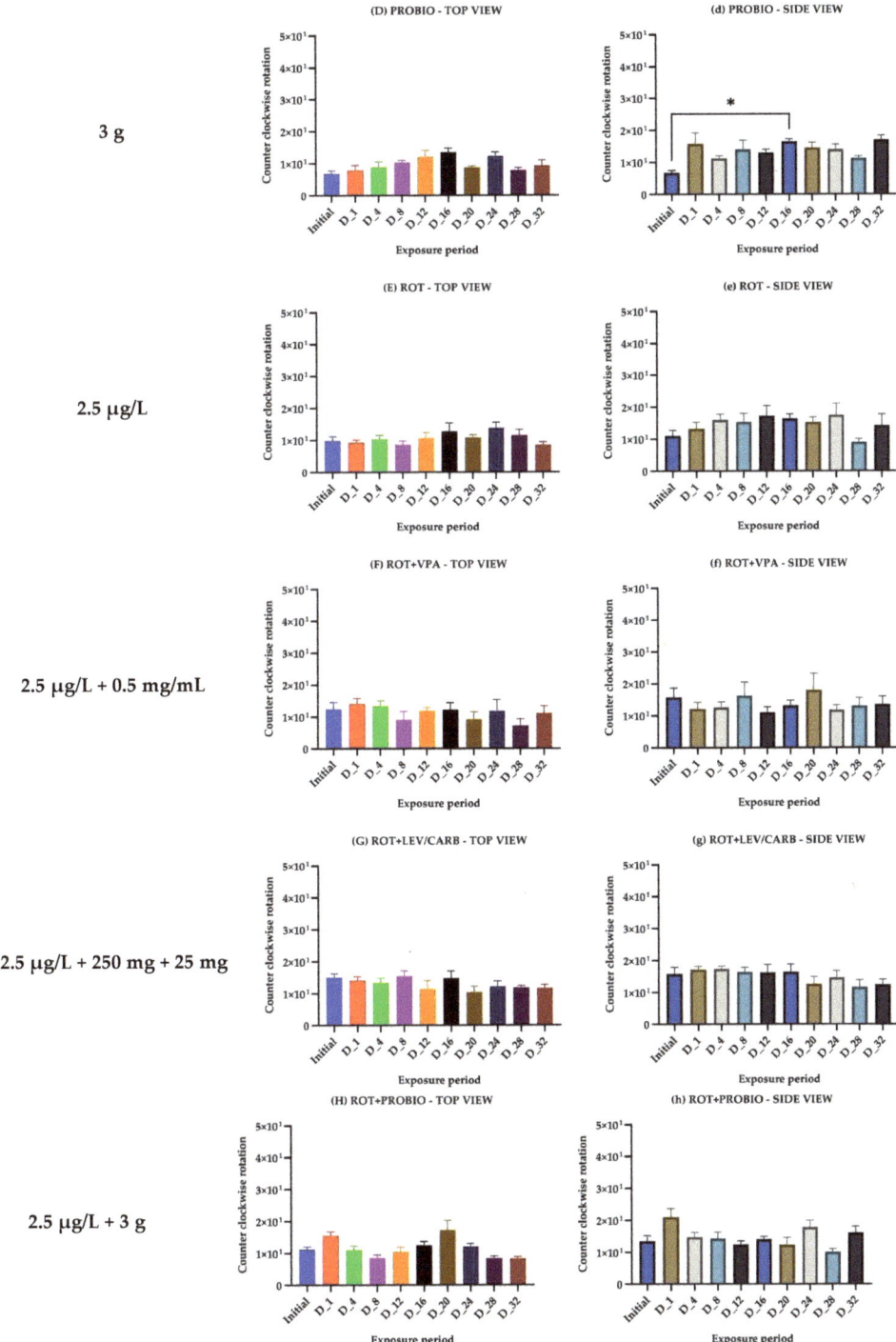

Figure 2. Counterclockwise rotation parameter in *Danio rerio* (n = 5) studied groups (values expressed as mean with SEM followed by Dunnett's test; * $p < 0.05$).

Statistically significant differences were noted on separate days following the centralization and analysis of data on the time spent in the right and the central arm. Thus, group (b) supplemented only with VPA recorded a preference toward the right arm in D_1—$p = 0.006$ and D_8—$p = 0.023$, while group (c) who was given LEV/CARB, only in D_12—$p = 0.008$. Regarding group (e) ROT and group (f) ROT + VPA, zebrafish exhibited anti-social behavior in D_1—$p = 0.002$ and D_4—$p = 0.012$. The exploratory capacity was somewhat influenced, as the behavior corresponded to a state of anxiety in D_4—$p = 0.005$, D_20—$p = 0.002$, D_28—$p = 0.004$, D_32—$p = 0.049$ (b) VPA, and in D_4—$p = 0.029$, D_24—$p = 0.021$, D_28 and D_32—$p < 0.001$ (c) LEV/CARB. As already mentioned in the case of the other arm, the groups exposed to (f) ROT + VPA and (g) ROT + LEV/CARB were the only ones compared to (e) ROT and (h) ROT + PROBIO in which there were visible changes; D_12—$p = 0.041$, D_16—$p = 0.005$ (e) (ROT) and D_8—$p = 0.008$, D_24—$p = 0.034$ (f) ROT + VPA. What is intriguing is the lack of efficacy of lactic acid strains administered in the (d) PROBIO and (h) ROT + PROBIO groups but also in (g) ROT + LEV/CARB ($p > 0.05$). The (a) CONTROL group maintained a linear trend throughout the entire experiment, as in the (d) PROBIO group. Even though in (g) ROT + LEV/CARB and (h) ROT + PROBIO these fluctuations were much more visible, there were still no significant differences when comparing the initial behavior with each day of testing (Figure 3).

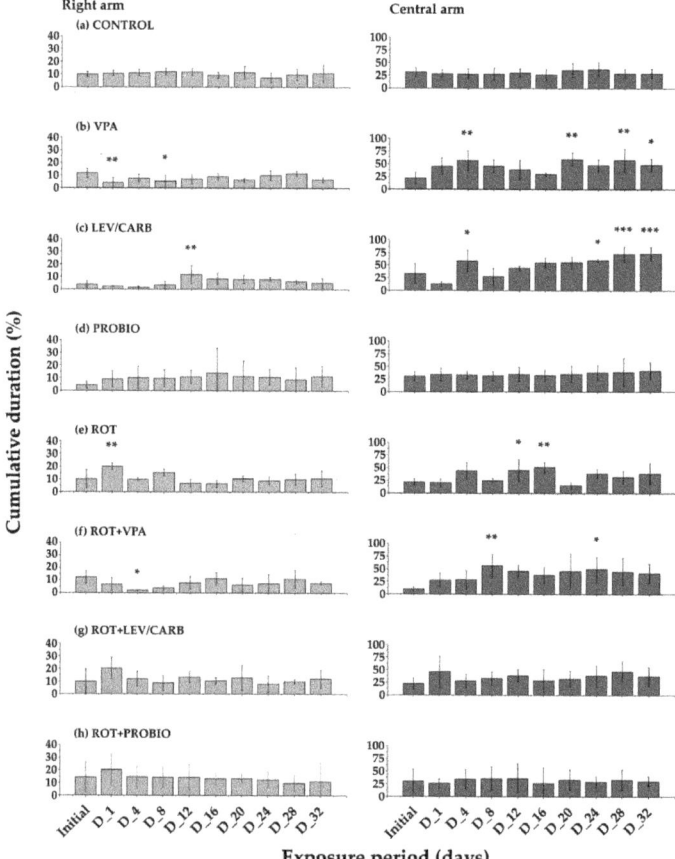

Figure 3. Anti-social pattern in *Danio rerio* (n = 5) studied groups and their tendencies toward both arms (values expressed as mean with SEM followed by Dunnett's test; * $p < 0.05$, ** $p < 0.005$, *** $p < 0.0005$).

Compared to the pre-treatment period, even in the (a) CONTROL group, a deductible phenotype was observed based on the test performed. Interestingly, there was no statistically significant difference ($p > 0.05$) in the baseline behavior and the exposure time to left arm time. Including the right and central arm in (a) CONTROL but also in those that received (b) VPA, (c) LEV/CARB, (d) PROBIO, or in combination with (e–h) ROT, specific patterns of aggressive behavior were recorded ($p < 0.05, 0.005$, and 0.001) either in relation to the initial stage or between different days. However, the lack of significance should be noted in group (d) PROBIO ($p > 0.05$) at the time spent in the left arm but also by comparison with pre-treatment ($p > 0.05$) in the other two arms. It can be concluded that the PROBIO administered did indeed have a beneficial effect, an argument, which is not valid in the case of group (h) ROT + PROBIO (Figure 4).

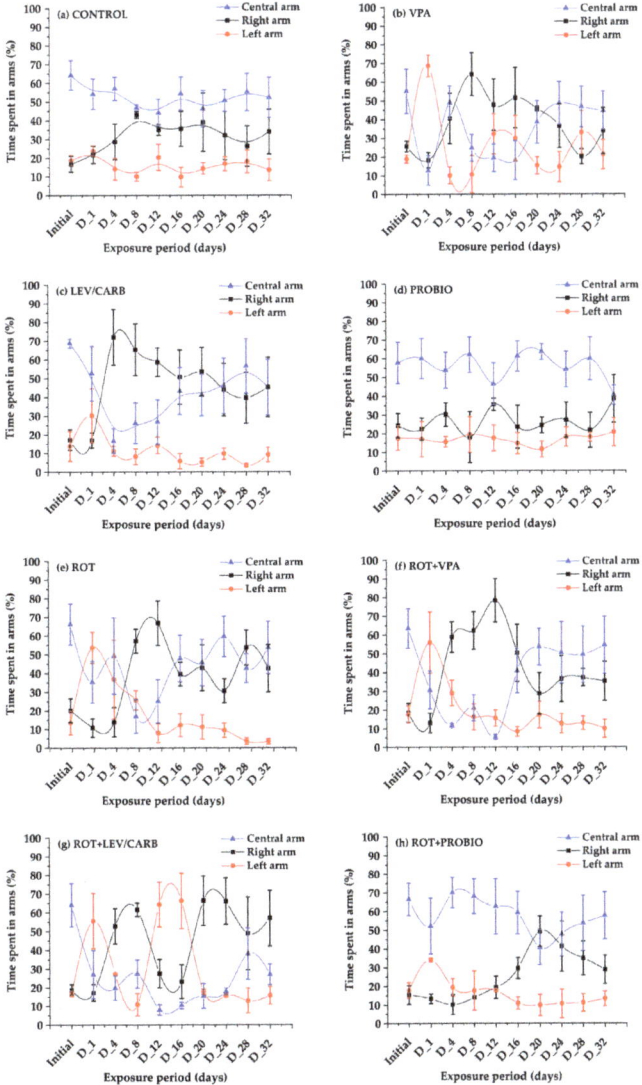

Figure 4. Aggressive-like patterns in *Danio rerio* (n = 5) studied groups and their tendencies toward all three arms (values expressed as mean with SEM followed by Dunnett's test).

4. Discussion

Zebrafish (*Danio rerio*) materialized as an optimal model to study a plethora of diseases [23]. It even outperformed rodent models, since their wide repertoire comprised normal and abnormal behaviors [24,25]. The social behavior might be attributed to their nature, living in shoals, being intrinsically collective creatures. They also portray well-documented expressions of fear and anxiety, and they can learn complex associations [26].

There are extensive data in the current literature describing the dose-time-dependent variable in inducing a PD-related phenotype in *Danio rerio*. Most of these studies, however, reflected the total distance swam, velocity, and freezing episodes reunited under the locomotion impairment umbrella rather than the social and aggressive components. Exposure to 2 µg/L ROT cause non-motor to mild symptoms [12,13], whereas 5 µg/L [14–17] up to 2 mg/L [27,28] might lead to excessive mortality, as in our case (unpublished data), or sufficient to induce a targeted phenotype.

VPA is nowadays an excellent stimulus for triggering symptoms that resembles autism spectrum disorder (ASD), demonstrating an inhibitory role following ROT exposure in rodents [29,30]. LEV/CARB are known to be dopaminergic agonists that, once ingested, cross the BBB in order to release dopamine, but in zebrafish, it seems to alleviate the cortisol level through the hypothalamic–pituitary–adrenal axis (HPA) [31]. Lastly, PROBIO proved to be the most powerful vehicle in restoring dysbacteriosis in fish, rodents, and humans [32].

Contrary to what we expected regarding the avoidance of chronic stress, we still observed a peculiar phenotype in the (a) CONTROL group and (c) LEV/CARB on the same day ($p < 0.05$). There was another instance when we noted a significant difference in behavior by comparison with the initial reference ($p < 0.05$) in the (d) PROBIO group. Notable phenotypical changes were absent in the counterclockwise rotation parameter in the groups exposed to ROT alone or a mixture, but relevant evidence occurred following the examination of anti-social behavior (Figure 2).

Groups (a) CONTROL, (d) PROBIO, (g) ROT + LEV/CARB, and (h) ROT + PROBIO did not register significant abnormal oscillations in behavior. Groups (b) VPA, (c) LEV/CARB, (e) ROT, and (f) ROT + VPA exhibited the most pronounced atypical behaviors with the most time spent in all three arms ($p < 0.05, 0.005, 0.0005$) (Figure 3). Afterward, we moved to evaluate the aggressivity level. The (a) CONTROL and (d) PROBIO groups exhibited a less pronounced level of aggressivity, comparable with the fluctuations displayed by the (b) VPA, (c) LEV/CARB, (e) ROT, (f) ROT + VPA, (g) ROT + LEV/CARB and (h) ROT + PROBIO groups ($p < 0.05, 0.005, 0.001$) (Figure 4).

It is noteworthy that we were not able to identify other teams whose purpose was to evaluate the harmful effect of ROT administration on the social and aggressive components. Considering that VPA is well known to induce symptoms that resemble the ASD, it was demonstrated on three distinct occasions that VPA may promote anxiety and hyperactivity, depending on the dose and exposure period.

Robea et al. [33] recently conducted a study on larvae zebrafish 6 days post-fertilization (dpf), aiming to expose them to 48 µM VPA for 24, 48, and 72 h. The group exposed to VPA for 72 h spent most of the time next to the mirror. There is also some controversy regarding this topic because Zimmermann et al. [34] contradict these findings, also using 48 µM. VPA influences the social component, anxiety, and locomotion rather than aggressive behavior. We highlighted the absence of any indicator pointing to a neurological disruption. This state was complementary to social behavior but correlated with high aggression. Liu et al. [35] brought solid evidence concerning how 20/100 µM VPA 7 h for 6 consecutive days caused social preference deficits in 24 h pf larvae, whereas acute exposure impaired locomotor activity. Neither intervention changed the behavioral response to light nor anxiety, considering that chronic exposure did not alter the locomotor activity.

There have been limited attempts to test LEV/CARB as triggers of aggressivity. Tan et al. [36] conducted a randomized controlled trial (RCT) in children diagnosed with Angelman Syndrome (AS) prophylactically treated with LEV. Per questionnaires applied and following the administration of 10 up to 15 mg/kg/day LEV, the cumulative data refute this possibility. However, an increase in dopamine (DA) level might exacerbate AS symptoms in a mouse model according to Riday et al. [37].

One possible explanation for the associated changes in human mood resides within the side effects. More specifically, the abrupt withdrawal or dose reduction in LEV increases the risk of neuroleptic malignant syndrome (NMS). NMS is also known as parkinsonism hyperpyrexia syndrome, which covers abnormal body temperature disturbance, spontaneous actions, and muscle rigidity. Patients might develop a dependence on LEV, which further explains the aggressive behavior [38].

Kutcher et al. [39] report marked interchanges, particularly in the aggressive-like reactions and submissive postures in LEV/CARB-exposed rats at 300 mg/kg subjected to intermittent semi-compulsory alcoholization and the joint kinetics of LEV/CARB. One method targeting the antioxidant balance stands in the use of antioxidants in L-DOPA mice as suggested by Hira et al. [40].

A regime based on lactic acid bacteria proved to promote improvements in the overall condition, but the interest congruent with our aim is lacking. Even though *Bifidobacterium longum* BB536 and *Lactobacillus rhamnosus* did not play a major role in the sociability of zebrafish exposed to 2 μg/L for 21 days [12], *Lactobacillus plantarum* and *rhamnosus* CECT8361/IMC 501 and *Bifidobacterium longum* CECT7347 are sufficient to alleviate anxiety-related behavior in larvae and adults [41–43].

5. Conclusions

In our studied animals, we observed an association in behavior in animals supplemented with ROT alone or a mixture and possible agonists. In this manuscript, the predetermined doses administered in zebrafish (*Danio rerio*) for 32 days were enough to cause social deficits coupled with elevated moods of aggression. PROBIO exerted a beneficial effect on both analyzed parameters, diminishing aggressive-like symptoms. There were also circumstances where (a) CONTROL also manifested an impaired behavior but comparably attenuated by comparison with the remaining experimental groups. Due to the scarcity of data in the current literature and without knowing what the outcome might be, we are limited to behavioral studies that could constitute the first phase of a possible branch of research, also based on the reliance on multiple animals. We consider this manuscript to be the first launching pad for analyses that aim to elucidate both aggressive and social-related dysfunctionalities, even translated to clinical practice for PD patients. As can be concluded, this approach benefits from substantial potential, since immunohistochemistry coupled with analyses showing neuroinflammation and subsequent impairment of the enzymes responsible for the antioxidant status could offer further insight.

Author Contributions: O.-D.I., R.D. (Raluca Duta), R.J. and I.-B.N.: Conceptualization, data curation, investigation, formal analysis, writing—original draft; M.N., C.F., A.C., R.D. (Romeo Dobrin), I.M. and B.D.: Conceptualization, methodology, supervision, validation, project administration, writing—review and editing. All authors have read and agreed to the published version of the manuscript.

Funding: This research received no external funding.

Institutional Review Board Statement: Not applicable.

Informed Consent Statement: Not applicable.

Data Availability Statement: The datasets used and analyzed in this study are available from the corresponding author on reasonable request.

Acknowledgments: Not applicable.

Conflicts of Interest: The authors declare no conflict of interest.

References

1. Robea, M.-A.; Balmus, I.-M.; Ciobica, A.; Strungaru, S.; Plavan, G.; Gorgan, L.D.; Savuca, A.; Nicoara, M. Parkinson's Disease-Induced Zebrafish Models: Focussing on Oxidative Stress Implications and Sleep Processes. *Oxid. Med. Cell. Longev.* **2020**, *2020*, 1370837. [CrossRef] [PubMed]
2. Sherer, T.B.; Betarbet, R.; Testa, C.M.; Seo, B.B.; Richardson, J.R.; Kim, J.H.; Miller, G.W.; Yagi, T.; Matsuno-Yagi, A.; Greenamyre, J.T. Mechanism of toxicity in rotenone models of Parkinson's disease. *J. Neurosci.* **2003**, *23*, 10756. [CrossRef] [PubMed]
3. Bové, J.; Prou, D.; Perier, C.; Przedborski, S. Toxin-induced models of Parkinson's disease. *NeuroRX* **2005**, *2*, 484–494. [CrossRef]
4. Lawana, V.; Cannon, J.R. Chapter Five—Rotenone neurotoxicity: Relevance to Parkinson's disease. In *Neurotoxicity of Pesticides*; Aschner, M., Costa, L.G., Eds.; Academic Press: Cambridge, MA, USA, 2020; Volume 4, pp. 209–254, ISBN 2468-7480.
5. Gupta, R.C. (Ed.) *Chapter 52—Rotenone*; Academic Press: Boston, MA, USA, 2012; pp. 620–623, ISBN 978-0-12-385926-6.
6. Gupta, R.C. *Veterinary Toxicology: Basic and Clinical Principles*; Elsevier: New York, NY, USA; Academic Press: London, UK, 2007; ISBN 9780123704672.
7. Bastías-Candia, S.; Zolezzi, J.M.; Inestrosa, N.C. Revisiting the Paraquat-Induced Sporadic Parkinson's Disease-Like Model. *Mol. Neurobiol.* **2019**, *56*, 1044–1055. [CrossRef]
8. Yurtsever, İ.; Üstündağ, Ü.V.; Ünal, İ.; Ateş, P.S.; Emekli-Alturfan, E. Rifampicin decreases neuroinflammation to maintain mitochondrial function and calcium homeostasis in rotenone-treated zebrafish. *Drug Chem. Toxicol.* **2020**, *45*, 1–8. [CrossRef]
9. Gao, F.; Chen, D.; Hu, Q.; Wang, G. Rotenone Directly Induces BV2 Cell Activation via the p38 MAPK Pathway. *PLoS ONE* **2013**, *8*, e72046.
10. Hijaz, B.A.; Volpicelli-Daley, L.A. Initiation and propagation of α-synuclein aggregation in the nervous system. *Mol. Neurodegener.* **2020**, *15*, 19. [CrossRef] [PubMed]
11. Reed, B.; Jennings, M. *Guidance on the Housing and Care of Zebrafish Danio rerio*; RSPCA: Horsham, UK, 2011.
12. Ilie, O.-D.; Paduraru, E.; Robea, M.-A.; Balmus, I.-M.; Jijie, R.; Nicoara, M.; Ciobica, A.; Nita, I.-B.; Dobrin, R.; Doroftei, B. The Possible Role of *Bifidobacterium longum* BB536 and *Lactobacillus rhamnosus* HN001 on Locomotor Activity and Oxidative Stress in a Rotenone-Induced Zebrafish Model of Parkinson's Disease. *Oxid. Med. Cell. Longev.* **2021**, *2021*, 9629102. [CrossRef]
13. Wang, Y.; Liu, W.; Yang, J.; Wang, F.; Sima, Y.; Zhong, Z.; Wang, H.; Hu, L.-F.; Liu, C.-F. Parkinson's disease-like motor and non-motor symptoms in rotenone-treated zebrafish. *Neurotoxicology* **2017**, *58*, 103–109. [CrossRef]
14. Khotimah, H.; Ali, M.; Sumitro, S.B.; Widodo, M.A. Decreasing α-synuclein aggregation by methanolic extract of Centella asiatica in zebrafish Parkinson's model. *Asian Pac. J. Trop. Biomed.* **2015**, *5*, 948–954. [CrossRef]
15. Ünal, İ.; Çalışkan-Ak, E.; Üstündağ, Ü.V.; Ateş, P.S.; Alturfan, A.A.; Altinoz, M.A.; Elmaci, I.; Emekli-Alturfan, E. Neuroprotective effects of mitoquinone and oleandrin on Parkinson's disease model in zebrafish. *Int. J. Neurosci.* **2020**, *130*, 574–582. [CrossRef] [PubMed]
16. Khotimah, H.; Sumitro, S.; Widodo, M. Zebrafish Parkinson's model: Rotenone decrease motility, dopamine, and increase α-synuclein aggregation and apoptosis of zebrafish brain. *Int. J. Pharm. Tech. Res.* **2015**, *8*, 614–621.
17. Cansız, D.; Ünal, İ.; Üstündağ, Ü.V.; Alturfan, A.A.; Altinoz, M.A.; Elmacı, İ.; Emekli-Alturfan, E. Caprylic acid ameliorates rotenone induced inflammation and oxidative stress in the gut-brain axis in Zebrafish. *Mol. Biol. Rep.* **2021**, *48*, 5259–5273. [CrossRef] [PubMed]
18. Strungaru, S.-A.; Robea, M.A.; Plavan, G.; Todirascu-Ciornea, E.; Ciobica, A.; Nicoara, M. Acute exposure to methylmercury chloride induces fast changes in swimming performance, cognitive processes and oxidative stress of zebrafish (*Danio rerio*) as reference model for fish community. *J. Trace Elem. Med. Biol.* **2018**, *47*, 115–123. [CrossRef]
19. Strungaru, S.-A.; Plavan, G.; Ciobica, A.; Nicoara, M.; Robea, M.A.; Solcan, C.; Petrovici, A. Toxicity and chronic effects of deltamethrin exposure on zebrafish (*Danio rerio*) as a reference model for freshwater fish community. *Ecotoxicol. Environ. Saf.* **2019**, *171*, 854–862. [CrossRef]
20. Kalueff, A.V. (Ed.) *Illustrated Zebrafish Neurobehavioral Glossary BT—The Rights and Wrongs of Zebrafish: Behavioral Phenotyping of Zebrafish*; Springer International Publishing: Cham, Switzerland, 2017; pp. 291–317, ISBN 978-3-319-33774-6.
21. Jijie, R.; Solcan, G.; Nicoara, M.; Micu, D.; Strungaru, S.-A. Antagonistic effects in zebrafish (*Danio rerio*) behavior and oxidative stress induced by toxic metals and deltamethrin acute exposure. *Sci. Total Environ.* **2020**, *698*, 134299. [CrossRef]
22. Paduraru, E.; Flocea, E.-I.; Lazado, C.C.; Simionov, I.-A.; Nicoara, M.; Ciobica, A.; Faggio, C.; Jijie, R. Vitamin C Mitigates Oxidative Stress and Behavioral Impairments Induced by Deltamethrin and Lead Toxicity in Zebrafish. *Int. J. Mol. Sci.* **2021**, *22*, 12714. [CrossRef]
23. Jijie, R.; Mihalache, G.; Balmus, I.-M.; Strungaru, S.-A.; Baltag, E.S.; Ciobica, A.; Nicoara, M.; Faggio, C. Zebrafish as a Screening Model to Study the Single and Joint Effects of Antibiotics. *Pharmaceuticals* **2021**, *14*, 578. [CrossRef]
24. Kalueff, A.V.; Gebhardt, M.; Stewart, A.M.; Cachat, J.M.; Brimmer, M.; Chawla, J.S.; Craddock, C.; Kyzar, E.J.; Roth, A.; Landsman, S.; et al. Towards a Comprehensive Catalog of Zebrafish Behavior 1.0 and Beyond. *Zebrafish* **2013**, *10*, 70–86. [CrossRef]
25. Faria, M.; Prats, E.; Rosas Ramírez, J.R.; Bellot, M.; Bedrossiantz, J.; Pagano, M.; Valls, A.; Gomez-Canela, C.; Porta, J.M.; Mestres, J.; et al. Androgenic activation, impairment of the monoaminergic system and altered behavior in zebrafish larvae exposed to environmental concentrations of fenitrothion. *Sci. Total Environ.* **2021**, *775*, 145671. [CrossRef] [PubMed]
26. Lieschke, G.J.; Currie, P.D. Animal models of human disease: Zebrafish swim into view. *Nat. Rev. Genet.* **2007**, *8*, 353–367. [CrossRef] [PubMed]

27. Ünal, İ.; Üstündağ, Ü.V.; Ateş, P.S.; Eğilmezer, G.; Alturfan, A.A.; Yiğitbaşı, T.; Emekli-Alturfan, E. Rotenone impairs oxidant/antioxidant balance both in brain and intestines in zebrafish. *Int. J. Neurosci.* **2019**, *129*, 363–368. [CrossRef] [PubMed]
28. Lv, D.; Li, L.; Chen, J.; Wei, S.-Z.; Wang, F.; Hu, H.; Xie, A.-M.; Liu, C.-F. Sleep deprivation caused a memory defects and emotional changes in a rotenone-based zebrafish model of Parkinson's disease. *Behav. Brain Res.* **2019**, *372*, 112031. [CrossRef] [PubMed]
29. Carriere, C.H.; Kang, N.H.; Niles, L.P. Neuroprotection by valproic acid in an intrastriatal rotenone model of Parkinson's disease. *Neuroscience* **2014**, *267*, 114–121. [CrossRef]
30. Monti, B.; Gatta, V.; Piretti, F.; Raffaelli, S.S.; Virgili, M.; Contestabile, A. Valproic Acid is Neuroprotective in the Rotenone Rat Model of Parkinson's Disease: Involvement of α-Synuclein. *Neurotox. Res.* **2010**, *17*, 130–141. [CrossRef]
31. Idalencio, R.; Lopes, T.M.; Soares, S.M.; Pompermaier, A.; de Alcantara Barcellos, H.H.; Kalichak, F.; Fagundes, M.; de Oliveira, C.M.; Barcellos, L.J.G. Effect of levodopa/carbidopa on stress response in zebrafish. *J. Comp. Physiol. A* **2021**, *207*, 393–399. [CrossRef]
32. Tan, A.H.; Hor, J.W.; Chong, C.W.; Lim, S.-Y. Probiotics for Parkinson's disease: Current evidence and future directions. *JGH Open* **2021**, *5*, 414–419. [CrossRef]
33. Robea, M.A.; Ciobica, A.; Curpan, A.-S.; Plavan, G.; Strungaru, S.; Lefter, R.; Nicoara, M. Preliminary Results Regarding Sleep in a Zebrafish Model of Autism Spectrum Disorder. *Brain Sci.* **2021**, *11*, 556. [CrossRef]
34. Zimmermann, F.F.; Gaspary, K.V.; Leite, C.E.; De Paula Cognato, G.; Bonan, C.D. Embryological exposure to valproic acid induces social interaction deficits in zebrafish (*Danio rerio*): A developmental behavior analysis. *Neurotoxicol. Teratol.* **2015**, *52*, 36–41. [CrossRef]
35. Liu, X.; Zhang, Y.; Lin, J.; Xia, Q.; Guo, N.; Li, Q. Social Preference Deficits in Juvenile Zebrafish Induced by Early Chronic Exposure to Sodium Valproate. *Front. Behav. Neurosci.* **2016**, *10*, 201. [CrossRef] [PubMed]
36. Tan, W.-H.; Bird, L.M.; Sadhwani, A.; Barbieri-Welge, R.L.; Skinner, S.A.; Horowitz, L.T.; Bacino, C.A.; Noll, L.M.; Fu, C.; Hundley, R.J.; et al. A randomized controlled trial of levodopa in patients with Angelman syndrome. *Am. J. Med. Genet. A* **2018**, *176*, 1099–1107. [CrossRef] [PubMed]
37. Riday, T.T.; Dankoski, E.C.; Krouse, M.C.; Fish, E.W.; Walsh, P.L.; Han, J.E.; Hodge, C.W.; Wightman, R.M.; Philpot, B.D.; Malanga, C.J. Pathway-specific dopaminergic deficits in a mouse model of Angelman syndrome. *J. Clin. Investig.* **2012**, *122*, 4544–4554. [CrossRef]
38. Newman, E.J.; Grosset, D.G.; Kennedy, P.G.E. The Parkinsonism-Hyperpyrexia Syndrome. *Neurocrit. Care* **2009**, *10*, 136–140. [CrossRef]
39. Kutcher, E.O.; Egorov, A.Y.; Chernikova, N.A.; Filatova, E.V. Long-Term Ethanol Alcoholization Decreases Levodopa-Induced Aggressive Behavior in Rats. *J. Evol. Biochem. Physiol.* **2018**, *54*, 216–220. [CrossRef]
40. Hira, S.; Saleem, U.; Anwar, F.; Ahmad, B. Antioxidants Attenuate Isolation- and L-DOPA-Induced Aggression in Mice. *Front. Pharmacol.* **2018**, *8*, 945. [CrossRef]
41. Valcarce, D.G.; Martínez-Vázquez, J.M.; Riesco, M.F.; Robles, V. Probiotics reduce anxiety-related behavior in zebrafish. *Heliyon* **2020**, *6*, e03973. [CrossRef] [PubMed]
42. Borrelli, L.; Aceto, S.; Agnisola, C.; De Paolo, S.; Dipineto, L.; Stilling, R.M.; Dinan, T.G.; Cryan, J.F.; Menna, L.F.; Fioretti, A. Probiotic modulation of the microbiota-gut-brain axis and behaviour in zebrafish. *Sci. Rep.* **2016**, *6*, 30046. [CrossRef] [PubMed]
43. Davis, D.J.; Bryda, E.C.; Gillespie, C.H.; Ericsson, A.C. Microbial modulation of behavior and stress responses in zebrafish larvae. *Behav. Brain Res.* **2016**, *311*, 219–227. [CrossRef]

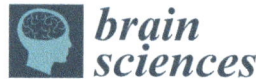 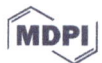

Article

Opicapone Improves Global Non-Motor Symptoms Burden in Parkinson's Disease: An Open-Label Prospective Study

Diego Santos García [1,2,*], Gustavo Fernández Pajarín [3], Juan Manuel Oropesa-Ruiz [4], Francisco Escamilla Sevilla [5], Raúl Rashid Abdul Rahim López [6] and José Guillermo Muñoz Enríquez [7]

1. CHUAC (Complejo Hospitalario Universitario de A Coruña), 15006 A Coruña, Spain
2. Hospital San Rafael, 15009 A Coruña, Spain
3. CHUS (Complejo Hospitalario Universitario de Santiago), Santiago de Compostela, 15706 A Coruña, Spain; gferpaj@gmail.com
4. Memory Unit, Hospital Universitario Juan Ramón Jiménez, 21005 Huelva, Spain; juaororui@gmail.com
5. Unidad de Trastornos del Movimiento, Servicio de Neurología, Hospital Universitario Virgen de las Nieves, Instituto de Investigación Biosanitaria (ibs.Granada), 18013 Granada, Spain; fescamilla@hotmail.com
6. Neurology Department, Puerta del Mar University Hospital, 11009 Cádiz, Spain; raulrashidlo@gmail.com
7. Complejo Público Asistencial de Zamora, 49022 Zamora, Spain; jgmeaadh6@hotmail.com
* Correspondence: diegosangar@yahoo.es; Tel.: +34-646173341

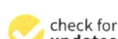

Citation: Santos García, D.; Fernández Pajarín, G.; Oropesa-Ruiz, J.M.; Escamilla Sevilla, F.; Rahim López, R.R.A.; Muñoz Enríquez, J.G. Opicapone Improves Global Non-Motor Symptoms Burden in Parkinson's Disease: An Open-Label Prospective Study. *Brain Sci.* 2022, 12, 383. https://doi.org/10.3390/brainsci12030383

Academic Editors: Patricia Martinez-Sanchez and Francisco Nieto-Escamez

Received: 16 February 2022
Accepted: 10 March 2022
Published: 12 March 2022

Publisher's Note: MDPI stays neutral with regard to jurisdictional claims in published maps and institutional affiliations.

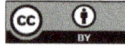

Copyright: © 2022 by the authors. Licensee MDPI, Basel, Switzerland. This article is an open access article distributed under the terms and conditions of the Creative Commons Attribution (CC BY) license (https://creativecommons.org/licenses/by/4.0/).

Abstract: Patients with Parkinson's disease (PD) can improve some non-motor symptoms (NMS) after starting treatment with opicapone. The aim of this study was to analyze the effectiveness of opicapone on global NMS burden in PD. OPEN-PD (Opicapone Effectiveness on Non-motor symptoms in Parkinson's Disease) is a prospective open-label single-arm study conducted in 5 centers from Spain. The primary efficacy outcome was the change from baseline (V0) to the end of the observational period (6 months ± 30 days) (V2) in the Non-Motor Symptoms Scale (NMSS) total score. Different scales were used for analyzing the change in motor, NMS, quality of life (QoL), and disability. Thirty-three patients were included between JUL/2019 and JUN/2021 (age 63.3 ± 7.91; 60.6% males; 7.48 ± 4.22 years from symptoms onset). At 6 months, 30 patients completed the follow-up (90.9%). The NMSS total score was reduced by 27.3% (from 71.67 ± 37.12 at V0 to 52.1 ± 34.76 at V2; Cohen's effect size = −0.97; $p = 0.002$). By domains, improvement was observed in sleep/fatigue (−40.1%; $p < 0.0001$), mood/apathy (−46.6%; $p = 0.001$), gastrointestinal symptoms (−20.7%; $p = 0.029$), and miscellaneous (−44.94%; $p = 0.021$). QoL also improved with a 18.4% reduction in the 39-item Parkinson's Disease Quality of Life Questionnaire Summary Index (from 26.67 ± 17.61 at V0 to 21.75 ± 14.9 at V2; $p = 0.001$). A total of 13 adverse events in 11 patients (33.3%) were reported, 1 of which was severe (not related to opicapone). Dyskinesias and nausea were the most frequent (6.1%). Opicapone is well tolerated and improves global NMS burden and QoL in PD patients at 6 months.

Keywords: effectiveness; non-motor symptoms; open-label study; opicapone; Parkinson's disease

1. Introduction

Parkinson's disease (PD), the second most common neurodegenerative disease after Alzheimer's disease, is a progressive neurodegenerative disorder causing motor and non-motor symptoms (NMS) that result in disability, loss of patient autonomy and caregiver burden [1]. The understanding of PD has changed over recent years, with the disease currently considered to be a neurodegenerative disorder involving a diversity of pathways and neurotransmitters that may explain, in part, the wide range of NMS that patients may have such as depression, anxiety, pain, cognitive impairment, apathy, gastrointestinal, urinary or cardiovascular symptoms, fatigue, or sleep problems [2,3]. NMS are frequent, disabling, and impact negatively on the quality of life (QoL) of PD patients [4], and strategies designed to improve NMS are necessary [5]. In clinical practice, the identification of NMS by the neurologist is very important, as well as knowing how they affect the patient.

The NMS burden can be high even in the early stages of PD and impact patients' QoL [6]. Moreover, NMS burden progresses over time in PD [7] and, very importantly, it is strongly correlated to motor complications [8]. In this context, a decrease of daily OFF episodes could help to improve some NMS in PD patients and a drug with an only dopaminergic effect (e.g., COMT inhibitor) could improve NMS [9–11] or hypothetically even the global NMS burden in PD patients [8].

Opicapone is a novel, long-acting, peripherally selective, once-daily, third generation COMT inhibitor [12]. Up to 32 trials have been conducted on opicapone use (with >900 subjects exposed to opicapone) [13]. In two Phase III clinical trials, opicapone 50 mg demonstrated to be superior to placebos in OFF-time reduction without increasing ON-time with troublesome dyskinesias in PD patients with moderate end-of-dose motor fluctuations [14,15]. Opicapone at doses of 5–50 mg/day has been found to be safe and well tolerated. The most common reported adverse effect was dyskinesia (16–21%) [14–17]. Regarding NMS, the effect of opicapone over them is not clear. The efficacy of opicapone on NMS was explored analyzing the data of the Non-Motor Symptoms Scale (NMSS) in PD patients who were included in the BIPARK II study, both in the double-blind and open-label phases [12,18]. At the end the double-blind phase, the NMSS total score slightly improved for both opicapone and placebo groups without significant differences between them. Numerical differences in favor of opicapone was seen for the sleep/fatigue domain. At the end of the open-label phase, a mean improvement of −4.2 points in the NMSS total score was still observed, and no worsening of any particular domain was detected [18]. More recently, a significant mean reduction of 6.8 ± 19.7 points ($p < 0.0001$) in the NMSS in 393 out of 495 PD patients treated with opicapone was observed at 3 months in a prospective, open-label, single-arm trial conducted in Germany and the United Kingdom under clinical practice conditions (OPTIPARK study) [11].

The aim of the present prospective open-label single-arm study (**OPEN-PD**, **Op**icapone **E**ffectiveness on **N**on-motor symptoms in **P**arkinson's **D**isease) was to analyze the effectiveness of opicapone on global NMS burden (defined as the NMSS total score) in PD patients. Secondary objectives were to analyze the effectiveness of opicapone on the NMS burden of each domain of the NMSS, and also specifically on sleep, apathy, pain, health-related QoL, and autonomy for activities of daily living (ADL).

2. Material and Methods

OPEN-PD, Opicapone Effectiveness on Non-motor symptoms in Parkinson's Disease, is a multicenter, observational (phase IV), prospective, open-label, follow-up study conducted in 5 centers from Spain. A total of 40 PD patients were expected to be included in the study. Inclusion criteria were: (1) diagnosis of PD according to the United Kingdom Parkinson's Disease Society Brain Bank criteria [19]; (2) to be under levodopa therapy and have indication for receiving opicapone according to the neurologist criteria in his/her clinical practice; (3) NMSS total score at baseline > 40; (4) age > 30 years old; (5) voluntary participation and signed informed consent form. Exclusion criteria were: (1) to be taking opicapone at the inclusion evaluation moment or to have been taking opicapone before; (2) to be under other COMT inhibitor therapy (entacapone or tolcapone) at the inclusion evaluation moment or to have received it in the previous month; (3) any contraindication to be treated with opicapone according to product data; (4) incapacity to complete the questionnaires adequately; (5) other disabling concomitant neurological disease (stroke, severe head trauma, neurodegenerative disease, etc.); (6) other severe and disabling concomitant non-neurological disease (oncological, autoimmune, etc.); (7) expected impossibility of long-term follow-up; (8) to be participating in a clinical trial and/or other type of study. All the neurologists who participated in the study of each center were experts on PD/movement disorders.

The study visits included (1) V0 (baseline); (2) V1 (2 months ± 14 days); and (3) V2 (6 months ± 30 days, end of the Observational Period). At baseline (V0), subjects completed an assessment that included motor symptoms (Hoehn and Yahr [H&Y] [20];

Unified Parkinson's Disease Rating Scale [UPDRS] part III and part IV [21]; Freezing of Gait Questionnaire [FOGQ] [22]), NMS (NMSS [23]; Parkinson's Disease Sleep Scale [PDSS] [24]; Apathy Scale (AS) [25]; King's Parkinson's Disease Pain Scale (KPPS) [26]; VAS-PAIN [27]), disability (Schwab & England Activities of Daily Living Scale [ADLS] [28]), and health related QoL (the 39-item Parkinson's Disease Questionnaire [PDQ-39] [29]). The same assessment was performed at V1 and V2 except for H&Y and UPDRS-III (only at baseline). Moreover, Patient Global Impression of Change (PGIC) [30] was conducted at V1 and V2. Information on sociodemographic aspects, factors related to PD, comorbidity, and treatment was collected.

The primary objective was to analyze the effectiveness of opicapone on global NMS burden (defined as the NMSS total score) at V2 (6 months ± 30 days). The NMSS includes 30 items, each with a different non-motor symptom. The symptoms refer to the 4 weeks prior to assessment. The total score for each item is the result of multiplying the frequency (0, never; 1, rarely; 2, often; 3, frequent; 4, very often) x severity (1, mild; 2, moderate; 3, severe) and will vary from 0 to 12 points. The scale score ranges from 0 to 360 points. The items are grouped into 9 different domains: (1) Cardiovascular (items 1 and 2; score, 0 to 24); (2) Sleep/fatigue (items 3, 4, 5 and 6; score, 0 to 48); (3) Mood/apathy (items 7, 8, 9, 10, 11 and 12; score, 0 to 72); (4) Perceptual problems/hallucinations (items 13, 14 and 15; score, 0 to 36); (5) Attention/memory (items 16, 17 and 18; score, 0 to 36); (6) Gastrointestinal symptoms (items 19, 20 and 21; score 0 to 36); (7) Urinary symptoms (items 22, 23 and 24; score, 0 to 36); (8) Sexual dysfunction (items 25 and 26; score 0 to 24); (9) Miscellaneous (items 27, 28, 29 and 30; score, 0 to 48). Secondary objectives included: (1) to analyze the effectiveness of opicapone on NMS burden of each domain of the NMSS, and specifically also on sleep (PDSS), apathy (AS), and pain (KPPS); (2) to analyze the effectiveness of opicapone on motor complications (UPDRS-IV) and gait problems (FOGQ) including freezing of gait (FOG) (FOGQ-item 3); (3) to analyze the effectiveness of opicapone on health related QoL (PDQ-39) and functional capacity for ADL (ADLS); (4) to assess the clinical global impression of change according to the patient (PGIC); and (5) to analyze the safety and security of opicapone in PD patients.

Opicapone was administered as a once-daily 50 mg capsule. This study did not contemplate the switching of entacapone or tolcapone (COMT inhibitors) to opicapone. So, patients with PD who were being treated with another COMT inhibitor different from opicapone should take at least 1 month without taking a COMT inhibitor (entacapone and/or tolcapone) to be considered a candidate to participate in the study. During follow-up, any other medications different from opicapone should not have been modified (regimen, doses, etc.) except if the neurologist considered these changes absolutely necessary. All the changes including PD and not-PD related medications and levodopa-equivalent daily dose (LEDD) [31] of levodopa were recorded.

2.1. Data Analysis

Data were processed using SPSS 20.0 for Windows. Continuous variables were expressed as the mean ± SD or median and quartiles. Relationships between variables were evaluated using the Student's t-test, the Mann–Whitney U test, or Spearman's or Pearson's correlation coefficient as appropriate (distribution for variables was verified by one-sample Kolmogorov–Smirnov tests). NMS burden was defined as: mild (NMSS 1–20); moderate (NMSS 21–40); severe (NMSS 41–70); and very severe (NMSS > 70) [32]. The PDQ-39 was expressed as a summary index (PDQ-39SI): (score/156) × 100. Each domain of the NMSS and PDQ-39 was expressed as a percentage: (score/total score) × 100.

The primary efficacy outcome was the change from baseline (V0) to the end of the observational period (6 months; V2) in the NMSS total score. The change from V0 to V2 in NMSS domains, PDSS, AS, KPPS, VAS-PAIN, UPDRS-IV, FOGQ, PDQ-39SI, and ADLS were the secondary efficacy outcome variables. Analyses on efficacy variables were performed with the ITT data set (all subjects who receive at least one pill of opicapone and had a baseline and treatment observation for the primary efficacy outcome measure). A paired-sample *t*-test or Wilcoxon's rank sum test, as appropriate, was performed for testing the change from baseline. Cohen's d formula was applied for measuring the effect size. The following was considered: <0.2—Negligible; 0.2–0.49—Small; 0.50–0.79—Moderate; and ≥0.80—Large. McNemar's or marginal homogeneity tests were applied for comparing the frequency distribution of groups between V0 and V2. Values of $p < 0.05$ were considered significant.

The safety data set consists of all subjects for whom the study device was initiated. Safety analyses was assessed by adverse events (AEs). All AEs was coded using the current version of the Medical Dictionary for Regulatory Activities (MedDRA). The number and percentage of subjects with treatment emergent AEs by MedDRA system organ class and preferred term, by severity, and by relationship to study treatment as assessed by the investigator, was provided for overall subjects.

2.2. Standard Protocol Approvals, Registrations, and Patient Consents

For this study, we received approval from the *Comité de Ética de la Investigación Clínica de Galicia* from Spain (2017/475; 31/OCT/2017). Written informed consents from all participants in this study were obtained before the start of the study. OPEN-PD was classified by the AEMPS (*Agencia Española del Medicamento y Productos Sanitarios*) as a Post-authorization Prospective Follow-up study with the code DSG-OPI-2017-01.

2.3. Data Availability

The protocol and the statistical analysis plan are available on request. De-identified participant data are not available for legal and ethical reasons.

3. Results

A total of 33 out of 35 PD patients were included between July/2019 and June/2021 (age 63.3 ± 7.91; 60.6% males). Two patients selected finally refused to participate by their own decision. Data about sociodemographic aspects, comorbidities, antiparkinsonian drugs, and other therapies are shown in Table 1. The mean time from symptoms onset of PD was 7.48 ± 4.22 years. All patients were receiving oral levodopa, and none were under a second line therapy (pump infusion or deep brain stimulation). About two out of three patients were receiving a MAO-B inhibitor and/or a dopamine agonist and less than 10% amantadine or an anticholinergic agent. Benzodiazepines, antidepressant agents, and analgesic drugs were taken by 36.4%, 24.2%, and 21.2% of the patients, respectively. None were taking an antipsychotic agent. The mean LEDD was 820.89 ± 323.31 mg (range from 350 to 1812 mg).

At baseline (V0), 97% (32/33) of the patients presented with motor fluctuations and 42.4% (14/33) with dyskinesia. The mean UPDRS-III during the ON state was 21.61 ± 13.17. With regard to the NMS, the mean NMSS total score at baseline was 71.67 ± 37.12, presenting 69.7% (23/33) and 30.3% (10/33) of the patients with severe and with very severe NMS burden, respectively. Considering the different domains from the NMSS, the highest scores were in domains 2 (sleep/fatigue), 7 (urinary symptoms), and 3 (mood/apathy) (Table 2). Regarding QoL, the most affected domains were 3 (emotional well-being), 8 (bodily discomfort), and 6 (cognition) (Table 2).

Table 1. Data about sociodemographic aspects, comorbidities, antiparkinsonian drugs, and other therapies at baseline (N = 33).

Age	63.3 ± 7.91 (48–77)	Time from symptoms onset	7.48 ± 4.22 (2–20)
Gender (males) (%)	60.6		
Ethnicity (%)		Motor fluctuations (%)	97
- Caucasian	97	Dyskinesia (%)	42.4
- Other	3		
		Treatment for PD (%):	
Civil status (%):		- Levodopa	100
- Married	78.8	- MAO-B inhibitor	63.6
- Widowed	3	- Dopamine agonists:	66.7
- Single	6.1	* Pramipexole	33.3
- Divorced	9.1	* Ropinirole	12.1
- Other	3	* Rotigotine	21.2
		- Amantadine	9.1
Living style (%)		- Anticholinergic drug	3
- With the partner	75.8		
- With another family member	6.1	L-dopa daily dose (mg)	648.46 ± 372.44 (200–1792)
- With a son/daughter	6.1	DA daily dose (mg)	162.84 ± 161.03 (0–630)
- Other	12	LEDD (mg)	820.89 ± 323.31 (350–1812)
Habitat (%):		Other treatments (%):	
- Rural (<5.000)	21.2	- Antidepressant	24.2
- Semiurban (5.000–20.000)	24.2	- Benzodiazepine	36.4
- Urban (>20.000)	54.6	- Antipsychotic	0
		- Analgesic	21.2
Comorbidities (%):			
- Arterial hypertension	39.4	Number of anti-PD drugs	2.75 ± 1.14 (1–5)
- Diabetes mellitus	15.2	Number of non-PD drugs	2.51 ± 2.56 (0–9)
- Dyslipemia	27.3	Total number of drugs	5.24 ± 2.92 (1–11)
- Hiperuricemia	3	Number of pills for PD	5.82 ± 1.6 (3–9)
- Cardiomyopathy	6	N. of pills for other cause	2.54 ± 2.69 (0–9.5)
- Cardiac arrhythmia	12.1	Total number of pills	8.37 ± 3.24 (3–18.5)
- Smoking	9.1		
- Alcohol consumption	18.2		

The results represent % or mean ± SD (range).

At 6 months, 30 patients completed the follow-up (90.9%). The NMSS total score was reduced by 27.3% (from 71.67 ± 37.12 at V1 to 52.1 ± 34.76 at V2; Cohen's effect size = −0.97; p=0.002) (Table 2). Six out of 30 patients presented a higher NMSS total score at the end of the follow-up compared to baseline (20%), whereas in the rest of the patients the NMSS total score was lower (range of decrease from 7 to 83 points). Compared to the score at V0, the change at V1 was significant too (p = 0.001) (Figure 1). By domains, improvement was observed in sleep/fatigue (−40.1%; Cohen's effect size = −1.06; p < 0.0001), mood/apathy (−46.6%; Cohen's effect size = −0.87; p = 0.001), gastrointestinal symptoms (-20.7%; Cohen's effect size = −0.56; p = 0.029), and miscellaneous (−44.94%; Cohen's effect size = −0.65; p = 0.021) (Table 2 and Figure 2). Compared to baseline, a significant improvement in sleep/fatigue and mood/apathy was reported at V1 whereas no differences were detected in any domain between V1 and V2 (Table S1—Supplementary Material). At the end of the follow-up, the NMS burden by groups was 9.7% mild; 38.7% moderate; 25.8% severe; and 25.8% very severe (comparison to V1, p = 0.001) (Figure 3). Regarding other scales assessing NMS, no significant results were observed, although a trend of significance was detected for the KPPS (p = 0.075) (Table 2). A significant improvement was detected in item 27 of the NMSS (pain not explained for other known condition), changing the score from 4.15 ± 4.5 at V0 to 1.9 ± 3.39 at V2 (p = 0.007). With regard to motor symptoms, it was detected a significant reduction in the FOGQ (from 7.42 ± 5.62 at V0 to 6.03 ± 5.41 at V2; Cohen's effect size = −0.56; p = 0.018). FOG at baseline was reported by 48.5% of the patients and 43.3% at the end of the follow-up (p = 0.687).

Table 2. Change in the score of the NMSS and other scales of the study from V0 (baseline; N = 33) to V2 (6 months ± 30 days; N = 30).

	V0	V2	Cohen's d	Δ V0–V2	p
MOTOR ASSESSMENT					
H&Y-OFF	2.5 [2, 3]	N. A.	N. A.	N. A.	N. A.
H&Y-ON	2 [1.5, 2]	N. A.	N. A.	N. A.	N. A.
UPDRS-III-ON	21.61 ± 13.17	N. A.	N. A.	N. A.	N. A.
UPDRS-IV	4.48 ± 2.09	3.87 ± 2.5	−0.38	−13.6%	0.083
FOGQ	7.42 ± 5.62	6.03 ± 5.41	−0.56	−18.7%	0.018
NON MOTOR ASSESSMENT					
NMSS total score	71.67 ± 37.12	52.1 ± 34.76	−0.97	−27.3%	0.002
- Cardiovascular	5.3 ± 9.21	4.03 ± 6.03	−0.24	−23.9%	0.346
- Sleep/fatigue	33.08 ± 19.02	19.82 ± 16.4	−1.06	−40.1%	<0.0001
- Mood/apathy	22.22 ± 22.58	11.87 ± 14.82	−0.87	−46.6%	0.001
- Perceptual symptoms	1.59 ± 4.76	1.88 ± 4.5	+0.12	+18.2%	0.334
- Attention/memory	13.55 ± 15.8	8.6 ± 19.62	−0.32	−36.5%	0.091
- Gastrointestinal symptoms	19.44 ± 16.27	15.41 ± 16.36	−0.56	−20.7%	0.029
- Urinary symptoms	32.57 ± 26.01	34.49 ± 26.02	+0.09	+5.8%	0.726
- Sexual dysfunction	15.78 ± 26.2	22.98 ± 30.97	+0.43	+45.6%	0.099
- Miscellaneous	21.96 ± 18.56	12.09 ± 14.11	−0.65	−44.94%	0.021
PDSS	104.62 ± 22.51	108.48 ± 26.86	+0.24	+3.6%	0.267
AS	13.76 ± 8.4	14.6 ± 8.71	+0.11	+6.1%	0.801
KPPS	14.33 ± 13.5	10.47 ± 9.62	−0.44	−26.9%	0.075
- Musculoskeletal pain	4.06 ± 3.46	3.47 ± 3.53	−0.14	−14.5%	0.474
- Chronic pain	1.76 ± 3.51	0.63 ± 1.75	−0.12	−64.2%	0.073
- Fluctuation-related pain	2.7 ± 4.24	1.23 ± 2.55	−0.06	−54.4%	0.133
- Nocturnal pain	4.18 ± 6.44	2.93 ± 4.2	−0.34	−29.9%	0.266
- Oro-facial pain	0.52 ± 1.46	0.43 ± 1.61	−0.09	−17.3%	0.524
- Discoloration, edema/swelling	0.18 ± 0.72	0.53 ± 1.47	+0.38	+194.4%	0.109
- Radicular pain	0.94 ± 2.35	1.23 ± 2.73	+0.09	+30.8%	0.878
VAS-PAIN	4.09 ± 3.11	4.55 ± 2.5	+0.41	+11.2%	0.187
QOL AND AUTONOMY					
PDQ-39SI	26.67 ± 17.61	21.75 ± 14.9	−0.99	−18.4%	0.001
- Mobility	26.74 ± 19.62	24.16 ± 24.68	−0.45	−9.6%	0.064
- Activities of daily living	26.01 ± 20.46	23.61 ± 19.82	−0.33	−8.9%	0.130

Table 2. Cont.

	V0	V2	Cohen's d	Δ V0–V2	p
- Emotional well-being	36.74 ± 26.95	26.94 ± 21.49	−0.83	−26.7%	0.004
- Stigmatization	22.72 ± 27.41	14.37 ± 20.77	−0.75	−36.7%	0.009
- Social support	12.37 ± 18.76	9.44 ± 15.43	−0.39	−23.6%	0.244
- Cognition	28.41 ± 19.45	24.16 ± 25.2	−0.25	−14.9%	0.306
- Communication	17.17 ± 20.61	16.94 ± 18.63	−0.09	−1.3%	0.895
- Pain and discomfort	34.34 ± 21.52	23.33 ± 19.98	−0.67	−32.1%	0.023
ADLS	80 ± 13.91	82.33 ± 14.54	−0.35	−2.9%	0.197

p values were computed using the Wilcoxon signed-rank test. The results represent mean ± SD or median [p25, p75]. Domains of the NMSS and PDQ-39SI were expressed as a percentage to be able to establish comparisons on their severity between them. Cohen's d formula was applied for measuring the effect size. It was considered: small effect = 0.2; medium effect = 0.5; large effect = 0.8. N. A., not applicable. ADLS, Schwab & England Activities of Daily Living Scale; FOGQ, Freezing of Gait Questionnaire; H&Y: Hoenh & Yahr; KPPS, King's PD Pain Scale; NMSS, Non-Motor Symptoms Scale; PDQ-39SI, 39-item Parkinson's Disease Quality of Life Questionnaire Summary Index; PDSS, Parkinson's disease Rating Scale; UPDRS, Unified Parkinson's Disease Rating Scale; VAS-Pain, Visual Analog Scale-Pain.

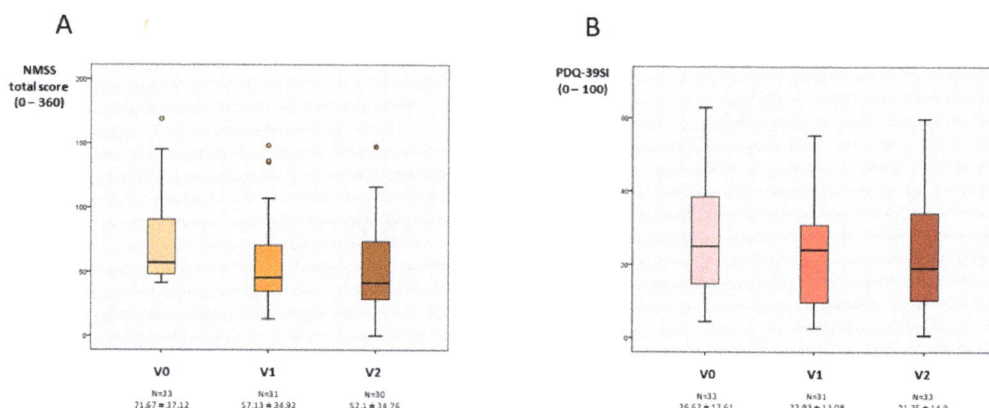

Figure 1. (**A**). NMSS total score at V0 (baseline), V1 (2 months ± 15 days), and V2 (6 months ± 30 days). V2 vs. V0, p = 0.002; V1 vs. V0, p = 0.001; and V2 vs. V1, p = 0.202. (**B**). PDQ-39SI at V0, V1, and V2. V2 vs. V0, p = 0.001; V1 vs. V0, p = 0.008; and V2 vs. V1, p = 0.496. Data are presented as box plots, with the box representing the median and the two middle quartiles (25–75%). p values were computed using the Wilcoxon signed-rank test. Mild outliers (O) are data points that are more extreme than Q1—1.5. NMS, non-motor symptoms; PDQ-39SI, 39-item Parkinson's Disease Questionnaire Summary Index.

QoL also improved at V2 with a 18.4% reduction in the PDQ-39SI (from 26.67 ± 17.61 at V0 to 21.75 ± 14.9 at V2; Cohen's effect size = -0.99; p = 0.001) compared to the score at baseline. Specifically, by domains, the difference between V0 and V2 was significant for PDQ-39SI-3 (Emotional well-being) (p = 0.004), PDQ-39SI-4 (Stigmatization) (p = 0.009), and PDQ-39SI-8 (Pain and discomfort) (p = 0.023) (Table 2). At 6 months, 17 patients out of 30 (56.7%) felt better regarding the PGIC: 1 very much improved; 9 much improved; 7 minimally improved; 10 had no changes; and 3 were minimally worse.

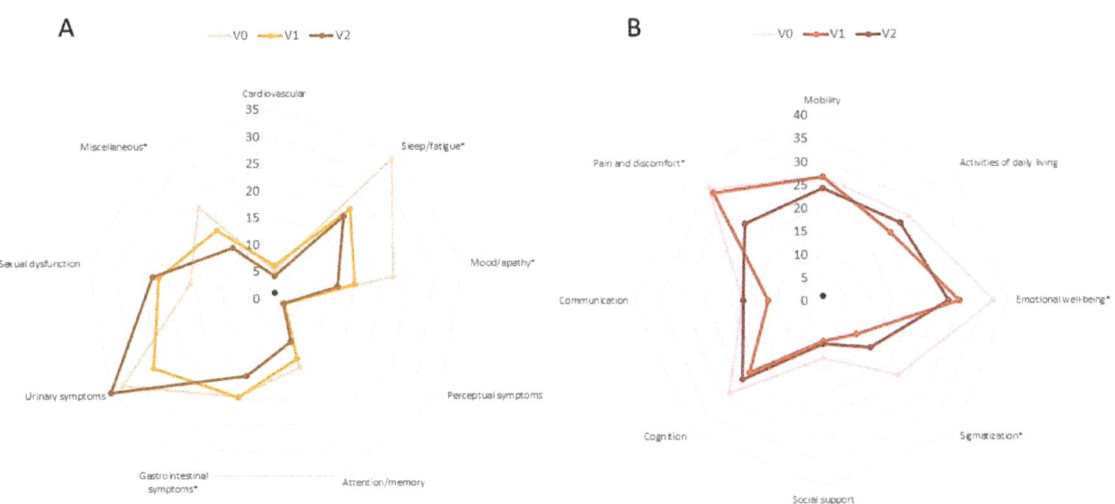

Figure 2. (**A**). Mean score on each domain of the NMSS scale at V0 (baseline), V1 (2 months ± 15 days), and V2 (6 months ± 30 days). The difference between V2 and V0 was significant for NMSS-2 (Sleep/fatigue) ($p < 0.0001$), NMSS-3 (Mood/apathy) ($p < 0.001$), NMSS-6 (Gastrointestinal symptoms) ($p = 0.029$), and NMSS-9 (Miscellaneous) ($p = 0.021$). (**B**). Mean score on each domain of the PDQ-39SI at V0, V1, and V2. The difference between V2 and V0 was significant for PDQ-39SI-3 (Emotional well-being) ($p = 0.004$), PDQ-39SI-4 (Stigmatization) ($p = 0.009$), and PDQ-39SI-8 (Pain and discomfort) ($p = 0.023$). p values were computed using the Wilcoxon signed-rank test.

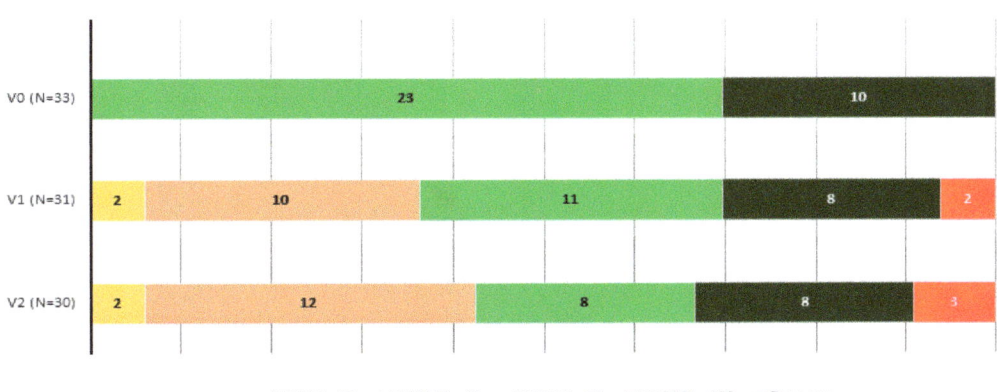

Figure 3. NMS burden with regard to the NMSS total score (0–20, slight burden; 21–40, moderate burden; 41–70, severe burden; 71–360 very severe burden) at V0, (baseline), V1 (2 months ± 14 days), and V2 (6 months ± 30 days). V2 vs. V0, $p = 0.001$; V1 vs. V0, $p = 0.001$; V2 vs. V1, $p = 0.366$.

A total of 13 adverse events in 11 patients (33.3%) were reported, 1 of which was severe (not related to opicapone) (Table 3). Dyskinesias and nausea were the most frequent (6.1%). Two patients discontinued due to an adverse event related to opicapone (nausea and insomnia), whereas in the third case it was a personal decision of the patient due to a lack of effect of the drug.

Table 3. Adverse events in patients from V0 to V2.

	N
Total AEs, N	13
- Dyskinesia	2
- Nausea	2
- Unrest	1
- Visual hallucinations	1
- Insomina	1
- Vivid dreams	1
- Tiredness	1
- Insomnia	1
- OFF time increase	1
- Arthritis in both wrists	1
- Supraspinatus tendonitis	1
Patients with at least one AE, N (%)	11 (33.3)
At least possibly related AEs, N	8
Patients with at least possibly* related to opicapone AEs, N (%)	7 (21.2)
Total SAEs, N	1
- Arthritis in both wrists	
Patients with al least one SAE, N (%)	1 (3)
At least possibly * related to opicapone SAEs, N	0
Patients with at least possibly related to opicapone SAEs, N (%)	0 (0)
Patients with at least one AE leading to discontinuation, N (%)	2 (6.1)
Patients with at least one possibly* related to opicapone AE leading to discontinuation N (%)	2 (6.1)
Deaths, N (%)	0 (0)

* Considered "possibly", "probably" or "definitely" related to treatment (opicapone). AE, adverse event; SAE, serious adverse event.

4. Discussion

The present study observed that global NMS burden (NMSS total score) improved in PD patients 6 months after starting with opicapone. Specifically, an improvement was detected in domains of the NMSS related to sleep, fatigue, mood, gastrointestinal symptoms, and pain. Moreover, the effect was significant at 2 months after starting with opicapone, and an improvement in QoL was observed as well. This is the first prospective study specifically designed for assessing the change in global NMS burden in PD patients after been treated with this drug.

NMS are frequent in PD, and their recognition is very important because of their negative impact on QoL [4,32]. In this study, PD patients had to present with severe or very severe NMS burden (NMSS total score > 40) at baseline for being included. Recently, it was observed that up to 30.5% and 44.9% of PD patients with a H&Y stage of 1 and 2, respectively, had severe or very severe NMS burden, and, importantly, patients with a lower H&Y stage may be more affected if they had a greater NMS burden than others with a higher H&Y stage [6]. Therefore, strategies designed to improve NMS are necessary [5]. In this context and considering that some NMS can be related to the deficit of other neurotransmitters different than dopamine (e.g., depression and serotonin), a key question is if NMS can improve with a drug with an only dopaminergic effect [33]. Increasing dopamine activity not only in the striatum but also in other areas of the brain could improve some NMS such as attention and executive functions, depression, anxiety, apathy, restless legs and periodic limb movements, urinary urgency, nocturia, dribbling of saliva, constipation, pain, or fatigue [33–37]. Specifically, some studies with first and second generation COMT inhibitors (entacapone and tolcapone) observed a benefit by the patients on some NMS [9,10,38,39], but really the evidence is scarce, possibly in part due to the fact that NMS are an emerging topic and have been much more studied in recent years. Moreover, if COMT inhibitors such as opicapone can improve ON time, non-motor fluctuations [40], NMS related to OFF episodes [41] and global NMS burden as a whole [8] could improve as well.

Opicapone is a third generation COMT inhibitor rationally designed to reduce the risk of toxicity and improve COMT inhibitory potency and peripheral tissue selectivity compared with other COMT inhibitors [42]. The efficacy and safety of opicapone in reducing OFF time in patients with PD and established motor fluctuations has been well established in three randomized, double-blind, placebo-controlled trials (BIPARK I; BIPARK II; COMFORT-PD) [14,15,43] and observational studies [11,44–46]. However, the effect of opicapone on NMS is a relatively unexplored aspect [42]. In the BIPARK II study, NMS were assessed with the NMSS at different time points, including baseline, the end of the double-blind phase, and the end of the open-label phase. At the end of the double-blind period, NMSS scores slightly improved across the opicapone and placebo groups, with no significant differences between them (placebo, -5.2; opicapone 25 mg, -2.0; opicapone 50 mg, -4.9) [16]. At the 1-year open-label endpoint, a mean improvement of -4.2 in NMSS total score was still maintained [16]. However, data about domains of the NMSS and even the NMSS total score at baseline was not provided in all groups. In those patients receiving opicapone 50 mg (N = 325), the mean baseline NMSS total score was 37.9 ± 28.7. In our study, the score was very much higher (71.67 ± 37.12) due to the inclusion criteria and aim proposed, which is important because the probability of having an improvement is related to the baseline score of the scale [47]. Similar results have previously been observed in the BIPARK I study (-5.7, placebo; -2, opicapone 50 mg). In the third pivotal study of opicapone conducted in Japan, NMS were not assessed [43]. In the only other published study analyzing how NMS changed in PD patients treated with opicapone, the OPTIPARK study [11], a decrease in the NMSS total score of 6.8 ± 19.7 points ($p < 0.0001$) at 3 months was observed. This was a prospective, open-label, single-arm trial conducted in Germany and the United Kingdom under clinical practice conditions, and data about NMS were collected in 393 PD patients. Again, the NMSS total score at baseline was lower than in our study (44.6 ± 30.3), and the change from baseline to the visit at 3 months in the NMS burden was not the primary efficacy outcome. In this study [11], Reichmann et al. reported a significant improvement in all domains of the NMSS except in domain 4 (perceptual problems/hallucinations), but the size effect was not calculated, and it is not clear whether it can be considered clinically relevant, with a decrease in the score that varied from 13.3% (cardiovascular symptoms; -0.2 from 1.5 ± 2.38 at baseline; $p = 0.0310$) to 22.4% (mood/apathy; -1.5 ± 6.82 from 6.7 ± 9.8; $p < 0.0001$). In our study, the greatest improvement was observed in the mood/apathy and sleep/fatigue domains, both with large effect. In the BIPARK II study, a significant signal was seen for the sleep/fatigue domain where the 50 mg dose reduced the NMSS sleep/fatigue score by -1.2 points versus -0.5 points with a placebo [42]. The small sample size of our cohort could explain why the change in sleep (PDSS) and pain (KPPS) scales was not significant. The PDSS was used in the BIPARK II study, but differences were not detected compared to a placebo [16]. In this line of research, studies such as OASIS (OpicApone Sleep dISorder; EudraCT number 2020-001176-15) and OCEAN (the OpiCapone Effect on motor fluctuations and pAiN; EudraCT number 2020-001175-32) are currently underway to evaluate the effect of opicapone 50 mg on sleep and pain, respectively. On the other hand, our study is the first prospective one exploring the effect of opicapone on motivation/apathy using a specific validated scale, but we did not find differences. A recent publication that reviewed data of small retrospective series of PD patients treated with opicapone in Spain suggests a possible positive effect of opicapone on NMS after 6 to 12 months, especially on sleep [48]. However, and in agreement with our findings, the frequency of apathy in 60 PD patients treated with opicapone in real clinical practice did not change at 6 months (32%) and 12 months (33%) compared to the baseline visit (32%) [48]. More studies designed to evaluate the effect of opicapone over NMS are really needed.

In addition to NMS, we observed in our study a trend of significant improvement in motor complications (UPDRS-IV; $p = 0.083$) and a significant improvement in gait problems ($p = 0.018$). Although the frequency of patients reporting FOG was similar before and after treatment with opicapone, gait problems as a whole may improve due to motor signs improvement and OFF time reduction [49]. Only two small studies looked at the effects of COMT inhibitors on gait parameters, providing support for tolcapone as an effective add-on to levodopa to prolong beneficial effects on gait speed [50,51]. In previously published studies of opicapone, its effect on gait was not analyzed. However, as we detected here, QoL improved significantly in PD patients treated with opicapone in real clinical practice [11]. We used the PDQ-39 and observed improvement in emotional well-being, stigmatization, and pain and discomfort. On the contrary, in the OPTIPARK study the brief version (PDQ-8) was used, and data about domains was not provided in the publication [11]. Contrary to this study, we did not find improvement in the autonomy for ADL.

Opicapone was not only effective but also safe and well-tolerated, with a very high drug maintenance rate at 6 months, above 90%. The rate was 79.4% (393/495) at 3 months and 85.3% (81/95) at 6 months for all the cohort and for the United Kingdom subgroup only, respectively, from the real clinical practice OPTIPARK cohort [11], and 92.2% (107/116) and 83.1% (128/154) in the double-blind phase of BIPARK I and BIPAK II studies, respectively [14,15]. The results about adverse events are in line with other studies [11,13–18,43–46], even with a lower percentage of events reported. Dyskinesia, as in some studies, was the most frequent adverse event in our study. The European public assessment report (EPAR) for opicapone states that dyskinesias were reported in more than 10% of participants receiving opicapone, in which case it may be necessary to reduce the levodopa dose within the first days to first weeks after starting opicapone to prevent severe dyskinesias [44]. This good tolerability of the drug was accompanied by an improvement according to the PGIC in almost 60% of the cases, in line with other reports [43,48].

Our study has some important limitations. The most important one is related to the study design itself, and since there is not a comparative arm with placebo, the results should be interpreted with caution. Second, the sample size is small, and it is possible that the changes observed in some variables are not significant due to this. In fact, due to different problems (i.e., administrative, commercial distribution of the drug in Spain, COVID-19 pandemic), the study was closed before reaching the initially planned sample size (N = 40). Third, the effect of opicapone on NMS was analyzed in PD patients with a severe or very severe NMS burden (NMSS total score > 40); therefore, the results cannot be extrapolated to patients with a mild or moderate NMS burden (NMSS total score $\leq$ 40). Fourth, mood was not assessed with a specific scale. On the other hand, this is the first study designed to assess the effect of opicapone on NMS burden in PD patients and the first one in which changes in some NMS such as pain, apathy, or sleep have been exhaustively analyzed. Despite some limitations, the results are novel and of great interest because there is a lack of knowledge about what benefits can opicapone produce over many symptoms in PD patients.

5. Conclusions

In conclusion, opicapone is well tolerated and improves global NMS burden and QoL in PD patients. Well-designed studies are necessary to analyze in detail the possible beneficial effect of opicapone on NMS in patients with PD.

Supplementary Materials: The following are available online at https://www.mdpi.com/article/10.3390/brainsci12030383/s1, Table S1: Change in the score of the NMSS and its domains between the visits of the study: V0 (N = 33), V1 (N = 31), V2 (N = 30).

Author Contributions: D.S.G.: conception, organization, statistical analysis, and execution of the project; G.F.P.: execution, review, and critique; J.M.O.-R.: execution, review, and critique; F.E.S.: execution, review, and critique; R.R.A.R.L.: execution, review, and critique; J.G.M.E.: execution, review, and critique. All authors have read and agreed to the published version of the manuscript.

Funding: The present study is a study promoted by an independent researcher (promoter: Diego Santos García). Bial Spain has financed its expenses.

Institutional Review Board Statement: The study was conducted according to the guidelines of the Declaration of Helsinki, and approved by the Comité de Ética de la Investigación Clínica de Galicia from Spain (2017/475; 31/OCT/2017).

Informed Consent Statement: Informed consent was obtained from all subjects involved in the study.

Data Availability Statement: The protocol and the statistical analysis plan are available on request. Deidentified participant data are not available for legal and ethical reasons.

Acknowledgments: We would like to thank all patients and caregivers who collaborated in this study. Many thanks also to *Fundación Degen* (https://fundaciondegen.org/, accessed on 16 February 2022), Alphabioresearch (https://www.alphabioresearch.com/, accessed on 16 February 2022), and Bial España.

Conflicts of Interest: The authors declare no conflict of interest.

Abbreviations

ADLS: Schwab & England Activities of Daily Living Scale; AS, Apathy Scale; CGI, Clinical Global Impressions; FOGQ, Freezing of Gait Questionnaire, H&Y: Hoenh & Yahr; KPPS, King's PD Pain Scale; NMS, non-motor symptoms; NMSS, Non-Motor Symptoms Scale; PD, Parkinson's disease; PDQ-39SI, 39-item Parkinson's Disease Quality of Life Questionnaire Summary Index; PDSS, Parkinson's Disease Sleep Scale; UPDRS, Unified Parkinson's Disease Rating Scale; VAS-Pain, Visual Analog Scale-Pain.

References

1. Dorsey, E.R.; Bloem, B.R. The Parkinson Pandemic—A Call to Action. *JAMA Neurol.* **2018**, *75*, 9–10. [CrossRef] [PubMed]
2. Tolosa, E.; Gaig, C.; Santamaría, J.; Compta, Y. Diagnosis and the premotor phase of Parkinson's disease. *Neurology* **2009**, *72* (Suppl. 7), 12–20. [CrossRef] [PubMed]
3. Bloem, B.R.; Okun, M.S.; Klein, C. Parkinson's disease. *Lancet* **2021**, *397*, 2284–2303. [CrossRef]
4. Santos García, D.; de Deus Fonticoba, T.; Suárez Castro, E.; Borrué, C.; Mata, M.; Solano Vila, B.; Cots Foraster, A.; Álvarez Sauco, M.; Coppadis Study Group. Non-motor symptoms burden, mood, and gait problems are the most significant factors contributing to a poor quality of life in non-demented Parkinson's disease patients: Results from the COPPADIS Study Cohort. *Parkinsonism Relat. Disord.* **2019**, *66*, 151–157. [CrossRef] [PubMed]
5. Seppi, K.; Weintraub, D.; Coelho, M.; Perez-Lloret, S.; Fox, S.H.; Katzenschlager, R.; Hametner, E.-M.; Poewe, W.; Rascol, O.; Goetz, C.G.; et al. The Movement Disorder Society Evidence-Based Medicine Review Update: Treatments for the non-motorsymptoms of Parkinson's disease. *Mov. Disord.* **2011**, *26* (Suppl. 3), S42–S80. [CrossRef]
6. Santos García, D.; De Deus Fonticoba, T.; Paz González, J.M.; Bartolome, C.C.; Aymerich, V.; Enriquez, M.; Suárez, E.; Jesus, S.; Aguilar, M.; Pastor, P.; et al. Staging Parkinson's Disease Combining Motor and Nonmotor Symptoms Correlates with Disability and Quality of Life. *Parkinsons Dis* **2021**, *2021*, 8871549. [CrossRef] [PubMed]
7. Santos-García, D.; de Deus, T.; Cores, C.; Canfield, H.; Paz González, J.M.; Miro, C.M.; Aymerich, L.V.; Suarez, E.; Jesus, S.; Coppadis Study Group; et al. Predictors of Global Non-Motor Symptoms Burden Progression in Parkinson's Disease. Results from the COPPADIS Cohort at 2-Year Follow-Up. *J. Pers. Med.* **2021**, *11*, 626. [CrossRef]
8. Santos-García, D.; de Deus Fonticoba, T.; Suárez Castro, E.; McAfee, D.; Catalán, F.; Alonso-Frech, C.; Villanueva, S.; Jesús, P.; Mir, M.; Aguilar, P.; et al. Non-motor symptom burden is strongly correlated to motor complications in patients with Parkinson's disease. *Eur. J. Neurol* **2020**, *27*, 1210–1223. [CrossRef]
9. Magalona, S.C.; Rasetti, R.; Chen, J.; Chem, Q.; Gold, I.; Decot, H.; Callicott, J.H.; Berman, K.F.; Apud, J.A.; Weinberger, D.R.; et al. Effect of tolcapone on brain activity during a variable attentional control task: A double-blind, placebo-controlled, counter-balanced trial in healthy volunteers. *CNS Drugs* **2013**, *27*, 663–673. [CrossRef]
10. Apud, J.A.; Mattay, V.; Chen, J.; Kolachana, B.S.; Callicot, J.H.; Rasetti, R.; Alce, G.; Iudicello, J.E.; Akbar, N.; Ega, M.F.; et al. Tolcapone improves cognition and cortical information processing in normal human subjects. *Neuropsychopharmacology* **2007**, *32*, 1011–1020. [CrossRef]
11. Reichmann, H.; Lees, A.; Rocha, J.F.; Magalhães, D.; Soares-da-Silva, P.; OPTIPARK investigators. Effectiveness and safety of opicapone in Parkinson's disease patients with motor fluctuations: The OPTIPARK open-label study. *Transl. Neurodegener.* **2020**, *9*, 9. [CrossRef] [PubMed]
12. Kiss, L.E.; Ferreira, H.S.; Torrão, L.; Bonifácio, M.J.; Palma, P.N.; Soares-da-Silva, P.; Learmonth, D.A. Discovery of a long-acting, peripherally selective inhibitor of catechol-O-methyltransferase. *J. Med. Chem.* **2010**, *53*, 3396–3411. [CrossRef] [PubMed]

13. Fabbri, M.; Rosa, M.M.; Ferreira, J.J. Clinical pharmacology review of opicapone for the treatment of Parkinson's disease. *Neurodegener. Dis. Manag.* **2016**, *6*, 349–362. [CrossRef] [PubMed]
14. Ferreira, J.J.; Lees, A.; Rocha, J.F.; Poewe, W.; Rascol, O.; Soares-da-Silva, P.; Bi-Park 1 Investigators. Opicapone as an adjunct to levodopa in patients with Parkinson's disease and end-of-dose motor fluctuations: A randomised, double-blind, controlled trial. *Lancet Neurol.* **2016**, *15*, 154–165. [CrossRef]
15. Lees, A.J.; Ferreira, J.; Rascol, O.; Poewe, W.; Rocha, J.-F.; McCrory, M.; Soares-da-Silva, P.; BIPARK-2 Study Investigators. Opicapone as Adjunct to Levodopa Therapy in Patients with Parkinson Disease and Motor Fluctuations: A Randomized Clinical Trial. *JAMA Neurol.* **2017**, *74*, 197–206. [CrossRef] [PubMed]
16. Costa, R.; Oliveira, C.; Pinto, R.; Lopes, N.; Nunes, T.; Rocha, F.; Soares-da-Silva, P. Opicapone long-term efficacy and safety in Parkinson´s disease BIPARK-II study: A one year open-label follow up. *J. Neurol.* **2014**, *261*, S119.
17. Gama, H.; Ferreira, J.; Lees, A. Evaluation of the safety and tolerability of opicapone in the treatment of Parkinson´s disease and motor fluctuations: Analysis of pooled Phase III studies. *Eur. J. Neurol.* **2015**, *22*, 611.
18. Oliveira, C.; Lees, A.; Ferreira, J. Evaluation of non-motor symptoms in opicapone treated Parkinson's disease patients: Results from a double-blind, randomized, controlled-study and open-label extention. *Eur. J. Neurol.* **2015**, *22*, 191.
19. Hughes, A.J.; Daniel, S.E.; Kilford, L.; Lees, A.J. Accuracy of clinical diagnosis of idiopathic Parkinson's disease: A clinico-pathological study of 100 cases. *J. Neurol. Neurosurg. Psychiatry* **1992**, *55*, 181–184. [CrossRef]
20. Hoehn, M.M.; Yahr, M.D. Parkinsonism: Onset, progression and mortality. *Neurology* **1967**, *17*, 427–442. [CrossRef]
21. Fahn, S.; Elton, R.L.; Members of the UPDRS Development Committee. *Unified Parkinson's Disease Rating Scale. Recent Developments in Parkinson's Disease*; Fahn, S., Marsden, C.D., Calne, D.B., Goldstein, M., Eds.; Macmillan Health Care Information: Florham Park, NJ, USA, 1987; Volume 2, pp. 153–164.
22. Giladi, N.; Shabtai, H.; Simon, E.S.; Biran, S.; Tal, J.; Korczyn, A.D. Construction of freezing of gait questionnaire for patients with Parkinsonism. *Parkinsonism Relat. Disord.* **2000**, *6*, 165–170. [CrossRef]
23. Chaudhuri, K.R.; Martinez-Martin, P.; Brown, R.G.; Sethi, K.; Stocchi, F.; Odin, P.; Abe, K.; MacPhee, G.; MacMahon, D.; Barone, P.; et al. The metric properties of a novel non-motor symptoms scale for Parkinson's disease: Results from an international pilot study. *Mov Disord.* **2007**, *22*, 1901–1911. [CrossRef] [PubMed]
24. Chaudhuri, K.R.; Pal, S.; DiMarco, A.; Whately-Smith, C.; Bridgman, K.; Mathew, R.; Pezzela, F.R.; Forbes, A.; Hög, B.; Trenkwalder, C. The Parkinson's disease sleep scale: A new instrument for assessing sleep and nocturnal disability in Parkinson's disease. *J. Neurol. Neurosurg. Psychiatry* **2002**, *73*, 629–635. [CrossRef] [PubMed]
25. Starkstein, S.E.; Mayberg, H.S.; Preziosi, T.J.; Andrezejewski, P.; Leiguarda, R.; Robinson, R.G. Reliability, validity, and clinical correlates of apathy in Parkinson's disease. *J. Neuropsychiatry Clin. Neurosci.* **1992**, *4*, 134–139.
26. Chaudhuri, K.R.; Rizos, A.; Trenkwalder, C.; Rascol, O.; Pal, S.; Martino, D.; Carrol, C.; Paviour, D.; Faluo-Pecurariou, C.; Kessel, B.; et al. King's Parkinson's disease pain scale, the first scale for pain in PD: An international validation. *Mov. Disord.* **2015**, *30*, 1623–1631. [CrossRef] [PubMed]
27. Burckhardt, C.S.; Jones, K.D. Adult measures of pain: The McGill Pain Questionnaire (MPQ), Rheumatoid Arthritis Pain Scale (RAPS), Short Form McGill Pain Questionnaire (SF-MPQ), Verbal Descriptive Scale (VDS), Visual Analog Scale (VAS), and West Haven-Yale Multidisciplinary Pain Inventory (WHYMPI). *Arthritis Rheum.* **2003**, *49*, S96–S104.
28. Schwab, R.S.; England, A.C. Projection Technique for Evaluating Surgery in Parkinson's Disease. In Proceedings of the Third Symposium on Parkinson's Disease, Edinburgh, UK, 20–22 May 1968; E. & S. Livingstone: Edinburgh, UK, 1969; pp. 152–157.
29. Jenkinson, C.; Fitzpatrick, R.; Peto, V.; Greenhall, R.; Hyman, N. The Parkinson's Disease Questionnaire (PDQ-39): Development and validation of a Parkinson's disease summary index score. *Age Ageing* **1997**, *26*, 353–357. [CrossRef]
30. Guy, W. *ECDEU Assessment Manual for Psychopharmacology*; National Institute of Mental Health. Psychopharmacology Research Branch, Division of Extramural Research Programs, Ed.; U.S. Deptartment of Health, Education and Welfare, Public Health Service, Alcohol, Drug Abuse and Mental Health Administration, National Institute of Mental Health, Psychopharmacology Research Branch, Division of Extramural Research Programs: Rockville, MD, USA, 1976; pp. 218–222.
31. Schade, S.; Mollenhauer, B.; Trenkwalder, C. Levodopa Equivalent Dose Conversion Factors: An Updated Proposal Including Opicapone and Safinamide. *Mov. Disord. Clin. Pract.* **2020**, *7*, 343–345. [CrossRef] [PubMed]
32. Martinez-Martin, P.; Rodriguez-Blazquez, C.; Kurtis, M.M.; Chaudhuri, K.R.; NMSS Validation Group. The impact of non-motor symptoms on health-related quality of life of patients with Parkinson's disease. *Mov. Disord.* **2011**, *26*, 399–406. [CrossRef] [PubMed]
33. Chaudhuri, K.R.; Schapira, A.H. Non-motor symptoms of Parkinson's disease: Dopaminergic pathophysiology and treatment. *Lancet. Neurol.* **2009**, *8*, 464–474. [CrossRef]
34. Mattay, V.; Tessitore, A.; Callicott, J.; Bertolino, A.; Goldberg, T.E.; Chase, T.N.; Daniel, H.; Weinberger, D.R. Dopaminergic modulation of cortical function in patients with Parkinson's disease. *Ann. Neurol.* **2002**, *51*, 156–164. [CrossRef] [PubMed]
35. Barone, P.; Scarzella, L.; Marconi, R.; Antonini, A.; Morgante, L.; Bracco, F.; Zappia, M.; Musch, B.; The Depression/Parkinson Italian Study Group. Pramipexole versus sertraline in the treatment of depression in Parkinson's disease: A national multicenter parallel group randomized study. *J. Neurol.* **2006**, *253*, 601–607. [CrossRef] [PubMed]
36. Fernández-Pajarín, G.; Sesar, Á.; Jiménez Martín, I.; Ares, B.; Castro, A. Continuous subcutaneous apomorphine infusion in the early phase of advanced Parkinson's disease: A prospective study of 22 patients. *Clin. Park. Relat. Disord.* **2021**, *6*, 100129. [CrossRef] [PubMed]

37. Trenkwalder, C.; Kies, B.; Rudzinska, M.; Fine, J.; Nikl, J.; Honczarenko, K.; Dioszeghy, P.; Hill, D.; Anderson, T.; Myllyla, V.; et al. Rotigotine effects on early morning motor function and sleep in Parkinson's disease: A double-blind, randomized, placebo-controlled study (RECOVER). *Mov. Disord.* **2011**, *26*, 90–99. [CrossRef] [PubMed]
38. Müller, T.; TANIMOS Study Investigators. Tolcapone addition improves Parkinson's disease associated nonmotor symptoms. *Ther. Adv. Neurol. Disord.* **2014**, *7*, 77–82. [CrossRef]
39. Artusi, C.A.; Sarro, L.; Imbalzano, G.; Fabbri, M.; Lopiano, L. Safety and efficacy of tolcapone in Parkinson's disease: Systematic review. *Eur. J. Clin. Pharmacol.* **2021**, *77*, 817–829. [CrossRef]
40. Martínez-Fernández, R.; Schmitt, E.; Martinez-Martin, P.; Krack, P. The hidden sister of motor fluctuations in Parkinson's disease: A review on nonmotor fluctuations. *Mov. Disord.* **2016**, *31*, 1080–1094. [CrossRef]
41. Witjas, T.; Kaphan, E.; Azulay, J.P.; Blin, O.; Ceccaldi, M.; Pouget, J.; Poncet, M.; Ali Chérif, A. Nonmotor fluctuations in Parkinson's disease: Frequent and disabling. *Neurology* **2002**, *59*, 408–413. [CrossRef]
42. Jenner, P.; Rocha, J.F.; Ferreira, J.J.; Rascol, O.; Soares-da-Silva, P. Redefining the strategy for the use of COMT inhibitors in Parkinson's disease: The role of opicapone. *Expert Rev. Neurother.* **2021**, *2*, 1019–1033. [CrossRef]
43. Takeda, A.; Takahashi, R.; Tsuboi, Y.; Nomoto, M.; Maeda, T.; Nishimura, A.; Yoshida, K.; Hattori, N. Randomized, controlled study of opicapone in Japanese Parkinson's patients with motor fluctuations. *Mov. Disord.* **2021**, *36*, 415–423. [CrossRef]
44. Lees, A.J.; Ferreira, J.; Rascol, O.; Reichmann, H.; Stocchi, F.; Tolosa, E.; Poewe, W. Opicapone for the management of end-of-dose motor fluctuations in patients with Parkinson's disease treated with L-DOPA. *Expert Rev. Neurother.* **2017**, *17*, 649–659. [CrossRef] [PubMed]
45. Fabbri, M.; Ferreira, J.J.; Lees, A.; Stocchi, F.; Poewe, W.; Tolosa, E.; Rascol, O. Opicapone for the treatment of Parkinson's disease: A review of a new licensed medicine. *Mov. Disord.* **2018**, *33*, 1528–1539. [CrossRef] [PubMed]
46. Scott, L.J. Opicapone: A review in Parkinson's disease. *CNS Drugs* **2021**, *35*, 121–131. [CrossRef] [PubMed]
47. Santos García, D.; Labandeira Guerra, C.; Yáñez Baña, R.; Cimas Hernando, M.I.; López, I.C.; Paz Gonález, J.M.; Alonso Losada, M.G.; González Palmás, M.J.; Miró, C.M. Safinamide Improves Non-Motor Symptoms Burden in Parkinson's Disease: An Open-Label Prospective Study. *Brain Sci.* **2021**, *11*, 316. [CrossRef] [PubMed]
48. López-Ariztegui, N.; Mata-Alvarez Santullano, M.; Tegel, I.; Almedia, F.; Sarasa, P.; Rojo, R.; Rico-Villademoros, F.; Abril Jaramillo, J.; Bermejo, P.; Borrúe, C.; et al. Opicapona para el tratamiento de la enfermedad de Parkinson: Datos de vida real en España (Opicapone for the treatment of Parkinson's disease: Real-life data in Spain). *Rev. Neurol.* **2021**, *73*, 1–14.
49. Smulders, K.; Dale, M.L.; Carlson-Kuhta, P.; Nutt, J.G.; Horak, F.B. Pharmacological treatment in Parkinson's disease: Effects on gait. *Parkinsonism Relat. Disord.* **2016**, *31*, 3–13. [CrossRef] [PubMed]
50. Napolitano, A.; Del Dotto, P.; Petrozzi, L.; Dell'Agnello, G.; Bellini, G.; Gambaccini, G.; Bonuccelli, U. Pharmacokinetics and pharmacodynamics of L-Dopa after acute and 6-week tolcapone administration in patients with Parkinson's disease. *Clin. Neuropharmacol.* **1999**, *22*, 24–29. [CrossRef]
51. Ondo, W.G.; Hunter, C.; Vuong, K.D.; Jankovic, J. The pharmacokinetic and clinical effects of tolcapone on a single dose of sublingual apomorphine in Parkinson's disease. *Parkinsonism Relat. Disord.* **2000**, *6*, 237–240. [CrossRef]

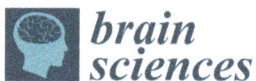 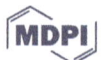

Article

Naturalistic Study of Depression Associated with Parkinson's Disease in a National Public Neurological Referral Center in Mexico

Reinhard Janssen-Aguilar [1], Patricia Rojas [2], Elizabeth Ruiz-Sánchez [2], Mayela Rodriguez-Violante [3], Yessica M. Alcántara-Flores [2], Daniel Crail-Meléndez [1], Amin Cervantes-Arriaga [3], Óscar Sánchez-Escandón [4] and Ángel A. Ruiz-Chow [1,5,*]

[1] Department of Psychiatry, National Institute of Neurology and Neurosurgery Manuel Velasco Suárez, Av. Insurgentes Sur No. 3877, Mexico City 14269, Mexico; rjanssen91@gmail.com (R.J.-A.); danielcrail@yahoo.com (D.C.-M.)
[2] Laboratory of Neurotoxicology, National Institute of Neurology and Neurosurgery Manuel Velasco Suárez, Av. Insurgentes Sur No. 3877, Mexico City 14269, Mexico; prcastane@hotmail.com (P.R.); elizabeth.ruiz@innn.edu.mx (E.R.-S.); fioremyr@gmail.com (Y.M.A.-F.)
[3] Movement Disorders Clinic, National Institute of Neurology and Neurosurgery Manuel Velasco Suárez, Av. Insurgentes Sur No. 3877, Mexico City 14269, Mexico; mrodriguez@innn.edu.mx (M.R.-V.); acervantes@innn.edu.mx (A.C.-A.)
[4] Clinic of Sleep Disorders, Metropolitan Autonomous University, Mexico City 14387, Mexico; oscarse@att.net.mx
[5] Liaison Psychiatry, Medical Center ABC, Av. Carlos Graef Fernández 154, Mexico City 05300, Mexico
* Correspondence: aaruizchow@gmail.com; Tel.: +52-55-5502-2820

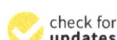

Citation: Janssen-Aguilar, R.; Rojas, P.; Ruiz-Sánchez, E.; Rodriguez-Violante, M.; Alcántara-Flores, Y.M.; Crail-Meléndez, D.; Cervantes-Arriaga, A.; Sánchez-Escandón, Ó.; Ruiz-Chow, Á.A. Naturalistic Study of Depression Associated with Parkinson's Disease in a National Public Neurological Referral Center in Mexico. *Brain Sci.* **2022**, *12*, 326. https://doi.org/10.3390/brainsci12030326

Academic Editors: Patricia Martinez-Sanchez and Francisco Nieto-Escamez

Received: 28 January 2022
Accepted: 24 February 2022
Published: 28 February 2022

Publisher's Note: MDPI stays neutral with regard to jurisdictional claims in published maps and institutional affiliations.

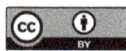

Copyright: © 2022 by the authors. Licensee MDPI, Basel, Switzerland. This article is an open access article distributed under the terms and conditions of the Creative Commons Attribution (CC BY) license (https://creativecommons.org/licenses/by/4.0/).

Abstract: Major depressive disorder (MDD) is a major health problem in Parkinson's disease (PD) patients. We described the clinical and sociodemographic factors of MDD among patients with PD at a national neurological referral center in Mexico. One hundred patients with PD + MDD were included in the study. All the patients were evaluated during the "ON" treatment phase of PD. Clinical scales for cognition (MMSE and MoCA) and MDD (MADRS) were applied. The mean age was 58.49 ± 11.02 years, and 57% of the sample was male. The most frequent symptom of PD was tremor (67%), and onset was more frequent on the right side (57%). Additionally, 49% of the patients with PD had moderate to severe (M/S) MDD. Selective serotonin reuptake inhibitors were the most frequent antidepressant treatment (69%). The scores of the scales were MADRS 21.33 ± 5.49, MoCA 21.06 ± 4.65, and MMSE 26.67 ± 1.20. The females had lower MMSE scores compared to the males ($p = 0.043$). The patients with M/S MDD had more rigidity at the beginning of PD ($p = 0.005$), fewer march alterations ($p = 0.023$), and a greater prevalence of left-side initial disease ($p = 0.037$). Rigidity was associated with M/S MDD (OR 3.75 $p = 0.013$). MDD was slightly more frequent in the males than in the females. The MDD symptoms and cognitive impairment were worse in the female population.

Keywords: Parkinson's disease; non-motor symptoms; neurodegenerative disease; major depressive disorder

1. Introduction

Parkinson's disease (PD) is a complex illness and the second most common neurodegenerative disorder, affecting 1% of the population over 60 and up to 4% over the age of 80 [1]. It is estimated that between 1 and 2% of the population in Mexico over the age of 60 suffers from PD [2], and the prevalence of the disease increases with age. The etiology of PD is currently unclear and no currently available treatment provides a cure [3]. In addition to classical motor symptoms (bradykinesia, rest tremor, or rigidity), the presence of non-motor features, such as hyposmia, sleep behavior disorder, cognitive impairment, pain, autonomic dysfunction, and psychiatric disturbances, are relevant. Psychiatric symptoms, such as major depressive disorder (MDD), anxiety, hallucination, delusion, apathy and anhedonia, impulsive and compulsive behavior, and cognitive dysfunction, appear to be present in most PD patients [4].

MDD is a major health problem in patients with PD. The predictors of MDD in PD are debatable and complex [3], although the prevalence of MDD in PD patients has been reported to be 20–35%, and the one-year incidence of minor MDD is 18%. It should also be mentioned that the prevalence and incidence of MDD in these patients vary depending on the diagnostic criteria [4]. However, MDD is not exclusive to the population over 60 years with PD and may occur in a population under 50 years of age, as in the case of early-onset and juvenile- and young-onset PD. In this population of onset before the age of 50, a prevalence of MDD up to 45.6% has been found [5]. This psychiatric disorder can manifest at any time, from the pre-motor stage to late stages of the disease [6], and generally involves apathy, anhedonia, and somatic and neurovegetative symptoms, such as fatigue, difficulty concentrating, and insomnia. Therefore, it may be challenging to identify clinical MDD in PD patients [7].

In particular, MDD appears to be one of the most important factors impairing both the subjective and objective quality of life, independent of motor deficits. It is likely that MDD in PD is multifactorial, and the triggers include motor deficits, disability, the burden on caregivers, economic strain, cognitive impairment, and the severity of the medical illness. Therefore, there is a need to study diverse associated factors, such as age, sex, disease severity, longer disease duration, a younger PD onset age, frequent falls, lower educational level, and regular use of non-aspirin bases (NSAIDs) or analgesics [3]. Then, this disease would not be underdiagnosed and undertreated in clinical practice. The aim of this study is to describe and examine the clinical and sociodemographic factors in major depressive disorder among patients with PD in the outpatient clinic of a national neurological referral center in Mexico. Evaluating MDD and identifying the risk factors for developing MDD is important for the Mexican population.

2. Materials and Methods

2.1. Participants

We carried out a cross-sectional observational study on 100 consecutive depressed PD subjects, evaluated for the first time at the Movement Disorders outpatient clinic at the National Institute of Neurology and Neurosurgery Manuel Velasco Suarez (INNNMVS) in Mexico City, Mexico. The study followed the principles of the Declaration of Helsinki and its later amendments. The protocol was approved by the ethics committee of INNNMVS (approval number 100/11). All participants signed informed consent for inclusion in the study.

Patients were recruited from 2016 to 2018. Diagnoses of PD were established by a specialist in movement disorders (according to the UK PD Brain Bank Criteria) [8], and diagnosis of MDD was made by a neuropsychiatrist (using the Montgomery–Asberg Depression Rating Scale, MADRS) [9]. Patients were excluded when they had a diagnosis of neurological diseases other than PD, had a follow-up of abnormal movements less than 1 year in the clinic, had a diagnosis of psychiatric diseases that were previously diagnosed, took antiparkinsonian medication with an antidepressant effect, or had modifications in antiparkinsonian drugs within 4 weeks of the start of antidepressant treatment.

In addition to standard assessment, a semi-structured interview was used to obtain information on the disease history (age of onset of PD, disease duration, family history of PD, symptoms at the beginning of PD, history of chronic degenerative diseases, PD treatment, previous MDD treatment, use of antidepressants at outpatient clinics, years on PD treatment, and history of psychiatric illness) and other sociodemographic data (age, gender, marital status, education level, alcohol use, caffeine use). All patients were assessed using the MDS-UPDRS (unified Parkinson's disease rating scale) part III scale for motor symptoms (completed in the "ON" period), MADRS, mini-mental state examination (MMSE), the Montreal cognitive assessment (MoCA), and the geriatric depression scale (GDS).

2.2. Clinical Instruments for Data Collection

MDS-UPDRS part III. This scale is used for the assessment of function in PD. UPDRS part III measures motor functions. It consists of 14 items with 27 questions, each scored from 0 to 4. Total scores for the UPDRS part III range from 0 to 108, with higher scores indicating greater motor symptoms/impairment [10].

MADRS. This scale is to evaluate MDD and includes nine items that the patient rates on a scale from 0 to 6: reported sadness, inner tension, reduced sleep, reduced appetite, concentration difficulties, lassitude, inability to feel, pessimistic thoughts, and suicidal thoughts. Higher scores indicate more severe MDD, and the maximum score is 54. MADRS is especially sensitive to changes and is, therefore, suitable for measuring the effect of treatments [11]. The scale has been validated in its Spanish language version, showing good psychometric properties, similar to those of the original scales [12].

MMSE. This is the most commonly used brief cognitive tool in the assessment of a variety of cognitive disorders. The tool comprises a short battery of 20 individual tests covering 11 domains with a maximum score of 30 points. Completion time is usually 8 min in cognitively unimpaired individuals and up to 15 min in patients with dementia. However, the main psychometric issue concerns MMSE's diagnostic validity against dementia, mild cognitive impairment, and delirium. Internal consistency appears to be moderate, and the test–retest reliability is good [13]. This scale has been validated in the Mexican population [14].

MoCA. This test has been shown to be a highly effective tracking tool for discriminating between normal cognitive function and mild cognitive impairment and early onset dementia [15]. The average time taken to administer the test is ten to fifteen minutes. The main advantage of MoCA is its sensitivity in detecting mild cognitive impairment (MCI) and mild Alzheimer's disease (90% and 100%, respectively) [15]. MoCA is a valid and reliable instrument for MCI and dementia-screening in the Mexican population, even after adjusting for age and education [16].

2.3. Statistical Analysis

The descriptive statistics, including the totals, proportions, and frequencies, were obtained from the categorical and ratio variables. In addition, central tendency and dispersion measures were obtained from the numerical variables. Statistical significance was evaluated using statistical hypothesis tests, by comparing proportions for nominal variables (chi-squared), and mean-comparison tests for numerical data (Student's t-test). Subsequently, logistic regression modeling was performed when dependent variables were binary, and the odds ratio (OR) was calculated [17]. All the statistical analyses were conducted using the Stata 14® program. Values with $p < 0.05$ were taken as statistically significant.

3. Results

3.1. Clinical and Sociodemographic Variables

Table 1 shows the clinical and sociodemographic variables in our study. As regards age, the mean was 58.49 ± 11.02 years and the mean age of onset of PD was 50.66 ± 11.86 years. This neurodegenerative disease was more frequent in men (57%, $n = 57$) than in women. Education beyond high school was reported in 35% of the patients ($n = 35$), 40% ($n = 40$) were economically productive, 68% ($n = 68$) were married, 30% ($n = 30$) had a history of psychiatric illness, 66% ($n = 66$) consumed caffeine, and 15% ($n = 15$) used tobacco. Regarding the years of evolution of PD, the mean was 7.83 ± 5.33 years, 13% ($n = 13$) had a family history of PD, and 67% ($n = 67$) had no comorbidities. Regarding diabetes type 2 (T2D) and arterial hypertension (AH), 11% ($n = 11$) had both T2D and AH. The most frequent symptom at the onset of the disease was tremors (67%, $n = 67$), and the most common side of onset was the right side (57%, $n = 57$). UPDRS part III, which measures motor functions in PD, resulted in a mean score of 33.67 ± 5.67. The mean score for MADRS was 21.33 ± 5.49. For cognitive assessment, the MoCA mean score was 21.06 ± 4.65, and MMSE was 26.67 ± 1.20. For the severity of MDD in the sample, using the MADRS score, 51% (n = 51) of the patients were classified as suffering from mild MDD, 44% (n = 44) with moderate MDD, and 5% (n = 5) with severe MDD.

Table 1. Sociodemographic variables of the general sample (n = 100).

Variables	Results
Age (years, average ± SD)	58.49 ± 11.02
Age at onset of PD (years, average ± SD)	50.66 ± 11.86
Years of PD evolution (average ± SD)	7.83 ± 5.33
UPDRS III (average ± SD)	33.67 ± 5.67
MADRS (average ± SD)	21.33 ± 5.49
MoCA (average ± SD)	21.06 ± 4.65
MMSE (average ± SD)	26.67 ± 1.20
Sex	
Male, % (n)	57 (57)
Female, % (n)	43 (43)
Diagnosis	
PD, % (n)	65 (65)
Early onset PD, % (n)	23 (23)
Youth PD, % (n)	3 (3)
Family PD, % (n)	6 (6)
Not defined, % (n)	2 (2)
Presence of family history	13 (13)
PPH	
None, % (n)	67 (67)
T2D, % (n)	11 (11)
AH, % (n)	11 (11)
Other, % (n)	18 (18)
Symptoms at the beginning of the disease	
Tremor, % (n)	67 (67)
Rigidity, % (n)	24 (24)
Gait disturbances, % (n)	7 (7)
Strength disturbances, % (n)	5 (5)
Bradykinesia, % (n)	2 (2)
Side of onset of the disease	
Right, % (n)	57 (57)
Left, % (n)	40 (40)
Bilateral, % (n)	2 (2)
Education higher than high school, % (n)	35 (35)
Economically productive, % (n)	40 (40)
Married, % (n)	68 868
History of psychiatric illness, % (n)	30 (30)
Consumes caffeine, % (n)	66(66)
Consumes tobacco, % (n)	15 (15)
Severity of MDD by MADRS	
Mild, % (n)	51 (51)
Moderate, % (n)	44 (44)
Severe, % (n)	5 (5)
Cases of moderate to severe depression, % (n)	49 (49)

PD: Parkinson's disease, UPDRS III: unified Parkinson´s disease rating scale, MADRS: Montgomery–Asberg depression rating scale, MoCA: Montreal cognitive assessment, MMSE: mini mental state examination, PPH: personal pathologic history, T2D: type 2 diabetes, AH: arterial hypertension, n: number of patients, SD: standard deviation. Some items do not add up to 100% because they could have more than one of the conditions.

3.2. Medication Variables

As seen in Table 2, selective serotonin reuptake inhibitors (SSRIs) were the most frequent antidepressant treatment (69%). To treat PD, levodopa/carbidopa (80%) and pramipexole (52%) were highly used. In our study, some subjects were under treatment with dual antidepressants, as well as more than one PD medication.

Table 2. Drug variables in the general sample ($n = 100$).

Variable	% (n)
Antidepressant management	
SSRIs	69 (69)
Dual antidepressant	20 (20)
Mirtazpine	5 (5)
Tricyclic antidepressant	13 (13)
Trazodone	1 (1)
PD management	
Donepezil	1 (1)
Pramipexole	52 (52)
Galantamine	1 (1)
Bromocriptine	4 (4)
Trihexiphenidyl	2 (2)
Leflunomide	1 (1)
Rotigotine	5 (5)
Levodopa	2 (2)
Levodopa/Carbidopa	80 (80)
Levodopa/Benserazide	5 (5)
Levodopa/Carbidopa/Entacapona	13 (13)
Selegiline	7 (7)
Rasagiline	1 (1)
Amantadine	22 (22)
Biperiden	13 (13)
Propanolol	3 (3)

SSRIs: selective serotonin reuptake inhibitors, PD: Parkinson's disease, n: number of patients. Some items do not add up to 100% because they could have more than one of the conditions.

3.3. Comparison between Mild and Moderate–Severe MDD Groups

Table 3 shows the results of the comparisons between the variables of both groups. The variables that showed statistically significant differences were rigidity (12.77% vs. 36.17%, $p = 0.005$), gait disturbances (12.77% vs. 2.13%, $p = 0.023$), left side of onset (31.91% vs. 48.94%, $p = 0.037$), and MADRS score (13.43 ± 3.79 vs. 25.44 ± 5.66).

3.4. Comparison between Sexes in General Sample

Table 3 shows the results of the hypothesis tests between the variables of both groups (male–female). The clinical variables that showed statistically significant differences were the MADRS score (18.41 ± 7.29 vs. 21.31 ± 8.10, $p = 0.028$) and the MMSE score (26.22 ± 2.97 vs. 25.03 ± 3.58, $p = 0.043$).

The sociodemographic variables that showed statistically significant differences were education superior to high school (43.64% vs. 23.08% $p = 0.043$), married status (80.00% vs. 51.28%, $p = 0.002$), and tobacco use (23.64% vs. 2.56%, $p = 0.003$). When the drug variables were compared, no statistically significant differences were found between the groups.

Table 3. Comparison between sexes and severity of MDD in general sample (*n* = 100) of patients with PD and MDD (hypothesis tests).

Variable	Male (*n* = 57)	Female (*n* = 43)	$p < 0.05$	Mild MDD (*n* = 51)	M/S MDD (*n* = 49)	$p < 0.05$
Age (years, average ± SD)	58.82 ± 11.42	58.05 ± 10.71	0.365	58.57 ± 10.75	57.92 ± 11.47	0.387
Age of onset PD (years, average ± SD)	50.65 ± 12.20	50.67 ± 11.68	0.496	50.96 ± 11.41	49.6 ± 12.47	0.291
Years of evolution PD (average ± SD)	8.18 ± 4.84	7.37 ± 6.00	0.230	7.62 ± 5.00	8.31 ± 5.84	0.268
UPDRS III (average ± SD)	29.80 ± 16.37	44.00 ± 16.03	0.188	28.35 ± 14.22	33.73 ± 18.1	0.134
MADRS (average ± SD)	18.41 ± 7.29	21.31 ± 8.10	**0.028**	13.43 ± 3.79	25.44 ± 5.66	**<0.001**
MOCA (average ± SD)	21.52 ± 4.51	20.41 ± 4.91	0.122	21.4 ± 4.51	20.77 ± 4.94	0.258
MMSE (average ± SD)	26.22 ± 2.97	25.03 ± 3.58	**0.043**	25.93 ± 2.92	25.51 ± 3.63	0.281
Sex						
Male	-	-	NA	62.75 (32)	51.06 (25)	0.085
Female	-	-	NA	37.25 (19)	48.94 (24)	0.085
PPH						
Presence of family history, % (*n*)	12.73 (7)	12.82 (6)	0.403	10.64 (5)	14.89 (7)	0.281
None, % (*n*)	69.09 (39)	64.10 (28)	0.288	61.70 (31)	72.34 (35)	0.202
T2D, % (*n*)	14.55(8)	5.13 (2)	0.134	10.64 (5)	10.64 (5)	0.347
AH, % (*n*)	7.27 (4)	15.38 (7)	0.070	8.51 (4)	12.77 (6)	0.395
Other, % (*n*)	14.55(8)	23.08 (10)	0.178	23.40 (12)	12.77 (6)	0.125
Symptoms at the onset of the disease						
Tremor, % (*n*)	36 (63.64)	71.79 (31)	0.154	74.47 (37)	59.57 (29)	0.072
Rigidity, % (*n*)	11 (20.00)	30.77 (13)	0.103	12.77 (6)	36.17 (18)	**0.005**
Gait disturbances, % (*n*)	7.27 (4)	7.69 (3)	0.497	12.77 (6)	2.13 (1)	**0.023**
Strength disturbances, % (*n*)	7.27 (4)	2.56 (1)	0.143	4.26 (2)	6.38 (3)	0.332
Bradykinesia, % (*n*)	1.82 (1)	2.56 (1)	0.420	2.13 (1)	2.13 (1)	0.494
Side of onset of the disease						
Right, % (*n*)	54.55 (31)	61.54 (26)	0.292	63.83 (32)	51.06 (25)	0.087
Left, % (*n*)	41.82 (24)	38.46 (17)	0.421	31.91 (16)	48.94 (24)	**0.037**
Bilateral, % (*n*)	3.64 (2)	0.00 (0)	0.107	4.26 (2)	0.00 (0)	0.074
Sociodemographic variables						
Education higher than high school, % (*n*)	43.64 (25)	23.08 (10)	**0.043**	29.79 (15)	40.43 (20)	0.158
Economically productive, % (*n*)	38.18 (22)	43.59 (19)	0.165	46.81 (23)	34.04 (17)	0.09
Married, % (*n*)	80.00 (46)	51.28 (22)	**0.002**	68.09 (34)	68.09 (33)	0.472
History of psychiatric illness, % (*n*)	23.64 (13)	38.46 (17)	0.086	23.40 (12)	36.17 (18)	0.1
Consumes caffeine, % (*n*)	69.09 (39)	61.54 (26)	0.250	65.96 (33)	65.96 (32)	0.471
Consumes tobacco, % (*n*)	23.64 (13)	2.56 (1)	**0.003**	21.28 (11)	8.51 (4)	0.073
Severity of MDD by MADRS						
Mild, % (*n*)	56.14 (32)	44.19 (19)	0.194	-	-	NA
Moderate, % (*n*)	40.35 (23)	48.84 (21)	0.163	-	-	NA
Severe, % (*n*)	3.51 (2)	6.98 (3)	0.188	-	-	NA
Drug variables						
SSRI, % (*n*)	70.18 (40)	72.09 (31)	0.417	74.51 (38)	67.35 (33)	0.215
Dual, % (*n*)	17.54 (10)	20.93 (9)	0.335	13.73 (7)	24.49 (12)	0.085
Mirtazapine, % (*n*)	8.77 (5)	2.33 (1)	0.090	9.80 (5)	2.04 (1)	0.051
Tricyclic, % (*n*)	10.53 (6)	13.95 (6)	0.301	11.76 (6)	12.24 (6)	0.471
Trazodone, % (*n*)	0.00 (0)	2.33 (1)	0.124	1.96 (1)	0.00 (0)	0.162
Donepezil, % (*n*)	0.00 (0)	2.33 (1)	0.124	1.96 (1)	0.00 (0)	0.162
Pramipexole, % (*n*)	47.37 (27)	53.49 (23)	0.272	45.10 (23)	55.10 (27)	0.159
Galantamine, % (*n*)	0.00 (0)	2.33 (1)	0.191	0.00 (0)	2.04 (1)	0.153
Bromocriptine, % (*n*)	3.51 (2)	4.65 (2)	0.386	5.88 (3)	2.04 (1)	0.164
Trihexiphenidyl, % (*n*)	1.75 (1)	2.33 (1)	0.580	0.00 (0)	4.08 (2)	0.073
Leflunomide, % (*n*)	0.00 (0)	2.33 (1)	0.124	1.96 (1)	0.00 (0)	1.000
Rotigotine, % (*n*)	7.02 (4)	6.98 (3)	0.503	5.88 (3)	8.16 (4)	0.328
Levodopa, % (*n*)	3.51 (2)	0.00 (0)	0.215	1.96 (1)	2.04 (1)	0.489
Levodopa/Carbidopa, % (*n*)	80.70 (46)	79.07 (34)	0.420	84.31 (43)	75.51 (37)	0.136
Levodopa/Benserazide, % (*n*)	5.26 (3)	74.42 (32)	0.445	3.92 (2)	67.35 (33)	0.307
Levodopa/Carbidopa/Entacapona, % (*n*)	12.28 (7)	13.95 (6)	0.403	13.73 (7)	12.24 (6)	0.413
Selegiline, % (*n*)	3.51 (2)	13.95 (6)	0.057	5.88 (3)	10.20 (5)	0.213
Rasagiline, % (*n*)	3.51 (2)	0.00 (0)	0.107	1.96 (1)	2.04 (1)	0.489
Amantadine, % (*n*)	19.30 (11)	25.58 (11)	0.226	23.53 (12)	20.41 (10)	0.353
Biperiden, % (*n*)	15.79 (9)	9.30 (4)	0.170	13.73 (7)	12.24 (6)	0.413
Propanolol, % (*n*)	3.51 (2)	2.33 (1)	0.366	1.96 (1)	4.08 (2)	0.267

MDD: major depressive disorder, M/S: moderate to severe, PD: Parkinson's disease, UPDRS III: unified Parkinson´s disease rating scale, MADRS: Montgomery–Asberg depression rating scale, MoCA: Montreal cognitive assessment, MSSE: mini mental state examination, PPH: personal pathologic history, T2D: type 2 diabetes, AH: arterial hypertension, SSRI: selective serotonin reuptake inhibitor, SD: standard deviation. Some items do not add up to 100% because they could have more than one of the conditions. Statistically significant results are shown in bold and cursive letters.

3.5. Comparison between Onset with Tremor and Onset with Other Symptoms

Supplementary Materials Table S1 shows the results of the hypothesis tests between the variables of both groups (onset with tremor–onset with other symptom). The clinical variables that showed statistically significant differences were age (60.33 ± 11.04 vs. 54.39 ± 10.16, *p = 0.006*), age of onset (52.91 ± 12.10 vs. 45.65 ± 9.95, *p = 0.002*), and AH

(14.49% vs. 3.23%, $p = 0.044$). No other variables showed statistically significant differences between groups.

3.6. Independent Logistic Regressions for Binary Dependent Variables

In the association analysis between M/S MDD and different variables, the only variable that was associated with moderate–severe MDD was rigidity at the onset of the disease (OR = 3.75, $p = 0.013$). This association persisted when the analysis was realized by sex and was done for the male group (OR = 4.39, $p = 0.047$).

4. Discussion

The current study reported the clinical and sociodemographic factors affecting MDD among patients with PD in the outpatient clinic of a national neurological referral center in Mexico.

Traditionally, MDD has been considered a predominantly female disease, with a two-fold greater prevalence than what is found in the male population. This observation is independent of country and culture [18]. In PD, depressive symptoms are reported in approximately 20% to 30% of the patients, and being female is a risk factor for presenting these symptoms [19]. In a large study that included more than 1400 patients, MDD was more common in the female than in the male patients and was more prevalent in individuals in the advanced stages of PD and those with dementia than in the patients with less severe disease [20]. In our study, we found a male predominance of PD with MDD (57%). However, most cases of MDD in male subjects were of a mild severity (56%) compared to female cases, which were moderate to severe (49% and 7%, respectively). This means that the severity of MDD in our subjects was greater in the female population compared to the male population, although, in comparing the groups, there were no statistically significant differences between them. In a study realized by Kahlil et al. (2018), similar findings were encountered. They found a male predominance of MDD in patients with PD (71.9%) [3].

Marital status has been addressed in various studies of PD-related MDD, without finding any association between this variable and the disease [3,21,22]. In our study, we encountered no association between the severity of the MDD and marital status. In addition, there was no difference between mild MDD and the moderate/severe groups when compared. However, when the male and female groups were compared, we encountered a statistically significant difference between the groups ($p = 0.002$), with the male group having a greater predominance of married status (80%) in comparison with the female group (51%). This variable should be addressed in future studies, especially in our population, since other factors, such as life expectancy and cultural beliefs, are different from those in other countries.

Another variable that has been studied and that contributes to the multifactorial nature of MDD in PD is educational level. The evidence encountered in some studies is controversial. In a study carried out by Eydivandi et al. (2021), an association was found between higher educational level and MDD ($p < 0.05$) [23]. On the other hand, Khalil et al. [3] reported no difference when comparing the educational levels of depressed and non-depressed groups ($p = 0.134$). In addition, no association was found between educational level and MDD in PD. In another study performed recently by Lian et al. (2019), when comparing the group without MDD with the depressed group in PD, the group with MDD showed a significantly lower education level [24]. In our study, no differences were found in educational level higher than high school when comparing the groups of mild MDD and moderate to severe MDD. On the other hand, when comparing the male and female groups, we found that the male group was more likely to have been educated beyond high school in comparison with the female group (43.64% vs. 23.08%, $p = 0.043$). This difference between the sexes could be attributable to cultural beliefs among the population, which limit access to adequate education for females.

Tremor corresponds to one of the cardinal symptoms of PD (stiffness, bradykinesia, and postural instability). Tremor is commonly the first symptom to appear in PD, being found in up to 90% of the patients throughout their lives [25]. In the present study, we found that 67% of the sample ($n = 67$) started PD with tremor. When we compared the groups of patients who started with tremor and those who started with other symptoms, we found that those who started with tremor were older at the time of the study and at the onset of the disease. Some studies, when comparing groups of tremor predominance vs. other motor symptoms, have not found statistically significant differences in terms of age and age of onset of the disease [26,27]. Similarly, when we made the comparison between onset with tremor (OWT) and onset with other symptoms (OWOS), we found that the group that begins only with tremor had a greater number of patients affected with AH (14.49%, $n = 10$). Some studies have tried to find some association between AH and the risk of developing PD; however, no association has been found between hypertension and PD [28,29]. These results could be attributed to the fact that the Mexican population is different from the populations of other studies, mainly in that this population has a high prevalence in AH, so this variable could behave as a risk factor in this particular population. Given the above, it would be interesting to address this variable as a possible risk factor in the Mexican population in subsequent studies.

Among the clinical variables that have been studied for their association with MDD and PD are rigidity and gait disturbances. In a study performed by Papapetropoulos et al. (2005), MDD was associated with severity of bradykinesia and axial rigidity [30]. In addition, another study carried out by Reijnders et al. (2009) showed that non-tremor-dominant PD, which is characterized by hypokinesia, rigidity, postural instability, and gait disorder, is associated with cognitive deterioration, MDD, apathy, and hallucinations [31]. In our study, when comparing the group of mild symptoms with the moderate to severe symptoms group, a statistically significant difference was found (12.77% vs. 36.17%, $p = 0.005$) in rigidity at the onset of disease. When realizing the logistic regressions for binary dependent variables, we found an association between rigidity at the onset of disease and moderate to severe MDD (OR = 3.75, $p = 0.013$). This association persisted in the analysis when adjusted for male sex (OR = 4.39, $p = 0.047$). There was no association with moderate to severe MDD in the females. Rigidity is an important symptom to assess because it can cause long-lasting psychological effects that could worsen MDD [32]. On the other hand, there are studies that have addressed gait disturbances. In a study carried out by Kincses et al. (2017), MDD in patients with PD was associated with gait components [33]. In our study, we only found differences between the groups of mild and moderate to severe depressed patients in gait disturbances at the onset of disease, with a predominance in the first group (12.77% vs. 2.13%, $p = 0.023$). These results may be associated with greater severity of rigidity in the late stages of PD, with a chronic evolution.

The side of onset of the disease has also been studied for its association with MDD in PD. In some studies, no differences were encountered between MDD in PD and side of onset of the disease (left, right, bilateral) when compared with patients with PD and no MDD [23,34]. In our sample, when comparing the group with mild MDD with the moderate to severe MDD group, a statistically significant difference was found between the groups for the left side of the onset variable (31.91% vs. 48.94%, $p = 0.037$). This means that, in our sample patients with PD and severe to moderate MDD, the onset was predominantly on the left side.

Another variable to take into account is tobacco consumption. In our study, when the female group was compared to the male group, the consumption of tobacco was greater in the male group, with statistically significant differences (23.64% vs. 2.56%, $p = 0.003$). In a study realized by Khalil et al. (2018), no differences were found between males when comparing the group with MDD in PD with a non-depressed PD group ($p = 0.415$) [3].

As regards cognitive evaluation with MoCA and MMSE, it has been reported in the literature that patients with PD can show normal scores in MMSE while having MoCA scores compatible with MCI and cognitive impairment. In a study carried out by Vásquez et al. [35], 80% of the studied sample had MCI, with an average score in the MoCA test of 20.7. However, the average score of the sample using the MMSE test was

26.7, which means that there was no cognitive impairment represented in this score. The authors concluded that MoCA may be a good screening test for patients with PD who do not present cognitive complaints with a normal score on an MMSE test. In our study, the average score for the MoCA test was 21.33, and, for the MMSE, it was 26.67. This means that, according to the MoCA scores, the sample showed mild cognitive impairment, which contrasted with the sample's average score using MMSE, which indicated no cognitive impairment. These findings are similar to those in the above-mentioned study and must be interpreted carefully because of the influence of age and level of education on the test scores, especially in the MMSE [36]. Additionally, our sample was diagnosed with co-morbid MDD, which can worsen the cognitive symptoms that accompany PD.

Selective serotonin reuptake inhibitors have traditionally been used for the treatment of MDD due to the adequate safety profile that these drugs provide. However, these drugs can worsen tremors in up to 5% of patients with PD [37]. On the other hand, dual antidepressants for the treatment of MDD in PD are considered "clinically useful" due to their superior effect compared to placebos in clinical trials [38]. In our study, 69% of the sample was under treatment with some selective serotonin reuptake inhibitor, and 20% were under treatment with dual antidepressants. From these results, we can see the tendency in our center is to treat MDD with selective serotonin reuptake inhibitors; however, a large portion of the patients were already starting to be treated with dual antidepressants. This last population will serve as the basis for future follow-up, response to treatment, and safety profile studies. In addition to dual antidepressants and selective serotonin reuptake inhibitors, the patients were also treated with tricyclic antidepressants and mirtazapine, as well as the respective antiparkinsonic treatment, the latter being highly variable between patients. When the drugs used for both MDD and PD were compared between the sexes (male–female) and MDD severity, no statistically significant difference was found.

This study has limitations that should be mentioned, such as the sample size. It is a study with a non-probabilistic sample. Similarly, various types of PD were included in the analysis, and the sample was obtained at a third level of attention, which limits the interpretation and generalization of the outcomes. Another limitation is that the comparison analyses were carried out between the sexes and severity of MDD and there was no comparison with a control group without MDD. Clinically, anxiety was not evaluated in this study, which is a limitation since it is a frequent comorbidity that could be exacerbating depressive symptoms. Considering the average age of onset (50.66 ± 11.86) and years of evolution (7.83 ± 5.33) of the sample, we must also take as a limitation what some authors have pointed out, that there could be an overlap between PD and progressive supranuclear palsy—parkinsonism predominance (PSP-P) if only clinical criteria are considered. Due to the above, there is a possibility that some cases of PSP-P were considered as PD [39,40].

5. Conclusions

In this study, we aimed to describe the sociodemographic and clinical variables of PD patients diagnosed with MDD at the outpatient clinic of a national neurological referral center. In our results, we found that the males were more prone to MDD than the females, although the severity was found to be higher in the female Mexican population. Cognitive impairment was worse in the females. The M/S MDD prevalence was as high as 49% in the PD patients. Rigidity at the onset of the disease was the only clinical variable that was associated with M/S MDD. The differences found between the sexes, as well as between the groups by severity of MDD, can be attributed to study limitations, such as the sample size. Therefore, it would be advisable for future studies to take this into account. However, our findings are important because they can serve as a guideline for further analyses, as well as for clinicians to consider populations that may be at risk for developing MDD in the context of PD. This is aimed at improving the quality of life of these patients, as well as their long-term results in the evolution of the disease. We stress the importance of raising awareness regarding MDD in PD.

Supplementary Materials: The following are available online at https://www.mdpi.com/article/10.3390/brainsci12030326/s1, Table S1: Comparison between patients who started with tremor and those who started with another symptom (Hypothesis test).

Author Contributions: Conceptualization, R.J.-A., P.R., E.R.-S. and Á.A.R.-C.; methodology, R.J.-A., Á.A.R.-C., Y.M.A.-F., M.R.-V., D.C.-M., A.C.-A. and Ó.S.-E.; validation, Á.A.R.-C. and M.R.-V.; formal analysis, R.J.-A., E.R.-S., P.R. and Y.M.A.-F.; investigation, R.J.-A., E.R.-S., P.R., M.R.-V. and Á.A.R.-C.; resources, P.R., E.R.-S., Á.A.R.-C. and M.R.-V.; data curation, E.R.-S. and P.R.; writing—original draft preparation, R.J.-A., E.R.-S., P.R. and Á.A.R.-C.; writing—review and editing, P.R., M.R.-V., Á.A.R.-C., A.C.-A., D.C.-M. and Ó.S.-E.; supervision, P.R. and Á.A.R.-C.; project administration, E.R.-S. and P.R.; funding acquisition, E.R.-S. and P.R. All authors have read and agreed to the published version of the manuscript.

Funding: This research was partially funded by the National Council of Science and Technology of Mexico (CONACyT) SALUD-2011-1-162087.

Institutional Review Board Statement: The study was conducted in accordance with the Declaration of Helsinki and approved by the Ethics Committee of National Institute of Neurology and Neurosurgery Manuel Velasco Suárez (protocol 100/11, 7 February 2012).

Informed Consent Statement: Informed consent was obtained from all subjects involved in the study.

Data Availability Statement: The data supporting the current study are available from the corresponding author upon reasonable request.

Conflicts of Interest: The authors declare no conflict of interest. The funders had no role in the design of the study; in the collection, analyses, or interpretation of data; in the writing of the manuscript, or in the decision to publish the results.

References

1. Lee, A.; Gilbert, R.M. Epidemiology of Parkinson Disease. *Neurol. Clin.* **2016**, *34*, 955–965. [CrossRef]
2. GBD 2016 Parkinson's Disease Collaborators. Global, regional, and national burden of Parkinson's disease, 1990–2016: A systematic analysis for the Global Burden of Disease Study 2016. *Lancet Neurol.* **2021**, *17*, 939–953, Erratum in *Lancet Neurol.* **2021**, *20*, e7. [CrossRef]
3. Khalil, M.I.; Rahman, M.R.; Munira, S.; Jahan, M. Risk Factors of Major Depressive Disorder in Parkinson's Disease. *Bangladesh Med. Res. Counc. Bull.* **2018**, *44*, 9–14. [CrossRef]
4. Han, J.W.; Ahn, Y.D.; Kim, W.S.; Shin, C.M.; Jeong, S.J.; Song, Y.S.; Bae, Y.J.; Kim, J.M. Psychiatric Manifestation in Patients with Parkinson's Disease. *J. Korean Med. Sci.* **2018**, *33*, e300. [CrossRef]
5. Kukkle, P.L.; Goyal, V.; Geetha, T.S.; Mridula, K.R.; Kumar, H.; Borgohain, R.; Ramprasad, V.L. Clinical Study of 668 Indian Subjects with Juvenile, Young, and Early Onset Parkinson's Disease. *Can. J. Neurol. Sci.* **2022**, *49*, 93–101, Erratum in *Nat. Rev. Neurosci.* **2017**, *18*, 509. [CrossRef] [PubMed]
6. Schapira, A.; Chaudhuri, K.R.; Jenner, P. Non-motor features of Parkinson disease. *Nat. Rev. Neurosci.* **2017**, *18*, 435–450. [CrossRef]
7. Torbey, E.; Pachana, N.A.; Dissanayaka, N.N. Depression rating scales in Parkinson's disease: A critical review updating recent literature. *J. Affect. Disord.* **2015**, *184*, 216–224. [CrossRef]
8. Marsili, L.; Rizzo, G.; Colosimo, C. Diagnostic Criteria for Parkinson's Disease: From James Parkinson to the Concept of Prodromal Disease. *Front. Neurol.* **2018**, *9*, 156. [CrossRef]
9. Williams, J.B.; Kobak, K.A. Development and reliability of a structured interview guide for the Montgomery Asberg Depression Rating Scale (SIGMA). *Br. J. Psychiatry* **2008**, *192*, 52–58. [CrossRef]
10. Movement Disorder Society Task Force on Rating Scales for Parkinson's Disease. The Unified Parkinson's Disease Rating Scale (UPDRS): Status and recommendations. *Mov. Disord.* **2003**, *18*, 738–750. [CrossRef]
11. Wikberg, C.; Pettersson, A.; Westman, J.; Björkelund, C.; Petersson, E.L. Patients' perspectives on the use of the Montgomery-Asberg depression rating scale self-assessment version in primary care. *Scand. J. Prim. Health Care* **2016**, *34*, 434–442. [CrossRef] [PubMed]
12. Lobo, A.; Chamorro, L.; Luque, A.; Dal-Ré, R.; Badia, X.; Baró, E.; Grupo de Validación en Español de Escalas Psicométricas (GVEEP). Validation of the Spanish versions of the Montgomery-Asberg depression and Hamilton anxiety rating scales. *Med. Clin.* **2002**, *118*, 493–499. [CrossRef]
13. Mitchell, A.J. The Mini-Mental State Examination (MMSE): Update on Its Diagnostic Accuracy and Clinical Utility for Cognitive Disorders. In *Cognitive Screening Instruments*, 2nd ed.; Larner, A.J., Ed.; Springer: Cham, Switzerland, 2017; pp. 37–48. [CrossRef]
14. Beaman, S.R.D.; Beaman, P.E.; Garcia-Peña, C.; Villa, M.A.; Heres, J.; Córdova, A.; Jagger, C. Validation of a modified version of the Mini-Mental State Examination (MMSE) in Spanish. *Aging Neuropsychol. Cogn.* **2004**, *11*, 1–11. [CrossRef]

15. Pinto, T.C.C.; Machado, L.; Bulgacov, T.M.; Rodrigues-Júnior, A.L.; Costa, M.L.G.; Ximenes, R.C.C.; Sougey, E.B. Is the Montreal Cognitive Assessment (MoCA) screening superior to the Mini-Mental State Examination (MMSE) in the detection of mild cognitive impairment (MCI) and Alzheimer's Disease (AD) in the elderly? *Int. Psychogeriatr.* **2019**, *31*, 491–504. [CrossRef] [PubMed]
16. Aguilar-Navarro, S.G.; Mimenza-Alvarado, A.J.; Palacios-García, A.A.; Samudio-Cruz, A.; Gutiérrez-Gutiérrez, L.A.; Ávila-Funes, J.A. Validity and Reliability of the Spanish Version of the Montreal Cognitive Assessment (MoCA) for the Detection of Cognitive Impairment in Mexico. *Rev. Colomb. Psiquiatr.* **2018**, *47*, 237–243. [CrossRef]
17. Juul, S. *An Introduction to STATA for Health Researchers*, 1st ed.; STATA Press: College Station, TX, USA, 2006; pp. 127–130.
18. Sadock, B.J.; Sadock, V.A. *Kaplan & Sadock's Synopsis of Psychiatry: Behavioral Sciences/Clinical Psychiatry*, 10th ed.; Lippincott Williams & Wilkins Publishers: Philadelphia, PA, USA, 2007; pp. 60–83.
19. Ray, S.; Agarwal, P. Depression and Anxiety in Parkinson Disease. *Clin. Geriatr. Med.* **2020**, *36*, 93–104. [CrossRef]
20. Riedel, O.; Heuser, I.; Klotsche, J.; Dodel, R.; Wittchen, H.U.; GEPAD Study Group. Occurrence risk and structure of depression in Parkinson disease with and without dementia: Results from the GEPAD Study. *J. Geriatr. Psychiatry Neurol.* **2010**, *23*, 27–34. [CrossRef]
21. Lubomski, M.; Davis, R.L.; Sue, C.M. Depression in Parkinson's disease: Perspectives from an Australian cohort. *J. Affect. Disord.* **2020**, *277*, 1038–1044. [CrossRef]
22. Cao, Y.; Li, G.; Xue, J.; Zhang, G.; Gao, S.; Huang, Y.; Zhu, A. Depression and Related Factors in Patients with Parkinson's Disease at High Altitude. *Neuropsychiatr. Dis. Treat.* **2021**, *17*, 1353–1362. [CrossRef]
23. Pir-hayati, M.; Eydivandi, N.; Khodashenas, M.; Fallah, H. Prevalence of Depression and Anxiety and Related Factors in Patients with Parkinson's Disease: Depression and Anxiety in Parkinson's Disease. *Int. Clin. Neurosci. J.* **2021**, *8*, 85–89. [CrossRef]
24. Lian, T.H.; Guo, P.; Zuo, L.J.; Hu, Y.; Yu, S.Y.; Liu, L.; Jin, Z.; Yu, Q.J.; Wang, R.D.; Li, L.X.; et al. An Investigation on the Clinical Features and Neurochemical Changes in Parkinson's Disease with Depression. *Front. Psychiatry* **2019**, *9*, 723. [CrossRef] [PubMed]
25. Zesiewicz Theresa, A. Parkinson disease. *Contin. Lifelong Learn. Neurol.* **2019**, *25*, 896–918. [CrossRef] [PubMed]
26. Lian, T.H.; Guo, P.; Zuo, L.J.; Hu, Y.; Yu, S.Y.; Yu, Q.J.; Zhang, W. Tremor-dominant in Parkinson disease: The relevance to iron metabolism and inflammation. *Front. Neurosci.* **2019**, *13*, 255. [CrossRef] [PubMed]
27. Youn, J.; Moon, J.K.; Cho, J.W.; Oh, E.; Kim, J.S.; Jang, W.; Park, J. The characteristics of non-motor symptoms in drug-naive Parkinson's disease: Analysis between tremor dominant and non-tremor dominant subtypes. *Mov. Disord.* **2014**, *11*, e0162254. [CrossRef]
28. Morano, A.; Jiménez-Jiménez, F.J.; Molina, J.A.; Antolín, M.A. Risk-factors for Parkinson's disease: Case-control study in the province of Caceres, Spain. *Acta Neurol. Scand.* **1994**, *89*, 164–170. [CrossRef] [PubMed]
29. Simon, K.C.; Chen, H.; Schwarzschild, M.; Ascherio, A. Hypertension, hypercholesterolemia, diabetes, and risk of Parkinson disease. *Neurology* **2007**, *69*, 1688–1695. [CrossRef]
30. Papapetropoulos, S.; Ellul, J.; Argyriou, A.A.; Chroni, E.; Lekka, N.P. The effect of depression on motor function and disease severity of Parkinson's disease. *Clin. Neurol. Neurosurg.* **2006**, *108*, 465–469. [CrossRef]
31. Reijnders, J.S.; Ehrt, U.; Lousberg, R.; Aarsland, D.; Leentjens, A.F. The association between motor subtypes and psychopathology in Parkinson's disease. *Parkinsonism Relat. Disord.* **2009**, *15*, 379–382. [CrossRef]
32. Zhu, J.; Lu, L.; Pan, Y.; Shen, B.; Xu, S.; Hou, Y.; Zhang, X.; Zhang, L. Depression and associated factors in nondemented Chinese patients with Parkinson's disease. *Clin. Neurol. Neurosurg.* **2017**, *163*, 142–148. [CrossRef]
33. Kincses, P.; Kovács, N.; Karádi, K.; Feldmann, Á.; Dorn, K.; Aschermann, Z.; Komoly, S.; Szolcsányi, T.; Csathó, Á.; Kállai, J. Association of Gait Characteristics and Depression in Patients with Parkinson's Disease Assessed in Goal-Directed Locomotion Task. *Parkinsons Dis.* **2017**, *2017*, 6434689. [CrossRef]
34. Yapici Eser, H.; Bora, H.A.; Kuruoğlu, A. Depression and Parkinson disease: Prevalence, temporal relationship, and determinants. *Turk. J. Med. Sci.* **2017**, *47*, 499–503. [CrossRef] [PubMed]
35. Vásquez, K.A.; Valverde, E.M.; Aguilar, D.V.; Gabarain, H.H. Montreal Cognitive Assessment scale in patients with Parkinson Disease with normal scores in the Mini-Mental State Examination. *Dement. Neuropsychol.* **2019**, *13*, 78–81. [CrossRef] [PubMed]
36. Llamas-Velasco, S.; Llorente-Ayuso, L.; Contador, I.; Bermejo-Pareja, F. Versiones en español del Minimental State Examination (MMSE). Cuestiones para su uso en la practica clinica [Spanish versions of the Minimental State Examination (MMSE). Questions for their use in clinical practice]. *Rev. Neurol.* **2015**, *61*, 363–371. [PubMed]
37. Seppi, K.; Weintraub, D.; Coelho, M.; Perez-Lloret, S.; Fox, S.H.; Katzenschlager, R.; Hametner, E.M.; Poewe, W.; Rascol, O.; Goetz, C.G.; et al. The Movement Disorder Society Evidence-Based Medicine Review Update: Treatments for the non-motor symptoms of Parkinson's disease. *Mov. Disord.* **2011**, *26* (Suppl. S3), S42–S80. [CrossRef]
38. Seppi, K.; Ray Chaudhuri, K.; Coelho, M.; Fox, S.H.; Katzenschlager, R.; Perez Lloret, S.; Weintraub, D.; Sampaio, C.; the collaborators of the Parkinson's Disease Update on Non-Motor Symptoms Study Group on behalf of the Movement Disorders Society Evidence-Based Medicine Committee. Update on treatments for nonmotor symptoms of Parkinson's disease-an evidence-based medicine review. *Mov. Disord.* **2019**, *34*, 180–198. [CrossRef]
39. Alster, P.; Madetko, N.; Koziorowski, D.; Friedman, A. Progressive Supranuclear Palsy—Parkinsonism Predominant (PSP-P)—A Clinical Challenge at the Boundaries of PSP and Parkinson's Disease (PD). *Front. Neurol.* **2020**, *11*, 180. [CrossRef]
40. Necpál, J.; Miroslav, B.; Jeleňová, B. "Parkinson's disease" on the way to progressive supranuclear palsy: A review on PSP-parkinsonism. *Neurol. Sci.* **2021**, *42*, 4927–4936. [CrossRef]

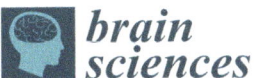

Communication

Zonisamide Ameliorates Microglial Mitochondriopathy in Parkinson's Disease Models

Satoshi Tada [1,†], Mohammed E. Choudhury [2,†], Madoka Kubo [1], Rina Ando [1], Junya Tanaka [2] and Masahiro Nagai [1,*]

1. Department of Clinical Pharmacology and Therapeutics, Ehime University Graduate School of Medicine, Toon 791-0295, Ehime, Japan; tada.satoshi.ia@ehime-u.ac.jp (S.T.); mkubo@m.ehime-u.ac.jp (M.K.); ando.rina.cn@ehime-u.ac.jp (R.A.)
2. Department of Molecular and Cellular Physiology, Graduate School of Medicine, Ehime University, Toon 791-0295, Ehime, Japan; mechoudh@m.ehime-u.ac.jp (M.E.C.); jtanaka@m.ehime-u.ac.jp (J.T.)
* Correspondence: mnagai@m.ehime-u.ac.jp; Tel.: +81-89-960-5095; Fax: +81-89-960-5938
† These authors contributed equally to this work.

Abstract: Mitochondrial dysfunction and exacerbated neuroinflammation are critical factors in the pathogenesis of both familial and non-familial forms of Parkinson's disease (PD). This study aims to understand the possible ameliorative effects of zonisamide on microglial mitochondrial dysfunction in PD. We prepared 1-methyl-4-phenyl-1,2,3,6-tetrahydropyridine and lipopolysaccharide (LPS) co-treated mouse models of PD to investigate the effects of zonisamide on mitochondrial reactive oxygen species generation in microglial cells. Consequently, we utilised a mouse BV2 cell line that is commonly used for microglial studies to determine whether zonisamide could ameliorate LPS-treated mitochondrial dysfunction in microglia. Flow cytometry assay indicated that zonisamide abolished microglial reactive oxygen species (ROS) generation in PD models. Extracellular flux assays showed that LPS exposure to BV2 cells at 1 μg/mL drastically reduced the mitochondrial oxygen consumption rate (OCR) and extracellular acidification rate (ECAR). Zonisamide overcame the inhibitory effects of LPS on mitochondrial OCR. Our present data provide novel evidence on the ameliorative effect of zonisamide against microglial mitochondrial dysfunction and support its clinical use as an antiparkinsonian drug.

Keywords: zonisamide; microglia; inflammation; mitochondria; Parkinson's disease

1. Introduction

Parkinson's disease (PD) is the second most common neurodegenerative disease, characterised by a progressive loss of dopaminergic neurones in the substantia nigra pars compacta [1]. Microglial cells are central to the pathophysiology of PD because they are potentially harmful to neurones when activated. Overwhelmed microglia can produce a range of reactive oxygen species (ROS), including nitric oxide and superoxide anions, and release proinflammatory cytokines that exacerbate dopaminergic degeneration and neurologic deficits in neurodegenerative diseases [2]. With respect to microglial phagocytosis, 1-methyl-4-phenyl-1,2,3,6-tetrahydropyridine (MPTP)-treated mice show a milieu of microglial phagocytosis, where microglia polarise and approach damaged dopaminergic neurones for phagocytosis [3]. Increased microglial phagocytosis is related to PD progression [4], and blocking microglial phagocytosis can rescue live neurones from inflammation-mediated neuronal death [5]. The expression of CD68, a microglial phagosome marker, has been found in the substantia nigra of patients with PD and PD animal models [6,7]. A recent study demonstrated that microglia depletion with CSF-1R inhibitors (GW2580) attenuated MPTP-induced dopaminergic neuronal loss and motor behavioural deficits [8]. Another study showed that a CSF-1R inhibitor (PLX3397) caused marked microglial ablation and ameliorated motor deficits in a transgenic mouse model of PD [9]. In contrast, PLX3397 exacerbates impaired motor activity, loss of dopaminergic neurones, and locomotor behavioural abnormalities [10]. In regard to microglia and inflammation, many cellular and animal studies using anti-inflammatory drugs have shown potentially ameliorative effects on PD symptoms, but their clinical use in terms of decelerating the progression of PD remains elusive [11]. Therefore, it is essential to identify a potent agent for microglial phenotype remodelling that is of important clinical use as an antiparkinsonian drug.

Zonisamide (ZNS) has beneficial effects on motor symptoms and sleep disorders in levodopa-treated patients with PD [12,13]. In our previous studies, ZNS showed an ameliorative effect against MPTP and a 6-OHDA-induced PD models of common marmosets, mice, and rats [14–17]. A recent post-mortem study on patients with PD showed that ZNS could suppress microglial Nav 1.6 [18], which has been demonstrated to be a significant contributor to microglial activation [19–21]. Additionally, ZNS improved neuropathic pain by inhibiting microglial activation in the spinal cord of a mouse model [22]. However, current studies have not revealed any evidence regarding the effects of ZNS on switching microglial functions in the milieu of PD. Therefore, we assess the effects of ZNS on mitochondrial activity using inflammatory in vivo and in vitro PD models. Considering the potential role of impaired microglial phagocytosis in the pathogenesis of PD [23], we specifically focus on the link between mitochondrial dysfunction and impaired phagocytosis in PD scenarios.

2. Materials and Methods

2.1. Animals

All experiments were performed in accordance with the guidelines of the Ethics Committee for Animal Experimentation of Ehime University, Japan. C57/BL6 mice (Clea Japan, Tokyo) were purchased, bred, and housed (4 mice/cage) at a temperature of $25 \pm 1\ °C$, with a relative humidity of $55\% \pm 5\%$, under a 12 h light (7:00–12:00)/12 h dark (19:00–7:00) cycle of automatic illumination at the Animal facility, Advanced Research Support Centre, Ehime University. For the present study, we selected mice that were 9 ± 0.5 weeks old with a body weight of 25 ± 2 g.

2.2. Cells

The murine microglial cell line BV2 and the neuronal cell line Neuro 2A were purchased from ATCC (Manassas, VA, USA). Both cell lines were maintained in DMEM (Wako, Osaka, Japan) supplemented with 10% foetal calf serum (Biowest, Nuaille, France) and antibiotics (Wako).

2.3. Flow Cytometry

For the in vivo study, mice received subcutaneous injections of MPTP (Sigma-Aldrich, St. Louis, MO, USA) and lipopolysaccharide (LPS) (Sigma-Aldrich), as described in Figure 1A. Mice were sacrificed under deep anaesthesia (CO_2 exposure, Matsuyama Nishi Sanso Company, Matsuyama, Japan), and whole brains were dissected out and subjected to flow cytometry analysis for multicolour immunofluorescence immuno-labelling (Brilliant Violet 570™ anti-mouse/human CD11b Antibody and Pacific Blue™ anti-mouse CD45 Antibody, BioLegend, San Diego, CA, USA) and mitochondrial ROS (MitoROS 520 (AAT Bioquest, Sunnyvale, CA, USA)) as described in earlier studies [24,25]. For the in vitro study, BV2 cells were exposed with or without LPS (1 µg/mL) and incubated with or without ZNS (100 µM) for 24 h. The cells were then processed for phagocytosis and mitROS assays as described in earlier studies [24,25]. The Gallios instrument (Beckman-Coulter, Brea, CA, USA) was used to perform flow cytometry of cells, and the results were analysed using FlowJo (Becton, Dickinson and Company, Franklin Lakes, NJ, USA).

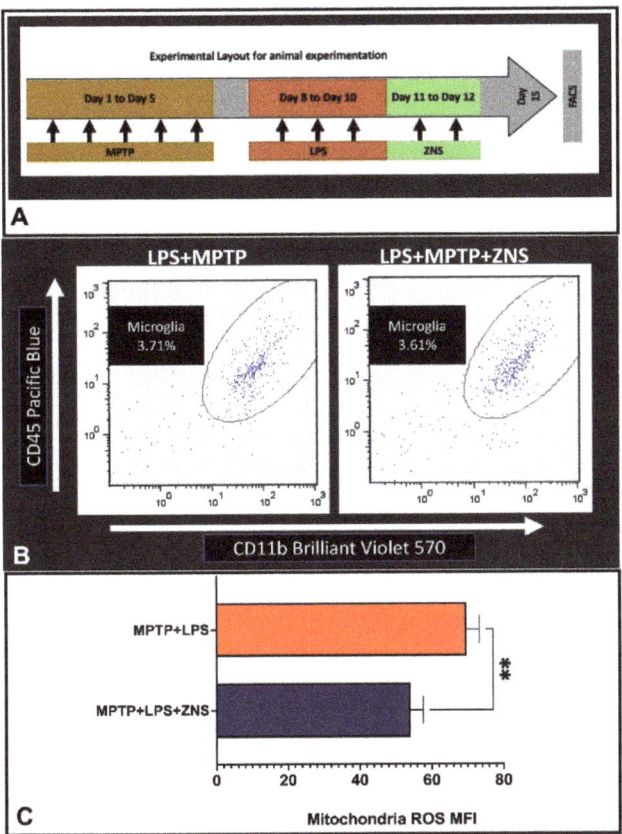

Figure 1. Effects of ZNS in MPTP and LPS-induced mice model of Parkinsonism. (**A**) Timeline of experiments. (**B**) Gating strategy and representative dot plot data where microglial cells were gated with CD45 and CD11b double-positive cells. (**C**) mitROS generation was assessed on microglia cell and presented with MFI where ZNS (40 mg/kg) suppressed microglia-derived mitROS in MPTP (25 mg/kg) and LPS (100 µg/kg) treated Parkinson's disease model mice. Data from four mice for each group were expressed as mean ± SD. Asterisks indicate ** 0.01, by student *t*-test. MPTP, 1-methyl-4-phenyl-1,2,3,6-tetrahydropyridine; LPS, lipopolysaccharide; FACS, fluorescence activated cell sorting; ZNS, zonisamide; ROS, reactive oxygen species; mitROS, mitochondrial reactive oxygen species; MFI, mean fluorescence intensity; SD, standard deviation.

2.4. Mitochondrial Bioenergetic Assay

The oxygen consumption rate (OCR) and extracellular acidification rate (ECAR) were measured to assess mitochondrial function in BV2 and Neuro 2A cells using the Seahorse XFp Extracellular Flux Analyser and XFp mito stress test kit (Agilent Technologies, Santa Clara, CA, USA), as described in an earlier study [24].

2.5. Quantitative Real-Time RT-PCR (qPCR)

Total RNA was extracted from cells using the Maxwell®® 16 Cell LEV Total RNA Purification Kit (Promega, Madison, WI, USA), and cDNA was synthesised using ReverTra Ace™ qPCR RT Master Mix with gDNA Remover (Toyobo, Osaka Japan). The cDNA samples were prepared from four separate culture samples and qPCR was performed as described before [26]. The primer sequences used in this study were purchased from (Hokkaido System Science Co., LTD, Hokkaido, Japan) and are listed as follows:

Timm23, forward (TATGGTGACTAGGCAAGGAG) and reverse (GCTACTGTGTTGAG-GTCATC); HIF-1α, forward (TAAATGTTCTGCCCACCCT) and reverse (GCGACAAAGT-GCATAAAACC); and GAPDH, forward (ACCCAGAAGACTGTGGATGG) and reverse (CACATTGGGGGTAGGAACAC).

2.6. Statistical Analysis

Data are expressed as mean ± standard deviation and were statistically analysed using Prism software (GraphPad Software, San Diego, CA, USA). Data were subjected to unpaired two-tailed *t*-tests or two ANOVA with Tukey's multiple comparison test, and significance was set at $p < 0.05$ [27].

3. Results

3.1. ZNS Inhibited mitROS Generation in the Microglia of In Vivo PD Models

Because aggravating immune responses play a central role in the pathogenesis of PD, the appropriate control of the immune system may be more important in the therapeutic view of this disease. Based on this concept, we evaluated whether ZNS induces any effects on microglial cells of a brain with PD. Considering the inflammatory features of a brain with PD, we developed a special inflammatory mouse PD model by challenging with two neurotoxins, MPTP and LPS, in which mice received MPTP for 5 days. Thereafter, these mice continued to receive LPS for 3 days (Figure 1A). Using flow cytometry, we gated microglial cells for microglial mitROS generation analysis, where ZNS exhibited suppressive effects. However, ZNS post-treatment did not significantly affect the number and morphological features, as shown by the dot plot (Figure 1B,C).

3.2. ZNS Abolished mitROS Generation and Phagocytic Activity in LPS-Treated BV2 Cells

Next, we assessed the effects of ZNS in BV2 mouse microglial cells in vitro. LPS exposure increased mitROS production and forward and side scatter values; however, when LPS was co-exposed with ZNS, the effects of LPS on mitROS were partially abolished (Figure 2B,E,F). Indeed, ZNS did not inhibit the effects of LPS on the side scatter value of BV2 cells, but it partially inhibited the effects of LPS on the forward scatter value of the cells (Figure 2G,H).

Excessive microglial phagocytosis in dopaminergic neuronal cells in the substantia nigra is considered one of the most important pathological events in PD progression. In the aspect of microglia phagocytosis, CD68 expression in brain tissues is an essential indicator of microglial phagocytosis [6]. In one of our previous studies, we showed that bromovaleryl-urea exhibited antiparkinsonian effects by inhibiting CD68 expression [23]. Similarly, another recent study demonstrated that a combined treatment of 1-deoxynojirimycin and ibuprofen decreased microglial phagocytosis and protected dopaminergic neuronal degeneration [28]. In this study, we demonstrate another antiparkinsonian feature of ZNS, which lowered the phagocytic activity of LPS-treated BV2 murine microglial cell lines (Figure 2A,C,D).

3.3. ZNS Ameliorated Mitochondrial Dysfunction of LPS-Treated BV2 Cells but Not MPP^+-Treated Neuro 2A Cells

Accumulating evidence has shown that impaired mitochondrial biogenesis is strongly linked to the pathogenesis of PD [29]. Using BV2 microglia cell lines, we prepared an in vitro PD model in which these cells were LPS-challenged. Of particular interest in this inflammatory PD model, LPS exposure decreased mitochondrial OCR and ECAR (Figure 3A). ZNS significantly prevented the development of the depressive effects of LPS on OCR (Figure 3B). Based on the effect of ZNS on BV2 cells, we extended our study to neuronal cells. In this approach, we used a murine neuronal cell line Neuro 2A, and used MPP^+ to prepare an additional in vitro cellular model of PD. Similar to LPS, MMP^+ exposure decreased mitochondrial OCR and ECAR in Neuro 2A cells (Figure 3C). However, in this case, ZNS did not exhibit any preventive effects (Figure 3D).

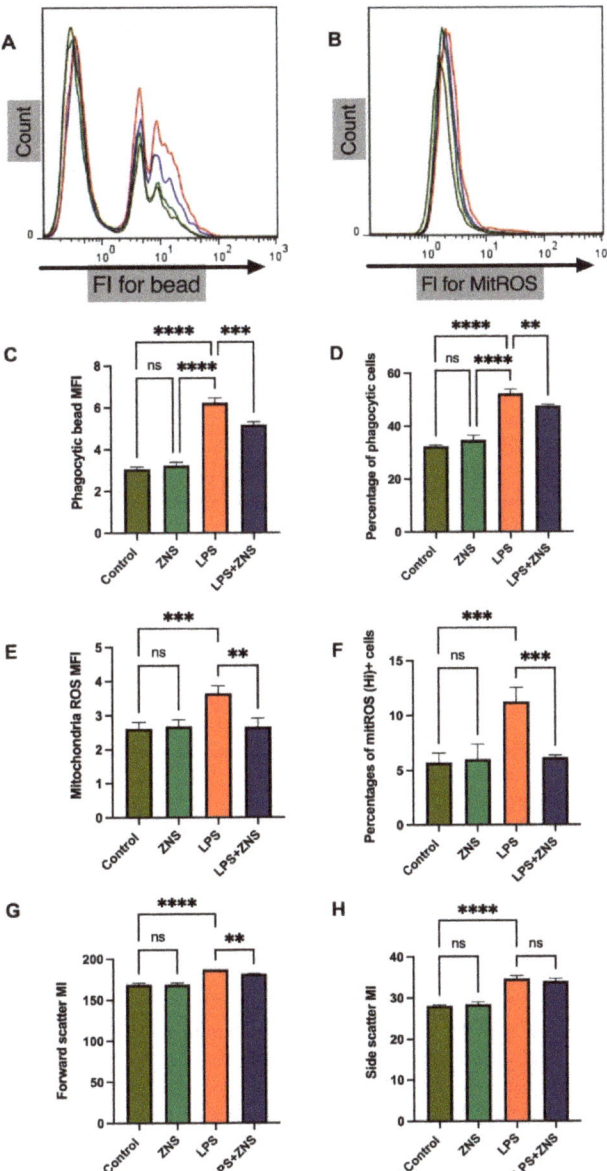

Figure 2. ZNS inhibits the phagocytic activity and mitochondrial reactive oxygen species generation of LPS-treated BV2 (murine microglial cell line). Cells were treated with or without LPS (1 μg/mL) and co-treated with or without ZNS (100 μM) overnight. (**A**) Representative histogram for phagocytic beads, (**B**) representative histogram for mitROS, (**C**) mean fluorescence intensity (MFI) for phagocytic bead, (**D**) percentages of phagocytic cells, (**E**) MFI for mitROS, (**F**) percentages of mitROS (high) positive cells, (**G**) mean intensity (MI) for forward scatter values, and (**H**) MI for side scatter values. Histogram peak colours: asparagus green for control, fern green for ZNS, maraschino red for LPS, and midnight blue for LPS + ZNS. Data are expressed as mean ± SD; (n-3). Asterisks indicate ** 0.01, *** 0.001, **** 0.0001 by two-way ANOVA. LPS, lipopolysaccharide; mitROS, mitochondrial reactive oxygen species; ZNS, zonisamide; SD, standard deviation.

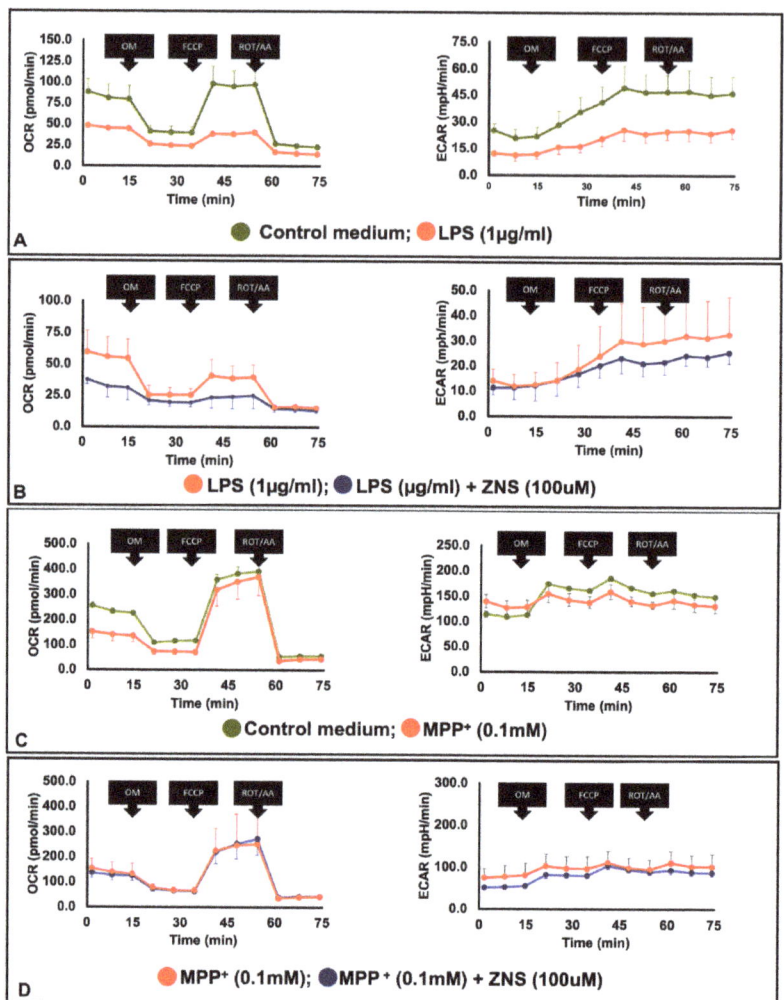

Figure 3. Ameliorative effect of ZNS on mitochondrial dysfunctions in LPS-induced in BV2 cells. (**A**) Cells were seeded in a Seahorse XF plate at 2.5×10^4 cells per well and treated with or without LPS (1 µg/mL) overnight. (**B**) Cells were treated with LPS in combination with or without ZNS overnight. (**C**) Cells were plated in a Seahorse XF plate at 2.5×10^4 cells per well and treated with or without MPP⁺ 100 µM for 1 h. (**D**) Cells were treated with MPP⁺ in combination with or without ZNS. The results are representative data from least three independent experiments. Representative bioenergetics profile data (n = 3) are shown as means ± SD, oxygen consumption rate (OCR, left) and extracellular acidification rate (ECAR, right). LPS, lipopolysaccharide; OM, oligomycin; FCCP, carbonyl cyanide-p-trifluoromethoxyphenylhydrazone; ROT/AA, rotenone and antimycin; ZNS, zonisamide; SD, standard deviation.

3.4. ZNS Reversed LPS Gene Expression in Treated BV2 Cells

Several studies have shown that the stabilisation of the hypoxia-inducible factor 1 α (HIF1α) plays a role in neuroprotection in PD brains [30]. Our qPCR data showed that treatment with LPS decreased the expression of mRNA encoding HIF1α, and ZNS partially abolished this LPS effect on BV2 cells (Figure 4A,C). Next, we assessed Timm23 mRNA expression, which has been shown to attenuate MPTP-induced denervation at the level of dopaminergic cell bodies in the substantia nigra pars compacta [31]. As shown in an endothelial cell study published earlier [32], we found that LPS treatment downregulated the expression of mRNA encoding Timm23 (Figure 4B). Similar to HIF1α, ZNS ameliorated the expression of Timm23 mRNA (Figure 4D). These data suggest that ZNS has ameliorative effects on microglial dysfunction in PD.

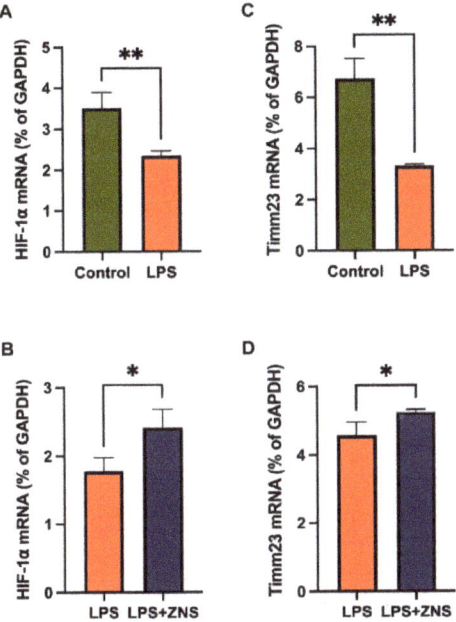

Figure 4. Ameliorative effect of ZNS on LPS-induced mitochondrial dysfunction-related genes in BV2 cells. (**A**) and (**C**) Cells were treated with or without LPS (1 μg/mL) overnight. (**B**) and (**D**) Cells were treated with LPS in combination with or without ZNS. mRNA expression of hypoxia inducible factor 1 α (HIF1α) (**A**) and (**B**), Timm23 (**C**) and (**D**). Data are expressed as mean ± SD. LPS, lipopolysaccharide; ZNS, zonisamide; SD, standard deviation. Asterisks indicate * 0.05, ** 0.01, by student *t*-test.

4. Discussion

Currently in Japan, ZNS is considered to be an adjunctive antiparkinsonian drug because of its beneficial effects on motor and sleep problems in patients with PD [13]. The antiparkinsonian effects of ZNS have been reported in our previous studies on MPTP and in a 6-OHDA-treated animal model of PD, where we found that ZNS acts as a neuroprotectant against MPTP-induced dopaminergic neuronal degeneration by acting directly on neurones and astrocytes [14–17]. In addition to our studies, several research studies published by different groups have highlighted the antiparkinsonian effects of ZNS [33]. A study showed that ZNS reduced neuroinflammation by inhibiting Nav1.6 and TNFα in microglial cells in an MPTP-treated mouse model of PD. The expression of Nav1.6 in microglial cells was found to be increased in patients with PD [18]. Microglial cells are believed to be involved in the progressive loss of dopaminergic neurones in PD through the release of potentially harmful substances. The depletion of the microglia with GW2580 (a CSF-1R inhibitor) attenuated MPTP-induced dopaminergic neuronal loss and motor behavioural deficits in a PD model [8]. We sought to determine whether ZNS has any effect on the remodelling of microglial cells in the LPS-primed MPTP murine model of PD. Our data revealed that ZNS inhibits mitROS generation by microglia in in vivo and in vitro PD models. MitROS is involved in microglial inflammatory responses by activating mitogen-activating proteins

(MAPs), as pharmacological inhibition of mitROS suppresses the activation of MAPs, NF-κB nuclear translocation, and TNFα release [34]. Related cellular and animal studies have demonstrated that NADPH oxidase is the main contributor to microglial ROS [35,36]. The glycoprotein gp91^{phox} is a critical catalytic subunit of NADPH oxidase, which modulates dopaminergic neuronal degeneration by releasing ROS and cytokines in the brain [37,38]. Increased NADPH oxidase in microglial cells has been documented in post-mortem studies, where an increased expression of gp91^{phox} has been observed [39]. Moreover, considering the inhibitory effects of ZNS on the expression of F4/80, a mature phagocytic cell marker in MPTP-treated mice [18], we identified the inhibitory effects of ZNS on the phagocytic activity of microglial cells.

In PD pathogenesis, mitochondrial dysfunction is characterised by overwhelmed oxidative stress, lack of respiratory chains, and defective mitophagy flux [40]. During inflammation, the maintenance of the normal mitochondrial function is critical for skewing from M1 type macrophages to M2 macrophages [41]. LPS is considered a potent M1 inducer, and exposure of LPS to BV2 suppressed mitochondrial bioenergetics, as revealed by the decreased OCR and ECAR. This is consistent with the findings of another study in which exposure of murine macrophages to LPS reduced both OCR and ECAR [42]. In terms of mitochondriopathy, as previously pointed out in striatal neurons, ZNS showed neuroprotective effects against mitochondrial impairment through complex I conservation [43]. In the present study, co-exposure to ZNS with LPS partially abolished the inhibitory effect of LPS on microglial OCR. However, similar to LPS-treated BV2 cells, MPP$^+$-treated Neuro 2A cells showed reduced mitochondrial OCR and EACR, but ZNS was not deemed to be effective in terms of reversing the respective MPP$^+$ effects in our present studies. A possible explanation for these apparently contradictory results could be attributed to variations in cellular models.

Patients with PD showed decreased expression of HIF1α, which is part of a highly conserved complex that governs the expression of several neuroprotective factors involved in cellular stress responses [30]. In the present study, LPS reduced the mRNA expression of HIF1α, whereas ZNS reversed this effect. The expression of another protein involved in the protein import machinery, Timm23, was found to be decreased in patients with PD, and mitochondrial complex I inhibition with MPP$^+$ also reduced the expression of Timm23 [31]. ZNS was found to be effective for mitochondrial complex I [43], and in the present study, ZNS partially reversed the mRNA expression of Timm23 in LPS-treated microglial cells.

Altogether, these findings underline the efficacy of ZNS as an antiparkinsonian drug because it was found to protect neurones in inflammatory PD brains by inhibiting mitROS generation and remodelling defective or detrimental microglia to supportive or beneficial ones. Therefore, these results suggest that ZNS may induce profound mitochondrial effects on related microglial dysfunction, and thus modify the risk of rapid PD progression.

Author Contributions: S.T. and M.K. performed the in vitro experiments and data analyses. M.E.C. conceptualised the research, directed the in vitro studies, performed in vivo experiments, and wrote the manuscript. M.K., R.A., and J.T. provided technical support. M.N. investigated the project and edited the manuscript. All authors have read and agreed to the published version of the manuscript.

Funding: This study was partly supported by Grants-in-Aid for Scientific Research from the Ministry of Education, Culture, Sports, Science and Technology of Japan (Grant-in-Aid for Scientific Research (C) to 20K06856 M.E.C).

Institutional Review Board Statement: Ethics Committee for Animal Experimentation of Ehime University, Japan (approval numbers; 05U29-2 and 05U30-2).

Acknowledgments: We are grateful to the staff of the Advanced Research Support Center (ADRES), Ehime University, for their generous support.

Conflicts of Interest: The authors declare no conflict of interest.

References

1. Emamzadeh, F.N.; Surguchov, A. Parkinson's Disease: Biomarkers, Treatment, and Risk Factors. *Front. Neurosci.* **2018**, *12*, 612. [CrossRef] [PubMed]
2. Hirsch, E.C.; Hunot, S. Neuroinflammation in Parkinson's disease: A target for neuroprotection? *Lancet Neurol.* **2009**, *8*, 382–397. [CrossRef]
3. Barcia, C.; Ros, C.M.; Annese, V.; Gomez, A.; Ros-Bernal, F.; Aguado-Llera, D.; Martinez-Pagan, M.E.; de Pablos, V.; Fernandez-Villalba, E.; Herrero, M.T. IFN-gamma signaling, with the synergistic contribution of TNF-alpha, mediates cell specific microglial and astroglial activation in experimental models of Parkinson's disease. *Cell Death Dis.* **2012**, *3*, e379. [CrossRef] [PubMed]
4. Barcia, C.; Ros, C.M.; Ros-Bernal, F.; Gomez, A.; Annese, V.; Carrillo-de Sauvage, M.A.; Yuste, J.E.; Campuzano, C.M.; de Pablos, V.; Fernandez-Villalba, E.; et al. Persistent phagocytic characteristics of microglia in the substantia nigra of long-term Parkinsonian macaques. *J. Neuroimmunol.* **2013**, *261*, 60–66. [CrossRef] [PubMed]
5. Fricker, M.; Oliva-Martin, M.J.; Brown, G.C. Primary phagocytosis of viable neurons by microglia activated with LPS or Abeta is dependent on calreticulin/LRP phagocytic signalling. *J. Neuroinflamm.* **2012**, *9*, 196. [CrossRef]
6. Aono, H.; Choudhury, M.E.; Higaki, H.; Miyanishi, K.; Kigami, Y.; Fujita, K.; Akiyama, J.I.; Takahashi, H.; Yano, H.; Kubo, M.; et al. Microglia may compensate for dopaminergic neuron loss in experimental Parkinsonism through selective elimination of glutamatergic synapses from the subthalamic nucleus. *Glia* **2017**, *65*, 1833–1847. [CrossRef]
7. Croisier, E.; Moran, L.B.; Dexter, D.T.; Pearce, R.K.; Graeber, M.B. Microglial inflammation in the parkinsonian substantia nigra: Relationship to alpha-synuclein deposition. *J. Neuroinflamm.* **2005**, *2*, 14. [CrossRef]
8. Neal, M.L.; Fleming, S.M.; Budge, K.M.; Boyle, A.M.; Kim, C.; Alam, G.; Beier, E.E.; Wu, L.J.; Richardson, J.R. Pharmacological inhibition of CSF1R by GW2580 reduces microglial proliferation and is protective against neuroinflammation and dopaminergic neurodegeneration. *FASEB J.* **2020**, *34*, 1679–1694. [CrossRef]
9. Qu, W.; Johnson, A.; Kim, J.H.; Lukowicz, A.; Svedberg, D.; Cvetanovic, M. Inhibition of colony-stimulating factor 1 receptor early in disease ameliorates motor deficits in SCA1 mice. *J. Neuroinflamm.* **2017**, *14*, 107. [CrossRef]
10. Yang, X.; Ren, H.; Wood, K.; Li, M.; Qiu, S.; Shi, F.D.; Ma, C.; Liu, Q. Depletion of microglia augments the dopaminergic neurotoxicity of MPTP. *FASEB J.* **2018**, *32*, 3336–3345. [CrossRef]
11. Hung, A.Y.; Schwarzschild, M.A. Approaches to Disease Modification for Parkinson's Disease: Clinical Trials and Lessons Learned. *Neurotherapeutics* **2020**, *17*, 1393–1405. [CrossRef] [PubMed]
12. Murata, M.; Hasegawa, K.; Kanazawa, I.; Fukasaka, J.; Kochi, K.; Shimazu, R.; The Japan Zonisamide on PD Study Group. Zonisamide improves wearing-off in Parkinson's disease: A randomized, double-blind study. *Mov. Disord.* **2015**, *30*, 1343–1350. [CrossRef] [PubMed]
13. Suzuki, K.; Fujita, H.; Matsubara, T.; Haruyama, Y.; Kadowaki, T.; Funakoshi, K.; Watanabe, Y.; Hirata, K. Zonisamide effects on sleep problems and depressive symptoms in Parkinson's disease. *Brain Behav.* **2021**, *11*, e02026. [CrossRef] [PubMed]
14. Yabe, H.; Choudhury, M.E.; Kubo, M.; Nishikawa, N.; Nagai, M.; Nomoto, M. Zonisamide increases dopamine turnover in the striatum of mice and common marmosets treated with MPTP. *J. Pharmacol. Sci.* **2009**, *110*, 64–68. [CrossRef] [PubMed]
15. Choudhury, M.E.; Moritoyo, T.; Yabe, H.; Nishikawa, N.; Nagai, M.; Kubo, M.; Matsuda, S.; Nomoto, M. Zonisamide attenuates MPTP neurotoxicity in marmosets. *J. Pharmacol. Sci.* **2010**, *114*, 298–303. [CrossRef]
16. Choudhury, M.E.; Moritoyo, T.; Kubo, M.; Kyaw, W.T.; Yabe, H.; Nishikawa, N.; Nagai, M.; Matsuda, S.; Nomoto, M. Zonisamide-induced long-lasting recovery of dopaminergic neurons from MPTP-toxicity. *Brain Res.* **2011**, *1384*, 170–178. [CrossRef]
17. Choudhury, M.E.; Sugimoto, K.; Kubo, M.; Iwaki, H.; Tsujii, T.; Kyaw, W.T.; Nishikawa, N.; Nagai, M.; Tanaka, J.; Nomoto, M. Zonisamide up-regulated the mRNAs encoding astrocytic anti-oxidative and neurotrophic factors. *Eur. J. Pharmacol.* **2012**, *689*, 72–80. [CrossRef]
18. Hossain, M.M.; Weig, B.; Reuhl, K.; Gearing, M.; Wu, L.J.; Richardson, J.R. The anti-parkinsonian drug zonisamide reduces neuroinflammation: Role of microglial Nav 1.6. *Exp. Neurol.* **2018**, *308*, 111–119. [CrossRef]
19. Black, J.A.; Liu, S.; Waxman, S.G. Sodium channel activity modulates multiple functions in microglia. *Glia* **2009**, *57*, 1072–1081. [CrossRef]
20. Hossain, M.M.; Sonsalla, P.K.; Richardson, J.R. Coordinated role of voltage-gated sodium channels and the Na^+/H^+ exchanger in sustaining microglial activation during inflammation. *Toxicol. Appl. Pharmacol.* **2013**, *273*, 355–364. [CrossRef]
21. Hossain, M.M.; Liu, J.; Richardson, J.R. Pyrethroid Insecticides Directly Activate Microglia through Interaction with Voltage-Gated Sodium Channels. *Toxicol. Sci.* **2017**, *155*, 112–123. [CrossRef] [PubMed]
22. Koshimizu, H.; Ohkawara, B.; Nakashima, H.; Ota, K.; Kanbara, S.; Inoue, T.; Tomita, H.; Sayo, A.; Kiryu-Seo, S.; Konishi, H.; et al. Zonisamide ameliorates neuropathic pain partly by suppressing microglial activation in the spinal cord in a mouse model. *Life Sci.* **2020**, *263*, 118577. [CrossRef] [PubMed]
23. Higaki, H.; Choudhury, M.E.; Kawamoto, C.; Miyamoto, K.; Islam, A.; Ishii, Y.; Miyanishi, K.; Takeda, H.; Seo, N.; Sugimoto, K.; et al. The hypnotic bromovalerylurea ameliorates 6-hydroxydopamine-induced dopaminergic neuron loss while suppressing expression of interferon regulatory factors by microglia. *Neurochem. Int.* **2016**, *99*, 158–168. [CrossRef] [PubMed]
24. Abe, N.; Choudhury, M.E.; Watanabe, M.; Kawasaki, S.; Nishihara, T.; Yano, H.; Matsumoto, S.; Kunieda, T.; Kumon, Y.; Yorozuya, T.; et al. Comparison of the detrimental features of microglia and infiltrated macrophages in traumatic brain injury: A study using a hypnotic bromovalerylurea. *Glia* **2018**, *66*, 2158–2173. [CrossRef]

25. Choudhury, M.E.; Mikami, K.; Nakanishi, Y.; Matsuura, T.; Utsunomiya, R.; Yano, H.; Kubo, M.; Ando, R.; Iwanami, J.; Yamashita, M.; et al. Insomnia and depressive behavior of MyD88-deficient mice: Relationships with altered microglial functions. *J. Neuroimmunol.* **2022**, *363*, 577794. [CrossRef]
26. Ando, R.; Choudhury, M.E.; Yamanishi, Y.; Kyaw, W.T.; Kubo, M.; Kannou, M.; Nishikawa, N.; Tanaka, J.; Nomoto, M.; Nagai, M. Modafinil alleviates levodopa-induced excessive nighttime sleepiness and restores monoaminergic systems in a nocturnal animal model of Parkinson's disease. *J. Pharmacol. Sci.* **2018**, *136*, 266–271. [CrossRef]
27. Islam, A.; Choudhury, M.E.; Kigami, Y.; Utsunomiya, R.; Matsumoto, S.; Watanabe, H.; Kumon, Y.; Kunieda, T.; Yano, H.; Tanaka, J. Sustained anti-inflammatory effects of TGF-beta1 on microglia/macrophages. *Biochim. Biophys. Acta Mol. Basis. Dis.* **2018**, *1864*, 721–734. [CrossRef]
28. Costa, T.; Fernandez-Villalba, E.; Izura, V.; Lucas-Ochoa, A.M.; Menezes-Filho, N.J.; Santana, R.C.; de Oliveira, M.D.; Araujo, F.M.; Estrada, C.; Silva, V.; et al. Combined 1-Deoxynojirimycin and Ibuprofen Treatment Decreases Microglial Activation, Phagocytosis and Dopaminergic Degeneration in MPTP-Treated Mice. *J. Neuroimmune Pharmacol.* **2021**, *16*, 390–402. [CrossRef]
29. Grunewald, A.; Kumar, K.R.; Sue, C.M. New insights into the complex role of mitochondria in Parkinson's disease. *Prog. Neurobiol.* **2019**, *177*, 73–93. [CrossRef]
30. Leston Pinilla, L.; Ugun-Klusek, A.; Rutella, S.; De Girolamo, L.A. Hypoxia Signaling in Parkinson's Disease: There Is Use in Asking "What HIF?". *Biology* **2021**, *10*, 723. [CrossRef]
31. Franco-Iborra, S.; Cuadros, T.; Parent, A.; Romero-Gimenez, J.; Vila, M.; Perier, C. Defective mitochondrial protein import contributes to complex I-induced mitochondrial dysfunction and neurodegeneration in Parkinson's disease. *Cell Death Dis.* **2018**, *9*, 1122. [CrossRef]
32. Luo, X.; Cai, S.; Li, Y.; Li, G.; Cao, Y.; Ai, C.; Gao, Y.; Li, T. Drp-1 as Potential Therapeutic Target for Lipopolysaccharide-Induced Vascular Hyperpermeability. *Oxid. Med. Cell Longev.* **2020**, *2020*, 5820245. [CrossRef] [PubMed]
33. Li, C.; Xue, L.; Liu, Y.; Yang, Z.; Chi, S.; Xie, A. Zonisamide for the Treatment of Parkinson Disease: A Current Update. *Front. Neurosci.* **2020**, *14*, 574652. [CrossRef]
34. Park, J.; Min, J.S.; Kim, B.; Chae, U.B.; Yun, J.W.; Choi, M.S.; Kong, I.K.; Chang, K.T.; Lee, D.S. Mitochondrial ROS govern the LPS-induced pro-inflammatory response in microglia cells by regulating MAPK and NF-kappaB pathways. *Neurosci. Lett.* **2015**, *584*, 191–196. [CrossRef] [PubMed]
35. Qin, L.; Liu, Y.; Wang, T.; Wei, S.J.; Block, M.L.; Wilson, B.; Liu, B.; Hong, J.S. NADPH oxidase mediates lipopolysaccharide-induced neurotoxicity and proinflammatory gene expression in activated microglia. *J. Biol. Chem.* **2004**, *279*, 1415–1421. [CrossRef] [PubMed]
36. Liu, Y.; Hao, W.; Dawson, A.; Liu, S.; Fassbender, K. Expression of amyotrophic lateral sclerosis-linked SOD1 mutant increases the neurotoxic potential of microglia via TLR2. *J. Biol. Chem.* **2009**, *284*, 3691–3699. [CrossRef]
37. Lull, M.E.; Block, M.L. Microglial activation and chronic neurodegeneration. *Neurotherapeutics* **2010**, *7*, 354–365. [CrossRef]
38. Qin, L.; Crews, F.T. NADPH oxidase and reactive oxygen species contribute to alcohol-induced microglial activation and neurodegeneration. *J. Neuroinflamm.* **2012**, *9*, 5. [CrossRef]
39. Wu, D.C.; Teismann, P.; Tieu, K.; Vila, M.; Jackson-Lewis, V.; Ischiropoulos, H.; Przedborski, S. NADPH oxidase mediates oxidative stress in the 1-methyl-4-phenyl-1,2,3,6-tetrahydropyridine model of Parkinson's disease. *Proc. Natl. Acad. Sci. USA* **2003**, *100*, 6145–6150. [CrossRef]
40. Franco-Iborra, S.; Vila, M.; Perier, C. The Parkinson Disease Mitochondrial Hypothesis: Where Are We at? *Neuroscientist* **2016**, *22*, 266–277. [CrossRef]
41. Van den Bossche, J.; Baardman, J.; Otto, N.A.; van der Velden, S.; Neele, A.E.; van den Berg, S.M.; Luque-Martin, R.; Chen, H.J.; Boshuizen, M.C.; Ahmed, M.; et al. Mitochondrial Dysfunction Prevents Repolarization of Inflammatory Macrophages. *Cell Rep.* **2016**, *17*, 684–696. [CrossRef] [PubMed]
42. Orihuela, R.; McPherson, C.A.; Harry, G.J. Microglial M1/M2 polarization and metabolic states. *Br. J. Pharmacol.* **2016**, *173*, 649–665. [CrossRef] [PubMed]
43. Costa, C.; Tozzi, A.; Luchetti, E.; Siliquini, S.; Belcastro, V.; Tantucci, M.; Picconi, B.; Ientile, R.; Calabresi, P.; Pisani, F. Electrophysiological actions of zonisamide on striatal neurons: Selective neuroprotection against complex I mitochondrial dysfunction. *Exp. Neurol.* **2010**, *221*, 217–224. [CrossRef] [PubMed]

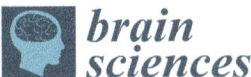

Systematic Review

Non-Immersive Virtual Reality to Improve Balance and Reduce Risk of Falls in People Diagnosed with Parkinson's Disease: A Systematic Review

Héctor García-López [1], Esteban Obrero-Gaitán [2], Adelaida María Castro-Sánchez [1], Inmaculada Carmen Lara-Palomo [1], Francisco Antonio Nieto-Escamez [3,4,*] and Irene Cortés-Pérez [2,5]

1. Department of Nursing, Physical Therapy and Medicine, University of Almeria, Road Sacramento s/n, 04120 Almeria, Spain; hector.garcia@ual.es (H.G.-L.); adelaid@ual.es (A.M.C.-S.); inma.lara.palomo@gmail.com (I.C.L.-P.)
2. Department of Health Sciences, University of Jaen, Paraje Las Lagunillas s/n, 23071 Jaen, Spain; eobrero@ujaen.es (E.O.-G.); icp00011@red.ujaen.es (I.C.-P.)
3. Department of Psychology, University of Almeria, Ctra. Sacramento s/n, 04120 Almeria, Spain
4. Center for Neuropsychological Assessment and Rehabilitation (CERNEP), Ctra. Sacramento s/n, 04120 Almeria, Spain
5. Granada Northeast Health District, Andalusian Health Service, Street San Miguel 2, 18500 Guadix, Spain
* Correspondence: pnieto@ual.es; Tel.: +34-950-214-628

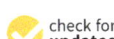

Abstract: (1) Objective: To evaluate the effectiveness of non-immersive virtual reality in reducing falls and improving balance in patients diagnosed with Parkinson's disease. (2) Methods: The following databases were searched: PUBMED, PEDro, Scielo, CINAHL, Web of Science, Dialnet, Scopus and MEDLINE. These databases were searched for randomized controlled trials published using relevant keywords in various combinations. The methodological quality of the articles was evaluated using the PEDro scale. (3) Results: A total of 10 studies with a total of 537 subjects, 58.7% of which (n = 315) were men, have been included in the review. The age of the participants in these studies ranged between 55 and 80 years. Each session lasted between 30 and 75 min, and the interventions lasted between 5 and 12 weeks. These studies showed that non-immersive virtual reality is effective in reducing the number of falls and improving both static and dynamic balance in patients diagnosed with Parkinson's disease. Results after non-immersive virtual reality intervention showed an improvement in balance and a decrease in the number and the risk of falls. However, no significant differences were found between the intervention groups and the control groups for all the included studies regarding balance. (4) Conclusions: There is evidence that non-immersive virtual reality can improve balance and reduce the risk and number of falls, being therefore beneficial for people diagnosed with Parkinson's disease.

Keywords: rehabilitation; Parkinson's disease; VR; virtual reality; non-immersive; risk of falls; balance

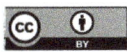

1. Introduction

Parkinson's disease (PD) is a chronic, progressive condition characterized by the loss of dopaminergic neurons located in the substantia nigra of the *Pars Compacta* (SNpc) of the midbrain, which eventually leads to depletion of the neurotransmitter dopamine in the basal ganglia [1,2]. It is considered the second most common neurodegenerative disorder, and affects 2%–3% of the population over 65 years of age [3,4]. The quality of life of patients with PD decreases considerably due to changes in both motor and non-motor functions. The resulting functional disability places a considerable physical and mental burden on family members and caregivers [5]. The clinical manifestations of PD are characterized by slow movements, resting tremor and rigidity, together with non-motor manifestations. The most common feature of PD is bradykinesia, a progressive slowness in carrying out movements, including difficulties for planning, initiating and executing tasks that require simultaneous and sequential movements, such as ambulation [6].

This leads to postural instability typical of PD, and largely contributes to the high risk of falls in PD patients [7]. Losing their ability to keep their balance while standing also undermines patients' quality of life and their functionality, and considerably increases the risk of falls [8]. As the disease progresses, PD patients lose postural stability, which in turn causes gait disorders and limitations in their basic, instrumental and advanced activities of daily living [9]. Although motor abnormalities such as resting tremor may improve with medication, other symptoms such as postural instability while standing do not respond to medication and require alternative therapeutic approaches [10].

Currently, the most widely used pharmacological treatment to manage the motor symptoms associated with PD is dopamine replacement and/or dopamine agonist therapy [11]. Treatment with L-Dopa improves patient quality of life by alleviating the motor symptoms associated with dopamine depletion [12]. However, since neuronal death continues, L-dopa must be successively up-dosed, and it usually loses its effectiveness after several years of chronic use. Chronic (5–10 years) treatment with L-Dopa also causes certain side effects, such as dyskinesia [13], hence the importance of introducing new therapeutic interventions that can diminish the impact of dyskinesia in PD [14].

Various therapies are being used as complement to pharmacological treatment in PD, such as: physical activity [15], deep brain stimulation (DBS) [16], transcranial magnetic stimulation (TMS) [17], cell replacement [18] or virtual reality therapy [19]. The latter is one of the latest techniques in the field of neurorehabilitation, ageing and disability [20].

Virtual reality (VR) is defined as a 3-dimensional (3D) computer generated environment in which the user is able to see, hear or manipulate the contents of such artificial environment [21]. The 3D environments can vary depending on their level of immersion. VR can be classified as immersive, semi-immersive and non-immersive [22]. The last two have been named "non-immersive" due to the lack of fully multisensory simulation, and the user still perceives some information from the real world [23]. Thus, in non-immersive VR systems (NIVR), subjects interact with a scenario displayed on a screen, but do not become completely immersed because they are able to perceive the real world together with the digital images. Most of these systems can use a joystick to interact with a PC or tablet [24]. Semi-immersive VR takes the subjects to a partially immersive scenario displayed on a screen, and frequently they able to interact with the digital scene through body movements. The disadvantage of this type of simulations is that users are susceptible to environmental distractions [25]. Some examples of devices used in semi-immersive VR are: Holobench, IMAX, DOMES and Inmersadesk [26].

Nevertheless, non-immersive systems traditionally have offered a number of advantages over immersive VR, such as low cost and user-friendliness, since they permit an individual to maintain contact with the real world [27].

One of the main advantages of VR systems is that they allow to develop different intervention protocols in which the therapist can change the content, duration, intensity and feedback. It is even possible to use VR technology in combination with other applications, such as brain-computer interface (BCI) technology that make possible to control avatars or objects in video games [28]. This training model is being used to promote neural reorganization and neuroplasticity, which is key during recovery from various neurological disorders, such as stroke, multiple sclerosis or infantile cerebral palsy (PCI), among others, and to improve balance and risk of falls [29].

The aim of this systematic review is to determine whether NIVR can be an effective complement to more conventional neurorehabilitation treatments in terms of improving postural stability while reducing the risk of falls in patients with PD.

The low cost and user-friendliness of non-immersive VR systems could result in a useful, and readily available tool for healthcare professionals in charge of rehabilitation of patients diagnosed with PD.

2. Materials and Methods

2.1. Study Design

This systematic review has been performed following the recommendations of the Preferred Reporting Items for Systematic Reviews and Meta-Analysis (PRISMA) (Moher, 2009) [30] and the Cochrane Handbook for Systematic Reviews of Interventions (Cumpston, 2019) [31]. The methodology of the review was registered in the International Prospective Register of Systematic Reviews (PROSPERO), under the following number: CRD42021266966 (11 August 2021). Available from: https://www.crd.york.ac.uk/prospero/display_record.php?ID=CRD42021266966.

2.2. Source Data and Search Strategy

We performed a literature search in PubMed Medline, PEDro (Physiotherapy Evidence Database), SciELO, CINAHL Complete, Web of Science, Dialnet, and Scopus between May 2021 and August 2021. We also searched the references of full text articles together with the grey literature (conference abstracts, expert papers and clinical practice guidelines) for studies published until the moment of the search. The Cochrane Collaboration PICOS strategy was used to formulate the research question [32]: Is non-immersive virtual reality an effective strategy for improving balance and reducing the number of falls in Parkinson's patients?, as shown in Table 1.

Table 1. PICOS: Participants, Interventions, Comparisons, Outcomes and Study design.

Participants	Interventions	Comparisons	Outcomes	Study Design
Patients with Parkinson's	NIVR	Fall prevention education, treadmill, conventional exercise, and sensory integration balance training	Index of falls, balance, functional mobility and motor status	Randomized clinical trials

Notes: PD = Parkinson's Disease; RVNI = non-immersive virtual reality; VR = virtual reality.

On this basis, we created a search strategy using Medline Medical Headings Subjects (MeSH) keywords, such as: "virtual reality", "virtual reality exposure therapy", "parkinson disease", "postural balance" and "accidental falls" and synonyms (entry terms). We only reviewed those articles we had access to the full text. Table 2 shows the search strategy used for each database.

Table 2. Search strategies used in each database.

Database	Search strategy
PubMed Medline	(parkinson disease[mh] OR parkinson disease[tiab] OR parkinson's disease[tiab] OR "parkinson"[tiab]) AND (virtual reality[mh] OR virtual reality[tiab] OR virtual reality exposure therapy[mh] OR "non-immersive virtual reality"[tiab] OR "Nintendo"[tiab] OR "Xbox" [tiab] OR videogam *[tiab] OR exergame *[tiab]) AND (postural balance[mh] OR postural balance[tiab] OR "balance"[tiab] OR postural control[tiab] OR accidental falls[mh] OR accidental falls[tiab] OR fall *[tiab] OR risk of fall *[tiab])
PEDro	Parkinson * virtual reality
Web of Science	TS = (Parkinson * AND (videogame * OR exergame * OR virtual reality) AND (balance or fall *))
SCOPUS	(TITLE-ABS-KEY (parkinson OR "Parkinson's disease")) AND (TITLE-ABS-KEY ("virtual reality" OR "exergames")) AND (TITLE-ABS-KEY ("balance" OR "fall"))
CINAHL	(MH "Parkinson Disease") AND ((MM "Virtual Reality Exposure Therapy") OR (MM "Virtual Reality") OR (MM "Exergames")) AND ((MM "Balance, Postural") OR (MM "Balance Training, Physical") OR (MM "Accidental Falls"))
DIALNET	Parkinson * AND ("virtual reality" OR exergame *) AND (balance OR fall *)
SciELO	Parkinson * AND ("virtual reality" OR exergame *) AND (balance OR fall *)

2.3. Study Design

We conducted a systematic review of the scientific literature by searching databases for published studies on the effectiveness of NIVR in preventing falls and improving balance in patients diagnosed with PD. This was followed by a critical analysis of the scientific literature retrieved from the literature search.

2.4. Study Screening: Inclusion and Exclusion Criteria

Three researchers performed the identification phase independently (F.A.N-E., I.C.L.-P, I.C.-P.). All studies selected by at least one of the investigators on the basis of the title and abstract were included for the final screening. Then, all the selected records were analyzed by two of these researchers. If consensus was not reached, the decision was made by a third researcher (A.M.C.-S.).

Studies included in the review had to meet the following inclusion criteria: (1) randomized clinical trial (RCT) or RCT pilot; (2) in which the effect of RVNI was analyzed; (3) compared to other interventions or simple observation; (4) on balance or risk of falls; (5) in Parkinson's patients; and (6) RCTs with a methodological quality >4 on the PEDro scale. Exclusion criteria were: (1) studies other than RCTs; (2) studies in which the sample included a range of neurological pathologies apart from Parkinson's and did not present their results disaggregated by pathology (3) single group studies.

2.5. Data Extraction

Two investigators (H.G.-L., E.O.-G.) extracted the data from the included studies, and discrepancies were resolved by consensus. Data were collected on the general characteristics of the study (authorship, year of publication, country and type of study), the characteristics of the sample (number of groups, participants per group and age of participants), the characteristics of the intervention (type of NIVR system, number of weeks, number of sessions per week, duration of each session and evaluation schedule).

2.6. Outcomes

The main outcome variables analyzed in this review were balance and risk of falls. Balance was analyzed using the Berg Balance Scale (BBS), the Activities-specific Balance and Confidence (ABC) scale, the Tinetti scale, and dynamic posturography performed using the balance master system (NeuroCom International Inc, Clackamas, OR). The risk of falls and balance confidence were analyzed using the Timed Up and Go Test (TUG) and the Functional Reach Test (FRT). These instruments have been used for such goal in previous studies [33,34]. The number of falls was also measured through self-report instruments, see Table 3.

2.7. Risk of Bias Assessment

The PEDro scale [35,36]—a checklist of 11 yes-or-no questions—was used to assess the methodological quality and risk of bias of the articles selected for the systematic review. The final score is the sum of answers 2 to 11, giving a score of between 0 and 10. A study is "excellent" if it has a score of 9–10; "good quality" if it has a score of 6 to 8 points; "moderate quality" if it scores between 4 and 5 points, and "low quality" if it scores less than 3. The eligibility criteria are not used to calculate the final score.

Table 3. Characteristics of the studies included in the systematic review.

Study	Participants (N)	Age (years)	Design	Evaluation	Outcomes	Measuring Instrument	Results
Del Din et al. (2020) [37]	128	71.68 ± 6.4	CG = 62 EG = 66	T0 = Baseline T1 = 6 wk	Number of falls	FRA	The FRA index decreased significantly in the CG and EG ($p \leq 0.035$).
Pelosin et al. (2020) [38]	24	71.9 ± 4.1	CG = 14 EG = 10	T0 = Baseline T1 = 6 w kT2 = 12 wk	Number of falls	Schedule	The EG and CG showed a significant time training interaction (F 1.33 = 7.39, $p = 0.012$). EG = TM + VR reduced the number of falls ($p < 0.001$) with respect to CG = TM.
Santos et al. (2019) [39]	45	64.3 ± 8.5	CG = 15 EG1 = 15 EG2 = 15	T0 = Baseline T1 = 8 wk	Balance Risk of falls	BBS TUG	No statistically significant differences between GG, EG1 and EG2 with respect to BBS ($p = 0.968$) and TUG ($p = 0.824$).
							Significant differences found in pre and post intervention analyses of all outcomes.
							The effect size was larger for EG2 = NW + CE in all functional tests.
Feng et al. (2019) [40]	28	66.93 ± 4.64 67.47 ± 4.79	CG = 14 EG = 14	T0 = Baseline T1 = 12 wk	Balance Risk of falls	BBS TUG	After Tx, BBS and TUG scores improved significantly in both groups ($p < 0.005$). The EG = VR showed improved performance compared to the CG = CP on BBS, TUG and Unified Parkinson's Disease Rating Scale ($p < 0.005$).
Gandolfi et al. (2017) [41]	76	69.84 ± 9.41 67.45 ± 7.18	CG = 38 EG = 38	T0 = Baseline T1 = 7 wk T2 = 11 wk	Balance Balance confidence activities Number of falls	BBS ABC Self-reported	There were significant differences between the groups, with the EG = home VR showing improvement in the BBS ($p = 0.04$).
							No significant differences between the groups for ABC and number of falls. Significant pre/post-test differences in EG = home VR with respect to the number of falls ($p = 0.034$).
Mirelman et al. (2016) [42]	130	73 ± 5 74 ± 5	CG = 64 EG = 66	T0 = Baseline T1 = 6 wk T2 = 30 wk	Number of falls	Incidence	The number of falls was lower in the EG = TM + VR than in the CG = TM in patients diagnosed with Parkinson's ($p = 0.001$).
Negrini et al. (2016) [43]	27	67 ± 9 66 ± 8	CG = 11 EG = 16	T0 = Baseline T1 = 5 wk T2 = 9 wk	Balance Risk of falls	BBS TT FRA	The post hoc analysis showed significant differences between groups in the pre-test, post-test and follow-up ($p < 0.02$) on BBS and FRA, but no significant difference between the pre-test and follow-up in the Tinetti test ($p = 0.2$) in the EG.
							No significant differences between the intervention groups ($p > 0.005$).
							The effect size was large in BBS ($d = 0.9$); moderate in TT ($d = 0.4$) and small in FRA ($d < 0.2$) after the intervention.

Table 3. Cont.

Study	Participants (N)	Age (years)	Design	Evaluation	Outcomes	Measuring Instrument	Results
Yang et al. (2016) [44]	23	72.5 ± 8.4 75.4 ± 6.3	CG = 12 EG = 11	T0 = Baseline T1 = 6 wk T2 = 8 wk	Balance Risk of falls	BBS TUG	Both groups obtained better results in relation to BBS and TUG after the intervention and at 8 weeks of follow-up ($p < 0.001$).
							No significant differences between the groups after the test and at 8 weeks of follow-up.
Lee et al. (2015) [45]	20	70.1 ± 3.3 68.4 ± 2.9	CG = 10 EG = 10	T0 = Baseline T1 = 6 wk	Balance	BBS	After 6 wk of Tx, BBS improved significantly in the EG (46.0 ± 1.3 to 48.1 ± 3.0; $p < 0.05$), but showed no significant improvement in the CG (45.0 ± 1.3 to 45.4 ± 1.5; $p > 0.05$).
Liao et al. (2015) [46]	36	64.6 ± 8.6 65.1 ± 6.7 67.3 ± 7.1	CG = 12 EG1 = 12 EG2 = 12	T0 = Baseline T1 = 6 wk T2 = 10 wk	Dynamic balance Sensory organization Risk of falls Number of falls	MV/SOT TUG FES-I	EG1 and EG2 showed significant improvements in MV/SOT compared to the CG after treatment and at 1 month of follow-up ($p < 0.001$).
							EG1 and EG2 showed significant improvements compared to the CG relative to follow-up ($p < 0.001$).
							No significant differences between EG1 and EG2 relative to FES-I.
							EG2 showed significant improvements in SOT, TUG, FES-I with respect to CG.

ABC = Activities-specific Balance Confidence Scale; BBS = Berg balance scale; CE = Conventional exercise; CG = Control group; CP = Conventional physiotherapy; EG = Experimental group; FES = Functional electrical stimulation; FES-I = Falls Efficacy Scale; FPE = Fall prevention education; FRA = fall rates relative to activity exposure index; HE = Healthy elderly patients; HT = Home training; IF = Idiopathic falls; MCI = Mild cognitive impairment; MV = Dynamic balance test; NDT = Neurodevelopmental treatment; NW = Nintendo Wii Fit; OA = Osteoarthritis; TM = Treadmill; TT = Tinetti Test; TUG = Timed Up and Go; Tx = Treatment; SIBT = Sensory Integration Balance Training; SOT = Sensory organization test; VR = virtual reality; WK = Weeks.

3. Results

3.1. Search Results

The initial search identified 609 potential articles (PubMed Medline, 130; Web of Science, 266; PEDro, 33; SCOPUS, 152; CINAHL, 18; SciELO, 7; Dialnet, 3), of which 278 were duplicates and therefore excluded, leaving 331 articles to review in full text. After reviewing the abstract, 270 articles were excluded, leaving 61 articles to be evaluated in full text due to their eligibility; 51 articles were excluded for the following reasons: different to RCT (13); does not use NIVR systems (17); and balance or risk of falls are not analyzed (21). Therefore, 10 studies were included in the systematic review. Figure 1 shows the PRISMA flow diagram with the different phases of the review [30] (eligibility and data synthesis. PRISMA flow diagram).

3.2. Characteristics of the Included Studies

A total of 537 participants were included in the 10 studies reviewed. The mean age of participants was 69 years; and there were 51 dropouts. Participants dropped out or were withdrawn for the following reasons: change in treatment; loss of interest or low motivation; personal reasons and adverse events; medical reasons; difficulty in travelling to the study site; and non-compliance with the treatment protocol. The mean number of participants in the intervention group after randomization was 28 subjects diagnosed with PD, with a range of between 10 and 66 subjects; three studies had more than 30 subjects in the intervention group [37,41,42].

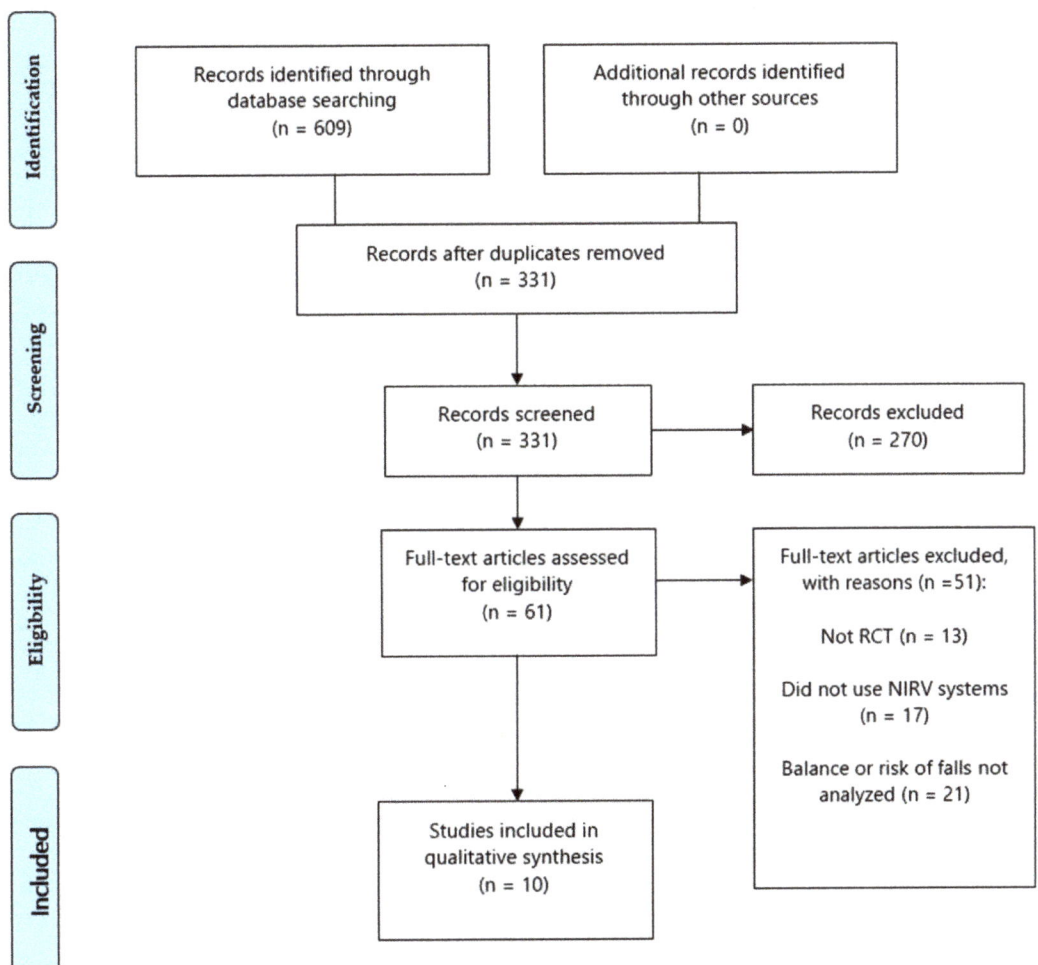

Figure 1. Eligibility and data synthesis: PRISMA flow diagram.

The NIVR rehabilitation protocols differed in terms of the device used, the time per session and frequency of treatment, and the duration of the intervention. The devices used were Nintendo Wii Fit [39–41,43,45,46], modified Microsoft Kinect connected to a large screen [37,38,42] and a custom-created non-immersive VR system consisting of a 22-inch touch screen and a balance board [44]. In one study, the frequency of treatment differed between the groups (twice a week for controls and three times a week for the experimental group) [43]; however, in the remaining nine studies [37–42,44–46] the average frequency of treatment was three times per week (range three to five times per week). The average session time using NIVR was 53.5 min (range 30–75 min). Table 4 summarizes interventions characteristics of the revised studies.

Table 4. Characteristics of interventions used in the included studies.

Study	Intervention	Type of NIVR	Time per Session	Frequency	Duration of Treatment
Del Din et al. (2020) [37]	CG = TM EG = TM + NIVR	Large screen Modified Microsoft Kinect	40 min	3/wk	6 wk
Pelosin et al. (2020) [38]	CG = TM EG = TM + NIVR	Large screen Modified Microsoft Kinect	45 min	3/wk	6 wk
Santos et al. (2019) [39]	CG = CE EG1 = NIVR EG2 = NIVR + CE	Nintendo Wii Fit	50 min	2/wk	8 wk
Feng et al. (2019) [40]	CG = CP EG = NIVR	Nintendo Wii Fit	45 min	5/wk	12 wk
Gandolfi et al. (2017) [41]	CG = clinical SIBT EG = home NIVR	Nintendo Wii Fit	50 min	3/wk	7 wk
Mirelman et al. (2016) [42]	CG = TM EG = TM + NIVR	Large screen Modified Microsoft Kinect	45 min	3/wk	6 wk
Negrini et al. (2016) [43]	CG = NIVR 10 ss EG = NIVR 15 ss	Nintendo Wii Fit	30 min	CG = 2/wk EG = 3/wk	5 wk
Yang et al. (2016) [44]	CG = CE EG = home NIVR	Touch screen Virtual balance training system	50 min	2/wk	6 wk
Lee et al. (2015) [45]	CG = NDT + FES EG = NDT + FES + NIVR	Nintendo Wii Fit	45 min 75 min	5/wk	6 wk
Liao et al. (2015) [46]	CG = FPE EG1 = CE + TM EG2 = NIVR + TM	Nintendo Wii Fit	60 min	2/wk	6 wk

ABC = Activities-specific Balance Confidence Scale; BBS = Berg balance scale; CE = Conventional exercise; CG = Control group; CP = Conventional physiotherapy; EG = Experimental group; FES = Functional electrical stimulation; FES-I = Falls Efficacy Scale; FPE = Fall prevention education; FRA = fall rates relative to activity exposure index; HE = Healthy elderly patients; HT = Home training; IF = Idiopathic falls; MCI = Mild cognitive impairment; MV = Dynamic balance test; NDT = Neurodevelopmental treatment; NW = Nintendo Wii Fit; OA = Osteoarthritis; TM = Treadmill; TT = Tinetti Test; TUG = Timed Up and Go; Tx = Treatment; SIBT = Sensory Integration Balance Training; SOT = Sensory organization test; VR = virtual reality; WK = Weeks.

In the experimental groups, NIVR consisted of a combination of treadmill training [37,38,42,46], conventional exercise programs [39], neurodevelopmental exercises [45] and functional electrical stimulation [45]. Treatment was carried out at home [41,44], and using NIVR alone [40,43]. In two studies, the NIVR program was applied at home [41,44], and in the remaining studies it took place in a clinical and experimental setting [37–40,42,43,45,46]. Several outcome measures were used to assess the efficacy of NIVR rehabilitation in the management of patients with PD. In five studies, the outcome measure was the number of falls [37,38,41,42,46]. There were significant differences in the number of patient-reported falls between the intervention and control groups in three of these studies [38,42,46].

3.3. Methodological Quality of Included Studies

The 10 studies [37–46] included in this systematic review were assessed for their methodological quality and risk of bias using the PEDro scale [35,36], as described in Table 5. The methodological quality of the included studies ranged from 4 to 8 on a scale of 11; criterion 1 of illegibility was not considered for the total score. The mean score was 6.1, which shows good overall methodological quality. No article showed low methodological quality, three studies were of moderate methodological quality [37,38,45], seven were moderate to high [39–44,46], and none was rated excellent.

Table 5. Assessment of methodological quality and risk of bias on the PEDro scale [35,36].

Study	Criterion											Total Score
	1	2	3	4	5	6	7	8	9	10	11	
Del Din et al. (2020) [37]	NO	YES	NO	YES	NO	NO	NO	NO	YES	YES	YES	5
Pelosin et al. (2020) [38]	YES	YES	YES	NO	NO	NO	YES	NO	NO	YES	NO	4
Santos et al. (2019) [39]	YES	YES	NO	YES	NO	NO	YES	YES	YES	YES	YES	7
Feng et al. (2019) [40]	YES	YES	NO	YES	NO	NO	YES	YES	YES	YES	YES	7
Gandolfi et al. (2017) [41]	YES	YES	NO	YES	NO	NO	YES	YES	NO	YES	YES	6
Mirelman et al. (2016) [42]	YES	YES	YES	YES	NO	NO	YES	YES	YES	YES	YES	8
Negrini et al. (2016) [43]	YES	NO	NO	NO	NO	YES	YES	YES	YES	YES	YES	6
Yang et al. (2016) [44]	YES	YES	NO	YES	NO	NO	YES	YES	YES	YES	YES	7
Lee et al. (2015) [45]	NO	YES	NO	YES	NO	NO	NO	NO	NO	YES	YES	4
Liao et al. (2015) [46]	YES	YES	YES	YES	NO	NO	YES	YES	NO	YES	YES	7

Data extracted from PEDro database. Criteria: 1, Eligibility criteria were specified (not used for score); 2, Subjects were randomly allocated to groups; 3, Allocation was concealed; 4, Groups were similar at baseline regarding the most important prognostic indicators; 5, There was blinding of all subjects; 6, There was blinding of all therapists who administered the therapy; 7, There was blinding of all assessors who measured at least one key outcome; 8, Measures of at least one key outcome were obtained from more than 85% of the subjects initially allocated to groups; 9, All subjects for whom outcome measures were available received the treatment or control condition as allocated or, where this was not the case, data for at least one key outcome was analyzed by 'intention-to-treat'; 10, The results of between-group statistical comparisons were reported for at least one key outcome; 11, The study provides both point measures and measures of variability for at least one key outcome). Yes criteria met; No: criteria not met.

3.4. Results of the Included Studies

3.4.1. Balance

Balance was analyzed using different scales in seven of the 10 studies [39–41,43–46]. The BBS was used to assess the static and dynamic balance skills of patients diagnosed with PD [39–41,43–45], the ABC scale was used to assess balance confidence in specific activities [41], one study used the Tinetti scale to assess balance and gait [43], and finally, one study tested sensory organization and dynamic balance using a dynamic posturography system called the Balance Master (NeuroCom International Inc., Clackamas, OR, USA) [46]. Three of the studies analyzed found no significant differences in balance between the intervention groups and the control group. [39,43,44].

Yang et al. [44] reported an improvement in balance in the group performing home NIVR compared to the group performing a traditional physical therapy program. This is consistent with the findings of Gandolfi et al., [41] who observed significantly greater improvement in the home NIVR group versus the group receiving sensory integration balance training.

After six weeks of treatment, Lee et al. [45] found significant improvement in balance in the group undergoing NIVR in combination with neurodevelopment therapy and functional electrical stimulation. In contrast, the control group that underwent combined neurodevelopmental therapy and functional electrical stimulation showed no statistically significant improvements.

Liao et al. [46] performed a study with three intervention groups. The experimental groups performed a conventional exercise program combined with treadmill training or NIVR combined with treadmill training, and were compared to a control group who only received a fall prevention educational program. The authors found significant differences between the experimental groups and the control group in terms of dynamic balance and sensory organization (evaluated using a clinical posturology instrument).

3.4.2. Risk of Falls

Pelosin et al., [38] similar to Mirelman et al., [42] reported an improvement in the number of falls in the experimental group after NIVR treatment combined with treadmill training compared to the treadmill-only group.

In a study with three intervention groups, Liao et al. [46] observed an improvement in the number of falls in the group performing NIVR in combination with treadmill training compared with the control group, which only received fall prevention education. However, they found no difference between the group performing NIVR combined with treadmill training and the group performing conventional exercises plus treadmill training.

Five studies [39,40,43,44,46] evaluated the risk of falls using the TUG test [39,40,44,46] and the functional range of motion test [43]. In three of these studies, the authors observed no significant differences in the risk of falls between the intervention and control groups [39,43,44].

Feng et al. [40] found significant differences between the intervention group performing NIVR compared to a traditional physiotherapy program.

Liao et al. [46] observed that the risk of falls in the group performing NIVR combined with treadmill training improved with respect to the control group receiving fall prevention education.

4. Discussion

Parkinson's disease is a movement disorder characterized by disordered communication between the visual, vestibular, and proprioceptive systems. Posture deficits are also frequently observed in these patients. Postural stability is known to depend on good coordination between the visual, vestibular and proprioceptive systems [47].

Since PD is a chronic progressive disease, rehabilitation is a long process that requires patient cooperation. One of the advantages of VR in the rehabilitation of PD patients is that it maintains patient motivation, resulting in a useful tool for long-term treatments and to maintain gait and postural performance in PD patients.

The present work has analyzed 10 CRT studies evaluating the effectiveness of NIVR as intervention strategy for risk of falls and balance rehabilitation in PD patients. The quality of these studies has been positively rated according to PEDro and comprised a total sample of 537 PD patients. Additionally, less than 10% of participants dropped out in the original studies, which can be considered a positive result regarding the adherence to the treatment. Despite the different approaches to NIVR described in the revised studies, this technique was found to be effective in improving static and dynamic balance in patients with PD, and for reducing the rate and risk of falls. The variety of approaches reported in the studies reviewed also illustrates the nature and diversity of NIVR procedures used in the treatment of this population and, therefore, supports the clinical validity of our findings.

NIVR has been shown to be more effective than conventional physical therapy for balance and gait rehabilitation in PD patients [40]. The authors referred that visual feedback from virtual activities is a relevant factor for PD patients during the rehabilitation process. Moreover, it has also been observed that NIVR combined with other therapeutic tools, such as treadmill training [37,38,42,46], conventional exercise [39] or functional electrical stimulation along with neurodevelopmental treatment [45], significantly improved balance and reduced falls in PD patients. In the same line, patients following NIVR programs at home have also shown an improvement in static and dynamic postural control, balance and walking function [41,44], showing that home-based VR might be a viable option for PD balance training.

Of the 10 studies included in this review, only Negrini et al. [43] used NIVR in both treatment groups, with 10 sessions in the control group and 15 in the experimental groups. These authors found significant differences in balance and fall rates between groups, but no significant differences in Tinetti test results.

The mean duration of NIVR treatment was 6.8 weeks (range 5 to 12 weeks), with between two to five sessions per week [37–46]. PD patients received an average of 25 NIVR sessions [37–46]. However, this treatment intensity places a considerable burden on financial and human resources.

The physiotherapy evidence database PEDro scores for 7 of the 10 articles included ranged from 6 to 8, indicating that they are of moderate to high methodological quality [39–44,46]; the remaining three studies were of moderate methodological quality [37,38,45].

Some authors have found that VR helps PD patients adjust segmental trunk alignment [40], while others have reported that VR games can also improve the patient's standing stability by improving organization and integration within the vestibular system [48]. Thus, VR games provide dynamic and static posture control activities that help PD patients improve control of their trunk and center of gravity, which in turn allows them to adjust their segmental trunk alignment. Visual feedback in VR games, therefore, allows patients to sense their own position and direction of movement in space based on visual tracking and to coordinate their body position. Some authors claims that multisensory perceptual feedback in VR rehabilitation promotes neural networking in cortical and subcortical areas of the brain [49]. Neuroimaging studies have shown that virtual motion can activate motion-related areas in the brain, a finding that supports its role in rewiring and reorganizing the affected brain circuits [50]. Thus, VR combined with immediate multisensory feedback facilitates task repetition and drives neural changes in the corresponding cortex. This reduces the fear of falling, and transfers this confidence into the real world through motor learning [51]. Amirthalingam et al. [52] recently suggested that task repetition using VR increases neural plasticity in both post-stroke patients and patients diagnosed with Parkinson's disease

It is imperative to mention that studies included in this review present several weaknesses and methodological limitations. The first concern is the reduced sample size, ranging between 20 and 130 patients. In addition, the method used to determine the sample size was not reported in some studies, thus limiting the external validity of their findings. In all but one of the studies, the treating therapists were not blinded [43]. In two studies, there was no confirmation that assessors measuring at least one of the key outcomes had been blinded [37,45], and there was no mention of patient blinding in any of the studies [37–46].

Although these shortcomings may have increased the risk of bias in these studies, it may not be feasible to blind participants or therapists in a clinical trial using this treatment tool. Furthermore, some important outcomes, such as balance or the number of falls, were not evaluated in all the studies reviewed.

We believe that more research is needed to evaluate the effectiveness of NIVR on these treatment outcomes in patients with PD. This systematic review also has certain limitations. We only included studies published in English; therefore, we cannot be sure that relevant scientific literature published in different languages was not overlooked. Furthermore, as we only included studies we had full access, relevant information about the effectiveness of NIVR in PD patients may have been overlooked. To the best of our knowledge, this is the first review of scientific evidence on the effectiveness of NIVR as a tool for improving balance and reducing the number and risk of falls in patients diagnosed with EP. Professionals in the field of neurorehabilitation should be aware of the outcomes achieved with NIVR devices in the treatment of PD, since evidence has shown that it can be a valuable tool in the context of rehabilitation programs. Thus, NIVR alone has shown to be more efficient than traditional intervention programs [40]. Additionally, NIVR increases the effectiveness of other therapies such as treadmill training [37,38,42,46], exercises programs [39,44] or functional electrical stimulation [45] producing a larger effect on the risk of falls and balance compared to their application alone.

5. Conclusions

The studies analyzed show that NIVR-based therapy programs lasting between 6 and 12 weeks can significantly reduce the number of falls in PD patients. Although the mixed results reported in these studies show that there is no clear evidence about the superiority of NIVR over other therapies, such as exercise programs or conventional physiotherapy.

NIVR combined with treadmill training has proven more effective than NIVR alone.

Home NIVR rehabilitation programs have shown to be effective in preventing falls and improving balance in PD patients.

Nevertheless, future studies about NIVR programs should be conducted in larger and more homogeneous samples. Moreover, studying patients following NIVR programs in isolation would help determine the effectiveness of this therapeutic approach. In the same line, the most efficient intervention protocol using NIVR should be defined, also comparing the effectiveness of different NIVR tools. Moreover, it will be fundamental that control protocols are carried out in a more homogeneous way and defined with more detail.

Author Contributions: Conceptualization, H.G.-L., F.A.N.-E. and I.C.L.-P.; methodology, H.G.-L. and E.O.-G.; data curation, H.G.-L., E.O.-G., A.M.C.-S., I.C.L.-P., F.A.N.-E. and I.C.-P.; writing—original draft preparation, H.G.-L.; writing—review and editing, H.G.-L., E.O.-G., A.M.C.-S., I.C.L.-P., F.A.N.-E. and I.C.-P.; supervision, F.A.N.-E. and E.O.-G. All authors have read and agreed to the published version of the manuscript.

Funding: This research received no external funding.

Institutional Review Board Statement: Not applicable.

Informed Consent Statement: Not applicable.

Data Availability Statement: All available data can be obtained by contacting the corresponding author.

Conflicts of Interest: The authors declare no conflict of interest.

References

1. Pringsheim, T.; Jette, N.; Frolkis, A.; Steeves, T.D. The prevalence of Parkinson's disease: A systematic review and meta-analysis. *Mov. Disord.* **2014**, *29*, 1583–1590. [CrossRef] [PubMed]
2. Berg, D.; Postuma, R.B.; Bloem, B.; Chan, P.; Dubois, B.; Gasser, T.; Goetz, C.G.; Halliday, G.; Hardy, J.; Lang, A.; et al. Time to redefine PD? Introductory statement of the MDS Task Force on the definition of Parkinson's disease. *Mov. Disord.* **2014**, *29*, 454–462. [CrossRef]
3. Poewe, W.; Seppi, K.; Tanner, C.M.; Halliday, G.M.; Brundin, P.; Volkmann, J.; Schrag, A.E.; Lang, A.E. Parkinson disease. *Nat. Rev. Dis. Prim.* **2017**, *3*, 17013. [CrossRef] [PubMed]
4. Marras, C.; Beck, J.C.; Bower, J.H.; Roberts, E.; Ritz, B.; Ross, G.W.; Abbott, R.D.; Savica, R.; Eeden, S.K.V.D.; Willis, A.W.; et al. Prevalence of Parkinson's disease across North America. *NPJ Park. Dis.* **2018**, *4*, 21. [CrossRef]
5. Crespo-Burillo, J.; Rivero-Celada, D.; Cabezón, A.S.-D.; Casado-Pellejero, J.; Alberdi-Viñas, J.; Alarcia-Alejos, R. Influencia de la estimulación cerebral profunda en la carga de cuidadores de pacientes con enfermedad de Parkinson. *Neurología* **2018**, *33*, 154–159. [CrossRef] [PubMed]
6. Vu, T.C.; Nutt, J.G.; Holford, N.H.G. Progression of motor and nonmotor features of Parkinson's disease and their response to treatment. *Br. J. Clin. Pharmacol.* **2012**, *74*, 267–283. [CrossRef] [PubMed]
7. Winser, S.J.; Kannan, P.; Bello, U.M.; Whitney, S.L. Measures of balance and falls risk prediction in people with Parkinson's disease: A systematic review of psychometric properties. *Clin. Rehabil.* **2019**, *33*, 1949–1962. [CrossRef] [PubMed]
8. Bloem, B.R.; Grimbergen, Y.A.M.; Cramer, M.; Willemsen, M.; Zwinderman, A.H. Prospective assessment of falls in Parkinson's disease. *J. Neurol.* **2001**, *248*, 950–958. [CrossRef] [PubMed]
9. Willemsen, M.D.; Grimbergen, Y.A.; Slabbekoorn, M.; Bloem, B.R. Falling in Parkinson disease: More often due to postural instability than to environmental factors. *Ned. Tijdschr. Geneeskd.* **2000**, *144*, 2309–2314. [PubMed]
10. Tomlinson, C.L.; Patel, S.; Meek, C.; Herd, C.; Clarke, C.; Stowe, R.; Shah, L.; Sackley, C.; Deane, K.; Wheatley, K.; et al. Physiotherapy intervention in Parkinson's disease: Systematic review and meta-analysis. *BMJ* **2012**, *345*, e5004. [CrossRef]
11. Obeso, A.J.; Oroz, M.C.R.; Goetz, C.G.; Marin, C.; Kordower, J.H.; Rodriguez, M.; Hirsch, E.; Farrer, M.; Schapira, A.; Halliday, G. Missing pieces in the Parkinson's disease puzzle. *Nat. Med.* **2010**, *16*, 653–661. [CrossRef] [PubMed]
12. Manson, A.; Stirpe, P.; Schrag, A. Levodopa-induced-dyskinesias clinical features, incidence, risk factors, management and impact on quality of life. *J. Park. Dis.* **2012**, *2*, 189–198. [CrossRef] [PubMed]
13. Ahlskog, J.E.; Muenter, M.D. Frequency of levodopa-related dyskinesias and motor fluctuations as estimated from the cumulative literature. *Mov. Disord.* **2001**, *16*, 448–458. [CrossRef]
14. Heumann, R.; Moratalla, R.; Herrero, M.T.; Chakrabarty, K.; Drucker-Colín, R.; Garcia-Montes, J.R.; Simola, N.; Morelli, M. Dyskinesia in Parkinson's disease: Mechanisms and current non-pharmacological interventions. *J. Neurochem.* **2014**, *130*, 472–489. [CrossRef]
15. Xu, X.; Fu, Z.; Le, W. Exercise and Parkinson's disease. *Int. Rev. Neurobiol.* **2019**, *147*, 45–74. [CrossRef] [PubMed]
16. Swann, N.C.; De Hemptinne, C.; Thompson, M.C.; Miocinovic, S.; Miller, A.M.; Gilron, R.; Ostrem, J.L.; Chizeck, H.J.; Starr, P.A. Adaptive deep brain stimulation for Parkinson's disease using motor cortex sensing. *J. Neural Eng.* **2018**, *15*, 046006. [CrossRef] [PubMed]
17. Elahi, B.; Chen, R.; Elahi, B. Effect of transcranial magnetic stimulation on Parkinson motor function-Systematic review of controlled clinical trials. *Mov. Disord.* **2008**, *24*, 357–363. [CrossRef]
18. Lindvall, O. Treatment of Parkinson's disease using cell transplantation. *Philos. Trans. R. Soc. B Biol. Sci.* **2015**, *370*, 20140370. [CrossRef] [PubMed]
19. Tuena, C.; Pedroli, E.; Trimarchi, P.D.; Gallucci, A.; Chiappini, M.; Goulene, K.; Gaggioli, A.; Riva, G.; Lattanzio, F.; Giunco, F.; et al. Usability issues of clinical and research applications of virtual reality in older people: A systematic review. *Front. Hum. Neurosci.* **2020**, *14*, 93. [CrossRef] [PubMed]
20. Lange, B.; Requejo, P.; Flynn, S.; Rizzo, A.; Valero-Cuevas, F.; Baker, L.; Winstein, C. The potential of virtual reality and gaming to assist successful aging with disability. *Phys. Med. Rehabil. Clin. N. Am.* **2010**, *21*, 339–356. [CrossRef] [PubMed]

21. Bohil, C.; Alicea, B.; Biocca, F.A. Virtual reality in neuroscience research and therapy. *Nat. Rev. Neurosci.* **2011**, *12*, 752–762. [CrossRef]
22. Mujber, T.; Szecsi, T.; Hashmi, M. Virtual reality applications in manufacturing process simulation. *J. Mater. Process. Technol.* **2004**, *156*, 1834–1838. [CrossRef]
23. Matijević, V.; Secić, A.; Mašić, V.; Sunić, M.; Kolak, Z.; Znika, M. Virtual reality in rehabilitation and therapy. *Acta Clin. Croat.* **2013**, *52*, 453–457. [PubMed]
24. Keshner, E.A.; Weiss, P.T. Introduction to the special issue from the proceedings of the 2006 International Workshop on Virtual Reality in Rehabilitation. *J. Neuroeng. Rehabil.* **2007**, *4*, 18. [CrossRef] [PubMed]
25. Moro, S.B.; Bisconti, S.; Muthalib, M.; Spezialetti, M.; Cutini, S.; Ferrari, M.; Placidi, G.; Quaresima, V. A semi-immersive virtual reality incremental swing balance task activates prefrontal cortex: A functional near-infrared spectroscopy study. *NeuroImage* **2014**, *85*, 451–460. [CrossRef] [PubMed]
26. De Miguel-Rubio, A.; Rubio, M.D.; Alba-Rueda, A.; Salazar, A.; Moral-Munoz, A.J.; Lucena-Anton, D. Virtual reality systems for upper limb motor function recovery in patients with spinal cord injury: Systematic review and meta-analysis. *JMIR Mhealth Uhealth* **2020**, *8*, e22537. [CrossRef] [PubMed]
27. Cameirão, M.S.; i Badia, S.B.; Oller, E.D.; Verschure, P.F. Neurorehabilitation using the virtual reality based Rehabilitation Gaming System: Methodology, design, psychometrics, usability and validation. *J. Neuroeng. Rehabil.* **2010**, *7*, 48. [CrossRef] [PubMed]
28. Paszkiel, S. Control based on brain-bomputer interface technology for video-gaming with virtual reality techniques. *J. Autom. Mob. Robot. Intell. Syst.* **2016**, *10*, 3–7. [CrossRef]
29. Téllez, P.D.; Moral-Munoz, J.A.; Fernández, E.C.; Couso, A.S.; Lucena-Anton, D. Efectos de la realidad virtual sobre el equilibrio y la marcha en el ictus: Revisión sistemática y metaanálisis. *Rev. Neurol.* **2019**, *69*, 223–234. [CrossRef]
30. Moher, D.; Liberati, A.; Tetzlaff, J.; Altman, D.G.; Group, T.P. Preferred reporting items for systematic reviews and meta-analyses: The PRISMA statement. *PLoS Med.* **2009**, *6*, e1000097. [CrossRef]
31. Higgins, J.; Thomas, J. *Cochrane Handbook for Systematic Reviews of Interventions*, 2nd ed.; Wiley-Blackwell: Chichester, UK, 2019.
32. Santos, C.M.D.C.; Pimenta, C.A.D.M.; Nobre, M.R.C. The PICO strategy for the research question construction and evidence search. *Rev. Lat. Am. Enferm.* **2007**, *15*, 508–511. [CrossRef] [PubMed]
33. Ba, L.J.V.; Perera, S.; Studenski, S.A. Is timed up and go better than gait speed in predicting health, function, and falls in older adults? *J. Am. Geriatr. Soc.* **2011**, *59*, 887–892. [CrossRef]
34. Barry, E.; Galvin, R.; Keogh, C.; Horgan, F.; Fahey, T. Is the Timed Up and Go test a useful predictor of risk of falls in community dwelling older adults: A systematic review and meta- analysis. *BMC Geriatr.* **2014**, *14*, 14. [CrossRef] [PubMed]
35. Sherringtonab, C.; Herbert, R.; Maher, C.; Mmoseleyad, A. PEDro. A database of randomized trials and systematic reviews in physiotherapy. *Man. Ther.* **2000**, *5*, 223–226. [CrossRef] [PubMed]
36. Macedo, L.G.; Elkins, M.; Maher, C.; Moseley, A.M.; Herbert, R.; Sherrington, C. There was evidence of convergent and construct validity of Physiotherapy Evidence Database quality scale for physiotherapy trials. *J. Clin. Epidemiol.* **2010**, *63*, 920–925. [CrossRef] [PubMed]
37. Del Din, S.; Galna, B.; Lord, S.; Nieuwboer, A.; Bekkers, E.M.J.; Pelosin, E.; Avanzino, L.; Bloem, B.R.; Rikkert, M.G.M.O.; Nieuwhof, F.; et al. Falls risk in relation to activity exposure in high-risk older adults. *J. Gerontol. Ser. A Boil. Sci. Med. Sci.* **2020**, *75*, 1198–1205. [CrossRef] [PubMed]
38. Pelosin, E.; Cerulli, C.; Ogliastro, C.; LaGravinese, G.; Mori, L.; Bonassi, G.; Mirelman, A.; Hausdorff, J.M.; Abbruzzese, G.; Marchese, R.; et al. A multimodal training modulates short-afferent inhibition and improves complex walking in a cohort of faller older adults with an increased prevalence of Parkinson's disease. *J. Gerontol. Ser. A Biol. Sci. Med. Sci.* **2019**, *75*, 722–728. [CrossRef]
39. Santos, P.; Machado, T.; Santos, L.; Ribeiro, N.; Melo, A. Efficacy of the Nintendo Wii combination with Conventional Exercises in the rehabilitation of individuals with Parkinson's disease: A randomized clinical trial. *Neurorehabilitation* **2019**, *45*, 255–263. [CrossRef] [PubMed]
40. Feng, H.; Li, C.; Liu, J.; Wang, L.; Ma, J.; Li, G.; Gan, L.; Shang, X.; Wu, Z. Virtual reality rehabilitation versus conventional physical therapy for improving balance and gait in Parkinson's Disease patients: A randomized controlled trial. *Med. Sci. Monit.* **2019**, *25*, 4186–4192. [CrossRef] [PubMed]
41. Gandolfi, M.; Geroin, C.; Dimitrova, E.; Boldrini, P.; Waldner, A.; Bonadiman, S.; Picelli, A.; Regazzo, S.; Stirbu, E.; Primon, D.; et al. Virtual reality telerehabilitation for postural instability in Parkinson's Disease: A multicenter, single-blind, randomized, controlled trial. *BioMed Res. Int.* **2017**, *2017*, 1–11. [CrossRef] [PubMed]
42. Mirelman, A.; Rochester, L.; Maidan, I.; Del Din, S.; Alcock, L.; Nieuwhof, F.; Rikkert, M.O.; Bloem, B.R.; Pelosin, E.; Avanzino, L.; et al. Addition of a non-immersive virtual reality component to treadmill training to reduce fall risk in older adults (V-TIME): A randomised controlled trial. *Lancet* **2016**, *388*, 1170–1182. [CrossRef]
43. Negrini, S.; Bissolotti, L.; Ferraris, A.; Noro, F.; Bishop, M.D.; Villafañe, J.H. Nintendo Wii Fit for balance rehabilitation in patients with Parkinson's disease: A comparative study. *J. Bodyw. Mov. Ther.* **2017**, *21*, 117–123. [CrossRef] [PubMed]
44. Yang, W.-C.; Wang, H.-K.; Wu, R.-M.; Lo, C.-S.; Lin, K.-H. Home-based virtual reality balance training and conventional balance training in Parkinson's disease: A randomized controlled trial. *J. Formos. Med. Assoc.* **2016**, *115*, 734–743. [CrossRef] [PubMed]
45. Lee, N.-Y.; Lee, D.-K.; Song, H.-S. Effect of virtual reality dance exercise on the balance, activities of daily living, and depressive disorder status of Parkinson's disease patients. *J. Phys. Ther. Sci.* **2015**, *27*, 145–147. [CrossRef] [PubMed]

46. Liao, Y.-Y.; Yang, Y.-R.; Cheng, S.-J.; Wu, Y.-R.; Fuh, J.-L.; Wang, R.-Y. Virtual reality–based training to improve obstacle-crossing performance and dynamic balance in patients with Parkinson's Disease. *Neurorehabil. Neural Repair* **2014**, *29*, 658–667. [CrossRef] [PubMed]
47. Lord, S.; Godfrey, A.; Galna, B.; Mhiripiri, D.; Burn, D.; Rochester, L. Ambulatory activity in incident Parkinson's: More than meets the eye? *J. Neurol.* **2013**, *260*, 2964–2972. [CrossRef]
48. Crosbie, J.H.; Lennon, S.; Basford, J.R.; McDonough, P.S.M. Virtual reality in stroke rehabilitation: Still more virtual than real. *Disabil. Rehabil.* **2007**, *29*, 1139–1146. [CrossRef]
49. Oh, Y.-B.; Kim, G.-W.; Han, K.-S.; Won, Y.H.; Park, S.-H.; Seo, J.-H.; Ko, M.-H. Efficacy of virtual reality combined with real instrument training for patients with stroke: A randomized controlled trial. *Arch. Phys. Med. Rehabil.* **2019**, *100*, 1400–1408. [CrossRef]
50. Ögün, M.N.; Kurul, R.; Yaşar, M.F.; Turkoglu, S.A.; Avci, Ş.; Yildiz, N. Effect of Leap Motion-based 3D Immersive Virtual Reality Usage on Upper Extremity Function in Ischemic Stroke Patients. *Arq. Neuro Psiquiatr.* **2019**, *77*, 681–688. [CrossRef] [PubMed]
51. Yeşilyaprak, S.S.; Yıldırım, M.S.; Tomruk, M.; Ertekin, Ö.; Algun, Z.C. Comparison of the effects of virtual reality-based balance exercises and conventional exercises on balance and fall risk in older adults living in nursing homes in Turkey. *Physiother. Theory Pr.* **2016**, *32*, 191–201. [CrossRef] [PubMed]
52. Amirthalingam, J.; Paidi, G.; Alshowaikh, K.; Jayarathna, A.I.; Salibindla, D.; Karpinska-Leydier, K.; Ergin, H.E. Virtual reality intervention to help improve motor function in patients undergoing rehabilitation for Cerebral Palsy, Parkinson's Disease, or Stroke: A systematic review of randomized controlled trials. *Cureus* **2021**, *13*, 16763. [CrossRef]

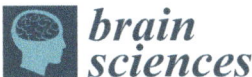

Review

Gastroparesis in Parkinson Disease: Pathophysiology, and Clinical Management

Heithem Soliman [1,2,*], Benoit Coffin [1,2] and Guillaume Gourcerol [3]

1. Centre de Recherche sur l'Inflammation, Université de Paris, Inserm UMRS 1149, 75018 Paris, France; benoit.coffin@aphp.fr
2. Département d'Hépato Gastro Entérologie, Hôpital Louis Mourier, DMU ESPRIT—GHU (AP-HP), 92700 Colombes, France
3. Centre Hospitalo-Universitaire de Rouen, INSERM UMR 1073, CIC-CRB 1404, 76000 Rouen, France; guillaume.gourcerol@chu-rouen.fr
* Correspondence: heithemsoliman90@hotmail.com

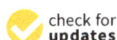

Citation: Soliman, H.; Coffin, B.; Gourcerol, G. Gastroparesis in Parkinson Disease: Pathophysiology, and Clinical Management. *Brain Sci.* **2021**, *11*, 831. https://doi.org/10.3390/brainsci11070831

Academic Editors: Patricia Martinez-Sanchez and Francisco Nieto-Escamez

Received: 19 May 2021
Accepted: 22 June 2021
Published: 23 June 2021

Publisher's Note: MDPI stays neutral with regard to jurisdictional claims in published maps and institutional affiliations.

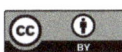

Copyright: © 2021 by the authors. Licensee MDPI, Basel, Switzerland. This article is an open access article distributed under the terms and conditions of the Creative Commons Attribution (CC BY) license (https://creativecommons.org/licenses/by/4.0/).

Abstract: Patients with Parkinson disease (PD) experience a range of non-motor symptoms, including gastrointestinal symptoms. These symptoms can be present in the prodromal phase of the disease. Recent advances in pathophysiology reveal that α-synuclein aggregates that form Lewy bodies and neurites, the hallmark of PD, are present in the enteric nervous system and may precede motor symptoms. Gastroparesis is one of the gastrointestinal involvements of PD and is characterized by delayed gastric emptying of solid food in the absence of mechanical obstruction. Gastroparesis has been reported in nearly 45% of PD. The cardinal symptoms include early satiety, postprandial fullness, nausea, and vomiting. The diagnosis requires an appropriate test to confirm delayed gastric emptying, such as gastric scintigraphy, or breath test. Gastroparesis can lead to malnutrition and impairment of quality of life. Moreover, it might interfere with the absorption of antiparkinsonian drugs. The treatment includes dietary modifications, and pharmacologic agents both to accelerate gastric emptying and relieve symptoms. Alternative treatments have been recently developed in the management of gastroparesis, and their use in patients with PD will be reported in this review.

Keywords: Parkinson disease; gastroparesis; alpha-synuclein; vagus nerve

1. Introduction

Parkinson disease (PD) is the second most common neurodegenerative disorder, after Alzheimer disease. It affects 2–3% of the population over 65 years and is more common in men [1]. The triad of parkinsonism is defined by motor symptoms that are rigidity, bradykinesia, and tremors [2]. However, the majority of patients with PD reveal a variety of non-motor symptoms, either as a specific complaint or upon specific questioning [3,4]. Gastrointestinal (GI) dysfunction in PD was already described by James Parkinson in 1817 in his first description of the disease [5]. Although historically overlooked [6], interest in GI manifestations has been increasing in the past decades. Several studies revealed five GI features—excess saliva, dysphagia, nausea (mainly related to delayed gastric emptying), decreased bowel movement frequency, and difficulty with defecation—as occurring more frequently in PD patients as compared to aged controls [7,8].

GI manifestations can occur at an early stage of PD and may precede motor symptoms in some cases by several years [9,10]. These disturbances impact the quality of life and are a common reason for emergency room visits and hospitalizations [11–13]. Gastroparesis, in particular, contributes to malnutrition and weight loss which is frequent in patients with PD [14]. In addition to its clinical aspect, the idea that PD may have its genesis in the gut has received increasing attention.

In this review, we aim to discuss the pathophysiological changes that might play a role in this GI dysfunction in PD. We will then discuss clinical manifestations linked to gastric dysmotility, namely gastroparesis, the diagnostic criteria of this disorder, and its management, regarding recent data.

2. Pathophysiology of GI Dysfunction in PD

Gastric motility and secretory functions are regulated by an extrinsic neuronal network composed of the sympathetic and parasympathetic systems, and an intrinsic neuronal semiautonomous network, the enteric nervous system (ENS). The ENS consists of myenteric (or Auerbach's) plexus and submucous (or Meissner's) plexus [15,16]. The myenteric plexus runs between circular and longitudinal muscle layers for the whole length of the gut and primarily provides motor innervation, whereas the submucous plexus plays a role in the control of secretion. The parasympathetic pathway is mainly driven by the vagus nerve, and by the sacral nerves for the distal part of the colon. The extrinsic system cooperates with the intrinsic network, and with the central nervous system. Intramural circuits of the ENS and efferent vagal nerves innervate motor neurons. Excitatory and inhibitory motor neurons drive the motility of the gastric smooth muscle. Interactions between the brainstem and ENS in the form of vago-vagal reflexes determine patterns of normal gastric motor activity [17].

The neuropathological hallmarks of PD are neuronal loss in the substantia nigra, leading to dopamine deficiency, and abnormal α-synuclein accumulation in the brain, with intracellular aggregates leading to the formation of Lewy bodies, or Lewy neurites [18]. The presence of Lewy bodies has been described in the GI tract and especially in the esophagus and colon since 1984 [19]. Mucosal biopsy samples harvested from the colon, stomach, and duodenum, have shown that misfolded α-synuclein is present in the ENS from the early stages in patients with PD and even 8 years before the onset of motor symptoms [20]. Myenteric neurons of the whole GI tract represent one of the earliest sites of α-synuclein accumulation, and this deposition occurs with a rostro-caudal gradient throughout the ENS [21]. High levels of Lewy bodies are also found in the central nervous system and in the dorsal motor nucleus of the vagus nerve (DMV) which has a strong influence on GI motility [22]. The causes of this distribution are unknown, although deposition follows the distribution of visceromotor projection neurons.

These observations led to the "Braak hypothesis", suggesting that the PD arises within the ENS, presumably triggered by a pathogen from within the gut lumen, and that the disease extends through the vagus nerve to the DMV in the brainstem, and then within the central nervous system [23]. Consistently, several studies revealed an alteration of intestinal permeability which could be the gateway for the disease [24,25]. This hypothesis is sustained by epidemiological studies, from Danish and Swedish registries, reporting that individuals who had undergone full truncal vagotomy were less likely to develop PD than individuals who had undergone selective vagotomy [26,27]. It also prompted investigations to assess enteric α-synuclein deposits, which are far more accessible than the brain as an early biomarker for PD [21]. However, conflicting results have been published, and autopsy studies on 417 patients did not confirm this gradient of deposition and did not find any case in which Lewy bodies and neurites were present in the peripheral autonomic network but not in the brain [28]. Thus, whether the disease spreads from the brain to the gut, or from the gut to the brain through the vagus nerve remains a matter of debate [29,30].

The role of α-synuclein on GI manifestations has not been established. Accumulation of those deposits could lead to a damaged neural network and impairment in gastric motility. Alterations of gastric motility in other synucleinopathies, such as multiple system atrophy, strengthens this hypothesis [31]. However, no neuronal loss has been described, and there has been no association between α-synuclein aggregates and GI symptoms [32,33]. The misfolded α-synuclein could thus play a role in modulating the synaptic pathway. A recent study interested in the spread of misfolded α-synuclein from the DMV to the substantia nigra, and provided the first evidence of an anatomically and functionally defined monosynaptic nigro-vagal pathway that modulates gastric motility [34,35]. This pathway has been shown to be dysfunctional in a rodent model of PD. Dopaminergic inputs to the DMV were then shown to modulate gastric motility, with a gastro-inhibitory response in the healthy model and a different response in PD models [36]. This pathway could thus be the link between the vagus and substantia nigra, and the misfolded α-synuclein in DMV could lead to maladaptive neural plasticity in vagal circuits regulating gastric motility.

Finally, impaired gastric motility in PD is multifactorial, and the ENS should not be considered as the only actor. A recent study revealed that GI dysfunction, specifically constipation, correlates with a reduction in dopamine transporter availability, implying a role for nigral degeneration or change in nigrostriatal dopamine function [37]. Moreover, there is evidence that treatment with levodopa could produce a worsening of gastric emptying, both in healthy volunteers and patients with advanced PD [38]. Alteration of hormone pathways involved in the control of gastric motility has also been documented, especially for cholecystokinin, a hormone known to inhibit gastric emptying [39]. Recent studies focus on the gut microbiome and reported its alteration in patients with PD, but its role in the genesis of the pathology or on GI symptoms remains unclear [40,41].

3. Gastroparesis

3.1. Prevalence in PD

Gastroparesis is a disorder defined by delayed gastric emptying of solid food in the absence of mechanical obstruction [42]. The main symptoms include early satiety after eating, postprandial fullness, nausea, vomiting, belching, and bloating. Severe forms lead to weight loss and impaired quality of life [43]. The prevalence of gastroparesis in PD has not been formally assessed. Impaired gastric emptying seems to be common reaching 70% to 100% of PD patients in a study using scintigraphy measurement [44]. However, this delayed emptying could be asymptomatic, with subjective symptoms present only in 25% to 45% of patients [45]. Interestingly, a recent study identified a subgroup of PD patients with accelerated gastric emptying [46]. Gastroparesis may occur in early and untreated PD, but its frequency seems to be higher in advanced disease [44,47]. The severity of gastroparesis is also correlated with the severity of motor impairment [48].

3.2. Pathophysiology

Delayed gastric emptying is associated with antral hypomotility and in some patients with pyloric sphincter dysfunction. Both mechanisms are caused by neuromuscular dysfunction. Extrinsic excitatory innervation is addressed from the vagus nerve and interacts with the intrinsic nerves of the ENS. In the smooth muscle layer, the interstitial cells of Cajal convey the signal to smooth muscle cells and are regarded as gastric pacemakers. These pacemaker cells do not seem to be altered in PD, suggesting that disturbance occurs either in the vagus nerve or in the myenteric plexus [49]. Alteration in a cholinergic anti-inflammatory pathway has also been demonstrated on an animal model of PD, which could lead to gastric muscular inflammation and muscular macrophage accumulation [50]. This muscular macrophage accumulation in the gastric wall has been described in idiopathic gastroparesis.

The neuropeptide ghrelin is another actor in gastric motility, secreted when the stomach is empty and increases gastric motility [51]. Only one study concerned the role of ghrelin in PD and revealed a decrease in serum concentration as compared with healthy volunteers [52]. Medications used to treat PD, such as anticholinergic or even levodopa, may also delay gastric emptying, which could explain the evolution of gastroparesis in the advanced stages of PD [53,54]. It is also important to remember that delayed gastric emptying might be responsible for medication failure since levodopa needs to reach the small intestine to be absorbed and might contribute to the on–off phenomenon with unpredictable motor symptoms [55].

3.3. Diagnostic Criteria

Clinical assessment of the symptoms should be performed with a reproducible and validated scale to allow a better follow-up and to standardize clinical trials on gastroparesis [56,57]. The Gastric Cardinal Symptom Index (GCSI) is to date the best validated score, based on the evaluation of nine items, scored from 0 to 5, (nausea, retching, vomiting, stomach fullness, early satiety, postprandial fullness, loss of appetite, bloating, stomach distension). The global score is then calculated on a range from 0 to 5, and is used to assess the effects of treatment, but not as a diagnostic tool to decide whether a patient should perform diagnostic tests.

Symptoms of gastroparesis are nonspecific and overlap with other sensory or motor upper GI disorders, in particular functional dyspepsia. Patients must first undergo an upper GI endoscopy to rule out any mechanical obstruction. Delayed gastric emptying must then be proven via a specific exam to confirm the diagnosis of gastroparesis. Gastric emptying scintigraphy is the most relevant test for functional and motility investigation. The patient will then take a solid radiomarked meal with a short life radioisotope, ^{99m}Tc. The content of the meal is an important factor and has been standardized, with sufficient calories and fat content adapted to Western-style meals; usually this consists of scrambled eggs [58]. The test should last at least 4 h, with image acquisition at 0, 1, 2, and 4 h. Gastroparesis is confirmed if the percent of retention is >60% at 2 h and/or >10% at 4 h [58,59].

The ^{13}C gastric emptying breathing test is a validated alternative for scintigraphic measurement and is more accessible with less radiation [60]. The principle of this test is that the rate of ^{13}C substrate incorporated in the solid meal is reflected by breath excretion of $^{13}CO_2$. The meal incorporates the stable isotope 13C in a substrate such as octanoic acid or spirulina platensis and is ingested after an 8-h fast. Breath samples are then collected before the meal, and at specified times, typically every 30 min, over 4 h [61]. However, this is an indirect test and could be altered by physical activity, by lung or liver disease, or cardiac failure, and by small intestinal absorption [62]. A systematic review on the evaluation of gastric emptying in PD revealed a large discrepancy between scintigraphy study and breath test study, with a higher rate of gastroparesis diagnosed in breath test studies [63]. Finally, the wireless motility capsule has been recently approved by the U.S. Food and Drug Administration (FDA) for gastric emptying measurement and has also been assessed in PD [64]. This single-use orally ingested data recording capsule measures pH, pressure, and temperature throughout the GI tract. It allows measurement of the transit time in the stomach, in the small intestine, and the colon [65]. However, the capsule does not seem to exit the stomach with the meal, as it is a large non-digestible object, but rather with powerful antral contractions of the migrating motor complex which aim to clear the stomach of indigestible material [66].

4. Treatment

4.1. Dietary Modifications

Therapeutic strategy first relies on dietary modification and is generally used for all patients. Patients are recommended to eat small meals and to avoid foods high in fat and indigestible fibers [67]. A small-particle-size diet has been shown to reduce upper GI symptoms in diabetic gastroparesis [68]. Thus, snacking and more frequent meals to maintain caloric intake are needed. Caloric liquids such as soups are also often well tolerated and recommended. In severe cases, vitamin deficiencies should be detected and supplemented. Rarely, feeding tube or parenteral nutrition can be necessary [69].

4.2. Pharmalogical Treatment

Most of the medical treatments used for gastroparesis have not been validated in the specific context of gastric dysmotility due to PD. Prokinetic drugs, and in the first step peripheral dopamine antagonist drugs, are the most commonly used medication. D2 receptor antagonists that cross the brain–blood barrier, including metoclopramide, are contraindicated in PD. By contrast, domperidone is a D2 receptor antagonist acting peripherally as it does not cross the brain–blood barrier, and it may be used to accelerate gastric emptying and relieve nausea and vomiting [70]. Of note, domperidone is associated with cardiac arrhythmia risks and is thus not approved by FDA [71,72]. However, recent data are reassuring on the safety profile of the drug used in the right settings, and domperidone should be considered as an option in gastroparetic PD patients [73]. Motilin receptor agonists, including erythromycin and azithromycin, are not appropriate for extended use owing to drug interactions (especially for erythromycin), to QT prolongation, and to their association with tachyphylaxis with loss of efficacy over a few weeks [74]. A selective 5-HT$_4$ receptor agonist, prucalopride, lacking cardiac side effects, is yet approved for the treatment of constipation and has been shown to improve gastric emptying in small open labeled studies in PD [75,76]. One small study reported improvement in gastric emptying with nizatidine, a histamine H2-receptor antagonist, in patients with PD [77]. This drug could also be used to treat some of the reflux symptoms associated with gastroparesis [78]. Finally, ghrelin antagonists such as relamorelin are being assessed as potential prokinetic agents and seem to be effective in improving symptoms and gastric emptying in patients with diabetic gastroparesis in two phase 2 trials [79,80].

Although proton-pump inhibitors (PPI) are often used to treat reflux symptoms that result from gastroparesis, they have been shown to delay gastric emptying and should thus be stopped when possible [81]. Moreover, some studies documented an association between long term use of PPI and cognitive decline even if controversial data have also been published [82,83]. Treatments used in the management of constipation, which is frequent in PD and can be associated with gastroparesis, can also impact gastric emptying. Bulk-forming products, such as psyllium or increasing dietary fiber may delay gastric emptying and cause bloating [84,85]. Osmotic laxatives, primarily polyethylene glycol, should be favored in the context of constipation associated with PD [86].

In case of failure of prokinetics, treatments addressing nausea and vomiting have been used in refractory gastroparesis, but they cannot be recommended in the context of PD. Commonly prescribed agents include prochlorperazine or chlorpromazine, but these treatments are contraindicated as they can worsen the evolution of PD by their action on the central nervous system [87]. Ondansetron, a 5-HT3 receptor antagonist, is considered a reasonable second-line medication in refractory gastroparesis [67]. This treatment is currently assessed as a potential target for psychosis and dyskinesia associated with PD, but its impact on nausea and vomiting in PD has not been specifically evaluated [88,89]. However, the association of ondansetron with apomorphine leads to several adverse effects (sedation, decreased blood pressure) and is contraindicated [90]. The impact of aprepitant, an NK-1 receptor antagonist used to treat chemotherapy-induced nausea, has still not been demonstrated in gastroparesis [91].

4.3. Interventional Techniques

Several instrumental techniques are now available for patients who do not respond to medical treatment. In some patients, gastroparesis is associated with pyloric sphincter dysfunction, and endoscopic therapies targeting the pylorus have thus been assessed. Botulinum toxin injections in the pyloric sphincter may alleviate gastroparesis, with data also presented in patients with PD [92]. However, two double-blinded studies failed to show improvement with this technique compared with placebo [93,94]. It may provide temporary relief, but not sustained improvement, lasting on average 3 months. Endoscopic pyloric dilation has been less commonly evaluated in gastroparesis, and not in PD, but could also allow a temporary relief in some patients [95]. Recently, gastric endoscopic pyloromyotomy has been developed for refractory patients, and reveals improvement in gastric emptying and symptomatic scores, with a more sustained relief in 66% of patients at 1 year [96,97]. This technique also has not been assessed in PD, and controlled trials are still missing.

Another approach that should not be forgotten is to circumvent the inconsistency in drug absorption that may result from gastroparesis. Other processes may interfere with response to levodopa and might be improved with these strategies, such as hiatal hernia, Helicobacter pylori infection, or small intestine bacterial overgrowth [98,99]. A variety of non-oral approaches to antiparkinsonian drug administration may be employed. Levodopa could be administered via transdermal patch, subcutaneous and sublingual apomorphine, or liquid infusion [55,100]. Deep brain stimulation of subthalamic nuclei may be required in PD. This technique has been shown to accelerate gastric emptying and to relieve other GI dysmotility symptoms, such as constipation [101,102].

5. Conclusions and Future Prospect

Gastroparesis is a frequent disorder in PD patients, and may lead to impaired quality of life, weight loss, and malnutrition. It may also impact drug absorption, and worsen the course of PD.

Much progress has been made in recent years in understanding the pathophysiology of digestive involvement in PD, with a growing role of α-synuclein deposits in the ENS and demonstration of its spreading through the vagus nerve, which interacts with the substantia nigra, and impacts gastric motility. New techniques are being developed to obtain adequate endoscopic biopsy samples from the neuromuscular layers of the stomach and the duodenum. These samples could help evaluate the pathological status of the ENS. Evaluation of pyloric dysfunction with specific endoscopic technique also appears as a promising strategy. Correlation between histological findings, new endoscopic technique evaluations, and treatment outcome could help personalize therapeutic strategy.

Gastroparesis can occur at a very early stage of PD and should be identified promptly and treated. Clinicians should also pay attention to its evolution at each evaluation, with symptomatic and nutritional evaluation. Prokinetics, including domperidone, and dietary modifications are the first line treatments. Newly developed prokinetic drugs require, however, larger validation trials in the context of PD. Endoscopic treatments are currently being developed, and may represent an alternative therapeutic strategy in the future to improve symptoms and gastric emptying. Whether acceleration of gastric emptying leads to a better control of PD symptoms remains, however, to be firmly established.

Author Contributions: Conceptualization, H.S. and G.G.; writing—original draft preparation H.S.; writing—review and editing B.C. and G.G.; All authors have read and agreed to the published version of the manuscript.

Funding: This research has received no external funding.

Conflicts of Interest: The authors declare no conflict of interest.

References

1. Tysnes, O.-B.; Storstein, A. Epidemiology of Parkinson's disease. *J. Neural. Transm.* **2017**, *124*, 901–905. [CrossRef]
2. Poewe, W.; Seppi, K.; Tanner, C.M.; Halliday, G.M.; Brundin, P.; Volkmann, J.; Schrag, A.-E.; Lang, A.E. Parkinson disease. *Nat. Rev. Dis. Primer.* **2017**, *3*, 17013. [CrossRef]
3. Poewe, W. Non-motor symptoms in Parkinson's disease. *Eur. J. Neurol.* **2008**, *15* (Suppl. 1), 14–20. [CrossRef]
4. Martinez-Martin, P.; Schapira, A.H.V.; Stocchi, F.; Sethi, K.; Odin, P.; MacPhee, G.; Brown, R.; Naidu, Y.; Clayton, L.; Abe, K.; et al. Prevalence of nonmotor symptoms in Parkinson's disease in an international setting; Study using nonmotor symptoms questionnaire in 545 patients. *Mov. Disord.* **2007**, *22*, 1623–1629. [CrossRef]
5. Parkinson, J. An essay on the shaking palsy. 1817. *J. Neuropsychiatry Clin. Neurosci.* **2002**, *14*, 223–236; discussion 222. [CrossRef]
6. Stacy, M.; Bowron, A.; Guttman, M.; Hauser, R.; Hughes, K.; Larsen, J.P.; LeWitt, P.; Oertel, W.; Quinn, N.; Sethi, K.; et al. Identification of motor and nonmotor wearing-off in Parkinson's disease: Comparison of a patient questionnaire versus a clinician assessment. *Mov. Disord. Off. J. Mov. Disord. Soc.* **2005**, *20*, 726–733. [CrossRef]
7. Edwards, L.L.; Pfeiffer, R.F.; Quigley, E.M.M.; Hofman, R.; Balluff, M. Gastrointestinal symptoms in Parkinson's disease. *Mov. Disord.* **1991**, *6*, 151–156. [CrossRef]
8. Khoo, T.K.; Yarnall, A.J.; Duncan, G.W.; Coleman, S.; O'Brien, J.T.; Brooks, D.J.; Barker, R.A.; Burn, D. The spectrum of nonmotor symptoms in early Parkinson disease. *Neurology* **2013**, *80*, 276–281. [CrossRef] [PubMed]
9. Cersosimo, M.G.; Benarroch, E.E. Neural control of the gastrointestinal tract: Implications for Parkinson disease. *Mov. Disord. Off. J. Mov. Disord. Soc.* **2008**, *23*, 1065–1075. [CrossRef] [PubMed]
10. Cersosimo, M.G.; Raina, G.B.; Pecci, C.; Pellene, A.; Calandra, C.R.; Gutiérrez, C.; Micheli, F.E.; Benarroch, E.E. Gastrointestinal manifestations in Parkinson's disease: Prevalence and occurrence before motor symptoms. *J. Neurol.* **2013**, *260*, 1332–1338. [CrossRef] [PubMed]
11. Li, H.; Zhang, M.; Chen, L.; Zhang, J.; Pei, Z.; Hu, A.; Wang, Q. Nonmotor symptoms are independently associated with impaired health-related quality of life in Chinese patients with Parkinson's disease. *Mov. Disord. Off. J. Mov. Disord. Soc.* **2010**, *25*, 2740–2746. [CrossRef] [PubMed]

12. Barone, P.; Antonini, A.; Colosimo, C.; Marconi, R.; Morgante, L.; Avarello, T.P.; Bottacchi, E.; Cannas, A.; Ceravolo, G.; Ceravolo, R.; et al. The PRIAMO study: A multicenter assessment of nonmotor symptoms and their impact on quality of life in Parkinson's disease. *Mov. Disord. Off. J. Mov. Disord. Soc.* **2009**, *24*, 1641–1649. [CrossRef] [PubMed]
13. Martinez-Martin, P. The importance of non-motor disturbances to quality of life in Parkinson's disease. *J. Neurol. Sci.* **2011**, *310*, 12–16. [CrossRef] [PubMed]
14. Bachmann, C.G.; Trenkwalder, C. Body weight in patients with Parkinson's disease. *Mov. Disord.* **2006**, *21*, 1824–1830. [CrossRef]
15. Pellegrini, C.; Antonioli, L.; Colucci, R.; Ballabeni, V.; Barocelli, E.; Bernardini, N.; Blandizzi, C.; Fornai, M. Gastric motor dysfunctions in Parkinson's disease: Current pre-clinical evidence. *Parkinsonism Relat. Disord.* **2015**, *21*, 1407–1414. [CrossRef] [PubMed]
16. Camilleri, M. Gastrointestinal motility disorders in neurologic disease. *J. Clin. Investig.* **2021**, *131*, e143771. [CrossRef]
17. Grundy, D.; Al-Chaer, E.D.; Aziz, Q.; Collins, S.M.; Ke, M.; Taché, Y.; Wood, J.D. Fundamentals of neurogastroenterology: Basic science. *Gastroenterology* **2006**, *130*, 1391–1411. [CrossRef]
18. Goedert, M.; Spillantini, M.G.; Del Tredici, K.; Braak, H. 100 years of Lewy pathology. *Nat. Rev. Neurol.* **2013**, *9*, 13–24. [CrossRef]
19. Qualman, S.J.; Haupt, H.M.; Yang, P.; Hamilton, S.R. Esophageal Lewy bodies associated with ganglion cell loss in achalasia. Similarity to Parkinson's disease. *Gastroenterology* **1984**, *87*, 848–856. [CrossRef]
20. Hilton, D.; Stephens, M.; Kirk, L.; Edwards, P.; Potter, R.; Zajicek, J.; Broughton, E.; Hagan, H.; Carroll, C. Accumulation of α-synuclein in the bowel of patients in the pre-clinical phase of Parkinson's disease. *Acta Neuropathol. (Berl.)* **2014**, *127*, 235–241.
21. Visanji, N.P.; Marras, C.; Hazrati, L.-N.; Liu, L.W.C.; Lang, A.E. Alimentary, my dear Watson? The challenges of enteric α-synuclein as a Parkinson's disease biomarker. *Mov. Disord.* **2014**, *29*, 444–450. [CrossRef]
22. Fasano, A.; Visanji, N.P.; Liu, L.W.C.; E Lang, A.; Pfeiffer, R.F. Gastrointestinal dysfunction in Parkinson's disease. *Lancet Neurol.* **2015**, *14*, 625–639. [CrossRef]
23. Braak, H.; de Vos, R.A.; Bohl, J.; Del Tredici, K. Gastric alpha-synuclein immunoreactive inclusions in Meissner's and Auerbach's plexuses in cases staged for Parkinson's disease-related brain pathology. *Neurosci. Lett.* **2006**, *396*, 67–72. [CrossRef]
24. Forsyth, C.B.; Shannon, K.M.; Kordower, J.H.; Voigt, R.M.; Shaikh, M.; Jaglin, J.A.; Estes, J.D.; Dodiya, H.B.; Keshavarzian, A. Increased intestinal permeability correlates with sigmoid mucosa alpha-synuclein staining and endotoxin exposure markers in early Parkinson's disease. *PLoS ONE* **2011**, *6*, e28032.
25. Clairembault, T.; Leclair-Visonneau, L.; Coron, E.; Bourreille, A.; Le Dily, S.; Vavasseur, F.; Heymann, M.-F.; Neunlist, M.; Derkinderen, P. Structural alterations of the intestinal epithelial barrier in Parkinson's disease. *Acta Neuropathol. Commun.* **2015**, *3*, 12. [CrossRef] [PubMed]
26. Svensson, E.; Horváth-Puhó, E.; Thomsen, R.; Djurhuus, J.C.; Pedersen, L.; Borghammer, P.; Sørensen, H.T. Vagotomy and subsequent risk of Parkinson's disease. *Ann. Neurol.* **2015**, *78*, 522–529. [CrossRef] [PubMed]
27. Liu, B.; Fang, F.; Pedersen, N.; Tillander, A.; Ludvigsson, J.F.; Ekbom, A.; Svenningsson, P.; Chen, H.; Wirdefeldt, K. Vagotomy and Parkinson disease. *Neurology* **2017**, *88*, 1996–2002. [CrossRef] [PubMed]
28. Adler, C.H.; Beach, T.G. Neuropathological basis of nonmotor manifestations of Parkinson's disease. *Mov. Disord. Off. J. Mov. Disord. Soc.* **2016**, *31*, 1114–1119. [CrossRef]
29. Lionnet, A.; Leclair-Visonneau, L.; Neunlist, M.; Murayama, S.; Takao, M.; Adler, C.H.; Derkinderen, P.; Beach, T.G. Does Parkinson's disease start in the gut? *Acta Neuropathol. (Berl.)* **2018**, *135*, 1–12. [CrossRef]
30. Leclair-Visonneau, L.; Neunlist, M.; Derkinderen, P.; Lebouvier, T. The gut in Parkinson's disease: Bottom-up, top-down, or neither? *Neurogastroenterol. Motil. Off. J. Eur. Gastrointest. Motil. Soc.* **2020**, *32*, e13777. [CrossRef]
31. Tanaka, Y.; Kato, T.; Nishida, H.; Yamada, M.; Koumura, A.; Sakurai, T.; Hayashi, Y.; Kimura, A.; Hozumi, I.; Araki, H.; et al. Is there delayed gastric emptying in patients with multiple system atrophy? An analysis using the (13)C-acetate breath test. *J. Neurol.* **2012**, *259*, 1448–1452. [CrossRef] [PubMed]
32. Annerino, D.M.; Arshad, S.; Taylor, G.M.; Adler, C.H.; Beach, T.G.; Greene, J.G. Parkinson's disease is not associated with gastrointestinal myenteric ganglion neuron loss. *Acta Neuropathol. (Berl.)* **2012**, *124*, 665–680. [CrossRef] [PubMed]
33. Cersosimo, M.G.; Benarroch, E.E. Pathological correlates of gastrointestinal dysfunction in Parkinson's disease. *Neurobiol. Dis.* **2012**, *46*, 559–564. [CrossRef] [PubMed]
34. Anselmi, L.; Toti, L.; Bove, C.; Hampton, J.; Travagli, R.A. A Nigro−Vagal Pathway Controls Gastric Motility and Is Affected in a Rat Model of Parkinsonism. *Gastroenterol.* **2017**, *153*, 1581–1593. [CrossRef]
35. Travagli, R.A.; Browning, K.N.; Camilleri, M. Parkinson disease and the gut: New insights into pathogenesis and clinical relevance. *Nat. Rev. Gastroenterol. Hepatol.* **2020**, *17*, 673–685. [CrossRef]
36. Bove, C.; Anselmi, L.; Travagli, R.A. Altered gastric tone and motility response to brain-stem dopamine in a rat model of parkinsonism. *Am. J. Physiol. Liver Physiol.* **2019**, *317*, G1–G7. [CrossRef]
37. Hinkle, J.T.; Perepezko, K.; Mills, K.A.; Mari, Z.; Butala, A.; Dawson, T.M.; Pantelyat, A.; Rosenthal, L.S.; Pontone, G.M. Dopamine transporter availability reflects gastrointestinal dysautonomia in early Parkinson disease. *Parkinsonism Relat. Disord.* **2018**, *55*, 8–14. [CrossRef]
38. Hardoff, R.; Sula, M.; Tamir, A.; Soil, A.; Front, A.; Badarna, S.; Honigman, S.; Giladi, N. Gastric emptying time and gastric motility in patients with Parkinson's disease. *Mov. Disord. Off. J. Mov. Disord. Soc.* **2001**, *16*, 1041–1047. [CrossRef]
39. Fujii, C.; Harada, S.; Ohkoshi, N.; Hayashi, A.; Yoshizawa, K.; Ishizuka, C.; Nakamura, T. Association between polymorphism of the cholecystokinin gene and idiopathic Parkinson's disease. *Clin. Genet.* **1999**, *56*, 394–399. [CrossRef]

40. Scheperjans, F.; Aho, V.; Pereira, P.A.B.; Koskinen, K.; Paulin, L.; Pekkonen, E.; Haapaniemi, E.; Kaakkola, S.; Eerola-Rautio, J.; Pohja, M.; et al. Gut microbiota are related to Parkinson's disease and clinical phenotype. *Mov. Disord.* **2015**, *30*, 350–358. [CrossRef] [PubMed]
41. Felice, V.D.; Quigley, E.M.; Sullivan, A.; O'Keeffe, G.W.; O'Mahony, S.M. Microbiota-gut-brain signalling in Parkinson's disease: Implications for non-motor symptoms. *Parkinsonism Relat. Disord.* **2016**, *27*, 1–8. [CrossRef] [PubMed]
42. Camilleri, M.; Chedid, V.; Ford, A.; Haruma, K.; Horowitz, M.; Jones, K.L.; Low, P.A.; Park, S.-Y.; Parkman, H.P.; Stanghellini, V. Gastroparesis. *Nat. Rev. Dis. Prim.* **2018**, *4*, 41. [CrossRef]
43. Yu, D.; Ramsey, F.V.; Norton, W.F.; Norton, N.; Schneck, S.; Gaetano, T.; Parkman, H.P. The Burdens, Concerns, and Quality of Life of Patients with Gastroparesis. *Dig. Dis. Sci.* **2017**, *62*, 879–893. [CrossRef]
44. Heetun, Z.S.; Quigley, E.M.M. Gastroparesis and Parkinson's disease: A systematic review. *Parkinsonism Relat. Disord.* **2012**, *18*, 433–440. [CrossRef] [PubMed]
45. Siddiqui, M.F.; Rast, S.; Lynn, M.J.; Auchus, A.P.; Pfeiffer, R.F. Autonomic dysfunction in Parkinson's disease: A comprehensive symptom survey. *Parkinsonism Relat. Disord.* **2002**, *8*, 277–284. [CrossRef]
46. Khoshbin, K.; Hassan, A.; Camilleri, M. Cohort Study in Parkinsonism: Delayed Transit, Accelerated Gastric Emptying, and Prodromal Dysmotility. *Neurol. Clin. Pract.* **2020**. [CrossRef]
47. Tanaka, Y.; Kato, T.; Nishida, H.; Yamada, M.; Koumura, A.; Sakurai, T.; Hayashi, Y.; Kimura, A.; Hozumi, I.; Araki, H.; et al. Is there a delayed gastric emptying of patients with early-stage, untreated Parkinson's disease? An analysis using the 13C-acetate breath test. *J. Neurol.* **2011**, *258*, 421–426. [CrossRef] [PubMed]
48. Goetze, O.; Nikodem, A.B.; Wieszcorek, J.; Banasch, M.; Przuntek, H.; Mueller, T.; Schmidt, W.E.; Woitalla, D. Predictors of gastric emptying in Parkinson's disease. *Neurogastroenterol. Motil. Off. J. Eur. Gastrointest. Motil. Soc.* **2006**, *18*, 369–375. [CrossRef]
49. Heimrich, K.G.; Jacob, V.Y.P.; Schaller, D.; Stallmach, A.; Witte, O.W.; Prell, T. Gastric dysmotility in Parkinson's disease is not caused by alterations of the gastric pacemaker cells. *Npj Park. Dis.* **2019**, *5*, 1–6. [CrossRef]
50. Zhou, L.; Zheng, L.; Zhang, X.; Zhu, J. Mo1541—Activating Alpha7 Nicotinic Acetylcholine Receptor on Macrophage Attenuates Gastric Inflamation and Gastroparesis in Parkinson's Disease Rats. *Gastroenterology* **2018**, *154*, S-746. [CrossRef]
51. Cheung, C.K.; Wu, J.C.-Y. Role of ghrelin in the pathophysiology of gastrointestinal disease. *Gut Liver* **2013**, *7*, 505–512. [CrossRef] [PubMed]
52. Unger, M.M.; Möller, J.C.; Mankel, K.; Eggert, K.M.; Bohne, K.; Bodden, M.; Stiasny-Kolster, K.; Kann, P.H.; Mayer, G.; Tebbe, J.J.; et al. Postprandial ghrelin response is reduced in patients with Parkinson's disease and idiopathic REM sleep behaviour disorder: A peripheral biomarker for early Parkinson's disease? *J. Neurol.* **2011**, *258*, 982–990. [CrossRef]
53. Parkman, H.P.; Trate, D.M.; Knight, L.C.; Brown, K.L.; Maurer, A.H.; Fisher, R.S. Cholinergic effects on human gastric motility. *Gut* **1999**, *45*, 346–354. [CrossRef] [PubMed]
54. Bestetti, A.; Capozza, A.; Lacerenza, M.; Manfredi, L.; Mancini, F. Delayed Gastric Emptying in Advanced Parkinson Disease: Correlation With Therapeutic Doses. *Clin. Nucl. Med.* **2017**, *42*, 83–87. [CrossRef] [PubMed]
55. Pfeiffer, R.F.; Isaacson, S.H.; Pahwa, R. Clinical implications of gastric complications on levodopa treatment in Parkinson's disease. *Parkinsonism Relat. Disord.* **2020**, *76*, 63–71. [PubMed]
56. Revicki, D.A.; Rentz, A.M.; Dubois, D.; Kahrilas, P.; Stanghellini, V.; Talley, N.J.; Tack, J. Gastroparesis Cardinal Symptom Index (GCSI): Development and validation of a patient reported assessment of severity of gastroparesis symptoms. *Qual. Life Res. Int. J. Qual. Life Asp. Treat. Care Rehabil.* **2004**, *13*, 833–844. [CrossRef]
57. Pasricha, P.J.; Camilleri, M.; Hasler, W.L.; Parkman, H.P. White Paper AGA: Gastroparesis: Clinical and Regulatory Insights for Clinical Trials. *Clin. Gastroenterol. Hepatol.* **2017**, *15*, 1184–1190. [CrossRef]
58. Tougas, G.; Eaker, E.Y.; Abell, T.L.; Abrahamsson, H.; Boivin, M.; Chen, J.; Hocking, M.P.; Quigley, E.M.; Koch, K.L.; Tokayer, A.Z.; et al. Assessment of gastric emptying using a low fat meal: Establishment of international control values. *Am. J. Gastroenterol.* **2000**, *95*, 1456–1462. [CrossRef]
59. Abell, T.L.; Camilleri, M.; Donohoe, K.; Hasler, W.L.; Lin, H.C.; Maurer, A.H.; McCallum, R.W.; Nowak, T.; Nusynowitz, M.L.; Parkman, H.P.; et al. Consensus recommendations for gastric emptying scintigraphy: A joint report of the American Neurogastroenterology and Motility Society and the Society of Nuclear Medicine. *J. Nucl. Med. Technol.* **2008**, *36*, 44–54. [CrossRef]
60. Szarka, L.A.; Camilleri, M.; Vella, A.; Burton, D.; Baxter, K.; Simonson, J.; Zinsmeister, A.R. A stable isotope breath test with a standard meal for abnormal gastric emptying of solids in the clinic and in research. *Clin. Gastroenterol. Hepatol. Off. Clin. Pract. J. Am. Gastroenterol. Assoc.* **2008**, *6*, 635–643.e1. [CrossRef]
61. Ghoos, Y.F.; Maes, B.D.; Geypens, B.J.; Mys, G.; Hiele, M.I.; Rutgeerts, P.J.; Vantrappen, G. Measurement of gastric emptying rate of solids by means of a carbon-labeled octanoic acid breath test. *Gastroenterology* **1993**, *104*, 1640–1647. [CrossRef]
62. van de Casteele, M.; Luypaerts, A.; Geypens, B.; Fevery, J.; Ghoos, Y.; Nevens, F. Oxidative breakdown of octanoic acid is maintained in patients with cirrhosis despite advanced disease. *Neurogastroenterol. Motil. Off. J. Eur. Gastrointest. Motil. Soc.* **2003**, *15*, 113–120.
63. Knudsen, K.; Szwebs, M.; Hansen, A.K.; Borghammer, P. Gastric emptying in Parkinson's disease—A mini-review. *Parkinsonism Relat. Disord.* **2018**, *55*, 18–25. [CrossRef]
64. Su, A.; Gandhy, R.; Barlow, C.; Triadafilopoulos, G. Utility of the wireless motility capsule and lactulose breath testing in the evaluation of patients with Parkinson's disease who present with functional gastrointestinal symptoms. *BMJ Open Gastroenterol.* **2017**, *4*, e000132.

65. Keller, J.; Bassotti, G.; Clarke, J.; Dinning, P.; Fox, M.; Grover, M.; Hellström, P.M.; Ke, M.; Layer, P.; Malagelada, C.; et al. Expert consensus document: Advances in the diagnosis and classification of gastric and intestinal motility disorders. *Nat. Rev. Gastroenterol. Hepatol.* **2018**, *15*, 291–308. [CrossRef]
66. Cassilly, D.; Kantor, S.; Knight, L.C.; Maurer, A.H.; Fisher, R.S.; Semler, J.; Parkman, H.P. Gastric emptying of a non-digestible solid: Assessment with simultaneous SmartPill pH and pressure capsule, antroduodenal manometry, gastric emptying scintigraphy. *Neurogastroenterol. Motil. Off. J. Eur. Gastrointest. Motil. Soc.* **2008**, *20*, 311–319. [CrossRef] [PubMed]
67. Camilleri, M.; Parkman, H.P.; A Shafi, M.; Abell, T.L.; Gerson, L. Clinical Guideline: Management of Gastroparesis. *Am. J. Gastroenterol.* **2013**, *108*, 18–38. [CrossRef]
68. Olausson, E.A.; Störsrud, S.; Grundin, H.; Isaksson, M.; Attvall, S.; Simrén, M. A small particle size diet reduces upper gastrointestinal symptoms in patients with diabetic gastroparesis: A randomized controlled trial. *Am. J. Gastroenterol.* **2014**, *109*, 375–385. [CrossRef] [PubMed]
69. Parkman, H.P.; Yates, K.P.; Hasler, W.L.; Nguyan, L.; Pasricha, P.J.; Snape, W.J.; Farrugia, G.; Calles, J.; Koch, K.L.; Abell, T.L.; et al. Dietary intake and nutritional deficiencies in patients with diabetic or idiopathic gastroparesis. *Gastroenterology* **2011**, *141*, 486–498.e1-7. [CrossRef] [PubMed]
70. Barone, J.A. Domperidone: A peripherally acting dopamine2-receptor antagonist. *Ann. Pharmacother.* **1999**, *33*, 429–440. [PubMed]
71. Soykan, I.; Sarosiek, I.; Shifflett, J.; Wooten, G.F.; McCallum, R.W. Effect of chronic oral domperidone therapy on gastrointestinal symptoms and gastric emptying in patients with Parkinson's disease. *Mov. Disord. Off. J. Mov. Disord. Soc.* **1997**, *12*, 952–957. [CrossRef]
72. Field, J.; Wasilewski, M.; Bhuta, R.; Malik, Z.; Cooper, J.; Parkman, H.P.; Parkman, H.P.; Schey, R. Effect of Chronic Domperidone Use on QT Interval: A Large Single Center Study. *J. Clin. Gastroenterol.* **2019**, *53*, 648–652. [CrossRef]
73. Ejaz, S.; Slack, R.; Kim, P.; Shuttlesworth, G.A.; Stroehlein, J.R.; Shafi, M. Sa1575—Cardiac Safety Profile of Patient Treated with Domperidone Using an Fda Approved Ind Protocol: A Prospective 5-Years Study. *Gastroenterology* **2018**, *154*, S-316. [CrossRef]
74. Thielemans, L.; Depoortere, I.; Perret, J.; Robberecht, P.; Liu, Y.; Thijs, T.; Carreras, C.; Burgeon, E.; Peeters, T.L. Desensitization of the human motilin receptor by motilides. *J. Pharmacol. Exp. Ther.* **2005**, *313*, 1397–1405. [CrossRef] [PubMed]
75. Asai, H.; Udaka, F.; Hirano, M.; Minami, T.; Oda, M.; Kubori, T.; Nishinaka, K.; Kameyama, M.; Ueno, S. Increased gastric motility during 5-HT4 agonist therapy reduces response fluctuations in Parkinson's disease. *Parkinsonism Relat. Disord.* **2005**, *11*, 499–502. [CrossRef] [PubMed]
76. Pinyopornpanish, K.; Soontornpun, A.; Kijdamrongthum, P.; Teeyasoontranon, W.; Angkurawaranon, C.; Thongsawat, S. The effect of prucalopride on gastric emptying in parkinson's disease patients, a pilot randomized, open-label study. *Thai J. Gastroenterol.* **2016**, *17*, 100–107. [CrossRef]
77. Doi, H.; Sakakibara, R.; Sato, M.; Hirai, S.; Masaka, T.; Kishi, M.; Tsuyusaki, Y.; Tateno, A.; Tateno, F.; Takahashi, O.; et al. Nizatidine ameliorates gastroparesis in Parkinson's disease: A pilot study. *Mov. Disord. Off. J. Mov. Disord. Soc.* **2014**, *29*, 562–566. [CrossRef]
78. Futagami, S.; Shimpuku, M.; Song, J.; Kodaka, Y.; Yamawaki, H.; Nagoya, H.; Shindo, T.; Kawagoe, T.; Horie, A.; Gudis, K.; et al. Nizatidine improves clinical symptoms and gastric emptying in patients with functional dyspepsia accompanied by impaired gastric emptying. *Digestion* **2012**, *86*, 114–121. [CrossRef] [PubMed]
79. Camilleri, M.; McCallum, R.W.; Tack, J.; Spence, S.C.; Gottesdiener, K.; Fiedorek, F.T. Efficacy and Safety of Relamorelin in Diabetics With Symptoms of Gastroparesis: A Randomized, Placebo-Controlled Study. *Gastroenterology* **2017**, *153*, 1240–1250.e2. [CrossRef] [PubMed]
80. Lembo, A.; Camilleri, M.; McCallum, R.; Sastre, R.; Breton, C.; Spence, S.; White, J.; Currie, M.; Gottesdiener, K.; Stoner, E. Relamorelin Reduces Vomiting Frequency and Severity and Accelerates Gastric Emptying in Adults With Diabetic Gastroparesis. *Gastroenterology* **2016**, *151*, 87–96.e6. [CrossRef]
81. Sanaka, M.; Yamamoto, T.; Kuyama, Y. Effects of proton pump inhibitors on gastric emptying: A systematic review. *Dig. Dis. Sci.* **2010**, *55*, 2431–2440. [CrossRef]
82. Wijarnpreecha, K.; Thongprayoon, C.; Panjawatanan, P.; Ungprasert, P. Proton pump inhibitors and risk of dementia. *Ann. Transl. Med.* **2016**, *4*, 240. [CrossRef]
83. Wod, M.; Hallas, J.; Andersen, K.; Rodríguez, L.A.G.; Christensen, K.; Gaist, D. Lack of Association Between Proton Pump Inhibitor Use and Cognitive Decline. *Clin. Gastroenterol. Hepatol. Off. Clin. Pract. J. Am. Gastroenterol. Assoc.* **2018**, *16*, 681–689. [CrossRef]
84. Ashraf, W.; Pfeiffer, R.F.; Park, F.; Lof, J.; Quigley, E.M. Constipation in Parkinson's disease: Objective assessment and response to psyllium. *Mov. Disord. Off. J. Mov. Disord. Soc.* **1997**, *12*, 946–951. [CrossRef] [PubMed]
85. Yu, K.; Ke, M.-Y.; Li, W.-H.; Zhang, S.-Q.; Fang, X.-C. The impact of soluble dietary fibre on gastric emptying, postprandial blood glucose and insulin in patients with type 2 diabetes. *Asia Pac. J. Clin. Nutr.* **2014**, *23*, 210–218. [PubMed]
86. Zesiewicz, T.A.; Sullivan, K.L.; Arnulf, I.; Chaudhuri, K.R.; Morgan, J.C.; Gronseth, G.S.; Miyasaki, J.; Iverson, D.J.; Weiner, W.J. Practice Parameter: Treatment of nonmotor symptoms of Parkinson disease: Report of the Quality Standards Subcommittee of the American Academy of Neurology. *Neurology* **2010**, *74*, 924–931. [CrossRef] [PubMed]
87. Barboza, J.L.; Okun, M.; Moshiree, B. The treatment of gastroparesis, constipation and small intestinal bacterial overgrowth syndrome in patients with Parkinson's disease. *Expert Opin. Pharmacother.* **2015**, *16*, 2449–2464. [CrossRef]

88. Fernandez, H.H.; Trieschmann, M.E.; Friedman, J.H. Treatment of psychosis in Parkinson's disease: Safety considerations. *Drug Saf.* **2003**, *26*, 643–659. [CrossRef] [PubMed]
89. Kwan, C.; Huot, P. 5-HT3 receptors in Parkinson's disease psychosis: A forgotten target? *Neurodegener. Dis. Manag.* **2019**, *9*, 251–253. [CrossRef]
90. Arnold, G.; Schwarz, J.; Macher, C.; Oertel, W.H. Domperidone is superior to ondansetron in acute apomorphine challenge in previously untreated parkinsonian patients—A double blind study. *Parkinsonism Relat. Disord.* **1997**, *3*, 191–193. [CrossRef]
91. Pasricha, P.J.; Yates, K.P.; Sarosiek, I.; McCallum, R.W.; Abell, T.L.; Koch, K.L.; Nguyen, L.A.B.; Snape, W.J.; Hasler, W.L.; Clarke, J.O.; et al. Aprepitant Has Mixed Effects on Nausea and Reduces Other Symptoms in Patients With Gastroparesis and Related Disorders. *Gastroenterology* **2018**, *154*, 65–76.e11. [CrossRef]
92. Triadafilopoulos, G.; Gandhy, R.; Barlow, C. Pilot cohort study of endoscopic botulinum neurotoxin injection in Parkinson's disease. *Parkinsonism Relat. Disord.* **2017**, *44*, 33–37. [CrossRef]
93. Arts, J.; Holvoet, L.; Caenepeel, P.; Bisschops, R.; Sifrim, D.; Verbeke, K.; Janssens, J.; Tack, J. Clinical trial: A randomized-controlled crossover study of intrapyloric injection of botulinum toxin in gastroparesis. *Aliment. Pharmacol. Ther.* **2007**, *26*, 1251–1258. [CrossRef]
94. Friedenberg, F.K.; Palit, A.; Parkman, H.P.; Hanlon, A.; Nelson, D.B. Botulinum toxin A for the treatment of delayed gastric emptying. *Am. J. Gastroenterol.* **2008**, *103*, 416–423. [CrossRef]
95. Murray, F.R.; Schindler, V.; Hente, J.M.; Fischbach, L.M.; Schnurre, L.; Deibel, A.; Hildenbrand, F.F.; Tatu, A.M.; Pohl, D. Pyloric dilation with the eosophgeal functional lumen imaging probe in gastroparesis improves gastric emptying, pyloric distensibility, and symptoms. *Gastrointest. Endosc.* **2021**. [CrossRef]
96. Gonzalez, J.M.; Benezech, A.; Vitton, V.; Barthet, M. G-POEM with antro-pyloromyotomy for the treatment of refractory gastroparesis: Mid-term follow-up and factors predicting outcome. *Aliment. Pharmacol. Ther.* **2017**, *46*, 364–370. [CrossRef]
97. Vosoughi, K.; Ichkhanian, Y.; Benias, P.; Miller, L.; Aadam, A.A.; Triggs, J.R.; Law, R.; Hasler, W.; Bowers, N.; Chaves, D.; et al. Gastric per-oral endoscopic myotomy (G-POEM) for refractory gastroparesis: Results from an international prospective trial. *Gut* **2021**. [CrossRef] [PubMed]
98. Fasano, A.; Bove, F.; Gabrielli, M.; Petracca, M.; Zocco, M.A.; Ragazzoni, E.; Barbaro, F.; Piano, C.; Fortuna, S.; Tortora, A.; et al. The role of small intestinal bacterial overgrowth in Parkinson's disease. *Mov. Disord. Off. J. Mov. Disord. Soc.* **2013**, *28*, 1241–1249. [CrossRef] [PubMed]
99. Maini Rekdal, V.; Bess, E.N.; Bisanz, J.E.; Turnbaugh, P.J.; Balskus, E.P. Discovery and inhibition of an interspecies gut bacterial pathway for Levodopa metabolism. *Science* **2019**, *364*, eaau6323. [CrossRef] [PubMed]
100. Chung, K.A.; Pfeiffer, R.F. Gastrointestinal dysfunction in the synucleinopathies. *Clin. Auton. Res.* **2021**, *31*, 77–99. [CrossRef]
101. Arai, E.; Arai, M.; Uchiyama, T.; Higuchi, Y.; Aoyagi, K.; Yamanaka, Y.; Yamamoto, T.; Nagano, O.; Shiina, A.; Maruoka, D.; et al. Subthalamic deep brain stimulation can improve gastric emptying in Parkinson's disease. *Brain J. Neurol.* **2012**, *135 Pt 5*, 1478–1485. [CrossRef]
102. Krygowska-Wajs, A.; Furgala, A.; Gorecka-Mazur, A.; Pietraszko, W.; Thor, P.; Potasz-Kulikowska, K.; Moskala, M. The effect of subthalamic deep brain stimulation on gastric motility in Parkinson's disease. *Parkinsonism Relat. Disord.* **2016**, *26*, 35–40. [CrossRef] [PubMed]

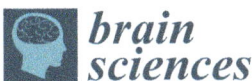

Systematic Review

Neurosonological Findings Related to Non-Motor Features of Parkinson's Disease: A Systematic Review

Cristina del Toro Pérez [1,†], Laura Amaya Pascasio [1,†], Antonio Arjona Padillo [1], Jesús Olivares Romero [1], María Victoria Mejías Olmedo [1], Javier Fernández Pérez [1], Manuel Payán Ortiz [1] and Patricia Martínez-Sánchez [1,2,*]

[1] Neurosonology Laboratory, Department of Neurology, Torrecárdenas University Hospital, 04009 Almería, Spain; cristinadeltoro@msn.com (C.d.T.P.); laura.amaya.pascasio@gmail.com (L.A.P.); aarjonap@gmail.com (A.A.P.); olivares.je@gmail.com (J.O.R.); v.mejiasolmedo@hotmail.com (M.V.M.O.); javifp1985@gmail.com (J.F.P.); payanortiz@hotmail.com (M.P.O.)
[2] Faculty of Health Sciences, CEINSA (Center of Health Research), University of Almería, La Cañada, 04120 Almería, Spain
* Correspondence: patrinda@ual.es
† The two authors have contributed equally to the manuscript.

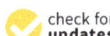

Citation: del Toro Pérez, C.; Amaya Pascasio, L.; Arjona Padillo, A.; Olivares Romero, J.; Mejías Olmedo, M.V.; Fernández Pérez, J.; Payán Ortiz, M.; Martínez-Sánchez, P. Neurosonological Findings Related to Non-Motor Features of Parkinson's Disease: A Systematic Review. *Brain Sci.* **2021**, *11*, 776. https://doi.org/10.3390/brainsci11060776

Academic Editor: Alicia M. Pickrell

Received: 8 May 2021
Accepted: 8 June 2021
Published: 11 June 2021

Publisher's Note: MDPI stays neutral with regard to jurisdictional claims in published maps and institutional affiliations.

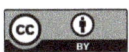

Copyright: © 2021 by the authors. Licensee MDPI, Basel, Switzerland. This article is an open access article distributed under the terms and conditions of the Creative Commons Attribution (CC BY) license (https://creativecommons.org/licenses/by/4.0/).

Abstract: Non-motor symptoms (NMS) in Parkinson's disease (PD), including neuropsychiatric or dysautonomic complaints, fatigue, or pain, are frequent and have a high impact on the patient's quality of life. They are often poorly recognized and inadequately treated. In the recent years, the growing awareness of NMS has favored the development of techniques that complement the clinician's diagnosis. This review provides an overview of the most important ultrasonographic findings related to the presence of various NMS. Literature research was conducted in PubMed, Scopus, and Web of Science from inception until January 2021, retrieving 23 prospective observational studies evaluating transcranial and cervical ultrasound in depression, dementia, dysautonomic symptoms, psychosis, and restless leg syndrome. Overall, the eligible articles showed good or fair quality according to the QUADAS-2 assessment. Brainstem raphe hypoechogenicity was related to the presence of depression in PD and also in depressed patients without PD, as well as to overactive bladder. Substantia nigra hyperechogenicity was frequent in patients with visual hallucinations, and larger intracranial ventricles correlated with dementia. Evaluation of the vagus nerve showed contradictory findings. The results of this systematic review demonstrated that transcranial ultrasound can be a useful complementary tool in the evaluation of NMS in PD.

Keywords: transcranial sonography; Parkinson's disease; non-motor symptoms; systematic review; depression; apathy; autonomic dysfunction; bladder dysfunction; restless legs syndrome; sleep disorders; cognitive disorders; dementia; hallucinations; apathy

1. Introduction

Parkinson's disease (PD) is a chronic progressive neurodegenerative disorder characterized not only by its motor aspects, but also by numerous non-motor symptoms (NMS) that encompass neuropsychiatric manifestation, sensory abnormalities, behavioral changes, sleep disturbances, and autonomic dysfunction. NMS may be the presenting clinical feature of PD in over 20% of individuals, which usually delays PD diagnosis and an early appropriate treatment [1]. Various studies have demonstrated that NMS have a greater impact on quality of life than motor manifestations, even during the first years after diagnosis. Moreover, hallucinations have been pointed out as the strongest predictor of nursing home placement for people with PD [2].

Depression and apathy are common in PD, with 40% of patients presenting apathy and 17% suffering from a major depressive disorder, occurring at any time during the course of the disease [3,4]. Common autonomic complaints are orthostatic hypotension, gastrointestinal dysfunction, and urinary symptoms. Together with REM sleep behavior disorder (RBD), they present a prevalence in the range of 25–50% [1].

During the last decades, there has been a growing use of transcranial sonography (TCS) to evaluate brainstem and subcortical brain structures as a complementary tool in the diagnosis of PD. TCS is reliable and sensitive in detecting basal ganglia abnormalities and has proven its potential to identify idiopathic PD from healthy controls based on substantia nigra (SN) hyperechogenicity, which is present in 67 to 95% PD patients compared to 3 to 9% in subjects without PD [5–7].

A review of TCS findings associated to NMS in PD performed by Walter et al. in 2010 showed evidence that some midbrain changes may be related to NMS and can contribute to their identification [8]. Since then, several studies exploring this topic have been published and new techniques have been developed.

The aim of the systematic review is to provide a clear view on the most relevant abnormalities identified with TCS and other ultrasound techniques that can be related to the presence of NMS in PD. The main NMS addressed are depression, anxiety, apathy, hallucinations, cognitive disorders, autonomic dysfunction, restless legs syndrome, sleep disorders, pain, fatigue, anosmia, ageusia, and libido alterations.

2. Materials and Methods

2.1. Search Strategy

This protocol follows the guidelines according to the preferred reporting items for systematic reviews and meta-analysis protocol (PRISMA-P) [9]. It was registered in the PROS PERO international database of prospectively registered systematic reviews (CRD 42021250195). PubMed, Scopus, and Web of Science electronic databases were searched for articles in English or Spanish, published up to January 2021, and with the following criteria: cross-sectional, case-control, and cohort observational studies including patients with Parkinson's disease, ultrasound assessment of neurological structures and evaluation of NMS, analyzing differences between echogenicity and/or size of the evaluated structures between PD suffering or not from a specific NMS. Case reports were excluded. The search query was: ("non-motor symptoms" OR "depression" OR "fatigue" OR "low blood pressure" OR "autonomic dysfunction" OR "orthostatic hypotension" OR "bladder dysfunction" OR "restless legs syndrome" OR "sleep disorders" OR "REM-sleep behavior disorder" OR "pain" OR "cognitive disorders" OR "anxiety" OR "hallucinations" OR "delusions" OR "anosmia" OR "apathy" OR "ageusia" OR "libido" OR "constipation") AND ("Parkinson's disease" OR "PD") AND ("transcranial sonography" OR "ultrasound" OR "transcranial ultrasonography").

In addition to the database search, a manual revision of the reference lists of all relevant articles was performed to identify additional studies of interest.

2.2. Selection of Studies

Two researchers (C.T. and L.A.) separately reviewed the titles and abstracts of the retrieved articles to determine the presence of the abovementioned criteria. Disagreements were solved by the consensus of a third author (P.M.). Duplicated entries, studies on diseases different from PD or evaluation techniques other than ultrasound, papers not written in English or Spanish, publications that were not research studies, and any other article that did not fit with the scope of the review were excluded.

2.3. Data Extraction

Upon manuscript selection, the following information was extracted: the number of participants and socio-demographic characteristics, the assessed NMS and the evaluation protocol or diagnostic strategies, the ultrasound modalities, and the major findings reported.

A limited number of studies were expected to be found by the systematic search and they were expected to be clinically and methodologically heterogeneous. Likewise, some of the results were based on qualitative findings. Therefore, conducting a meta-analysis was not included in this protocol.

2.4. Quality Assessment

The risk of bias of the included studies was evaluated using QUADAS-2 [10] for assessing the risk of bias recommendations by The Cochrane Collaboration. In this review, there is no gold standard test for comparison of the ultrasound findings. Consequently, we considered the proposed diagnosis criteria of the non-motor syndrome, based on validated scales or neurologist advice, for each study as the reference gold standard.

3. Results

After removing duplicates, the database search yielded 263 results. An additional 14 studies were identified through the references of the principal records. A total of 277 publications were screened for eligibility and 254 studies were excluded for the following reasons: publications involving different pathologies, symptoms evaluated in a population different from PD, systematic reviews, and animal experimental studies. The PRISMA Flow Diagram is shown in Figure 1. Eventually, 23 studies were included and are summarized in Table 1.

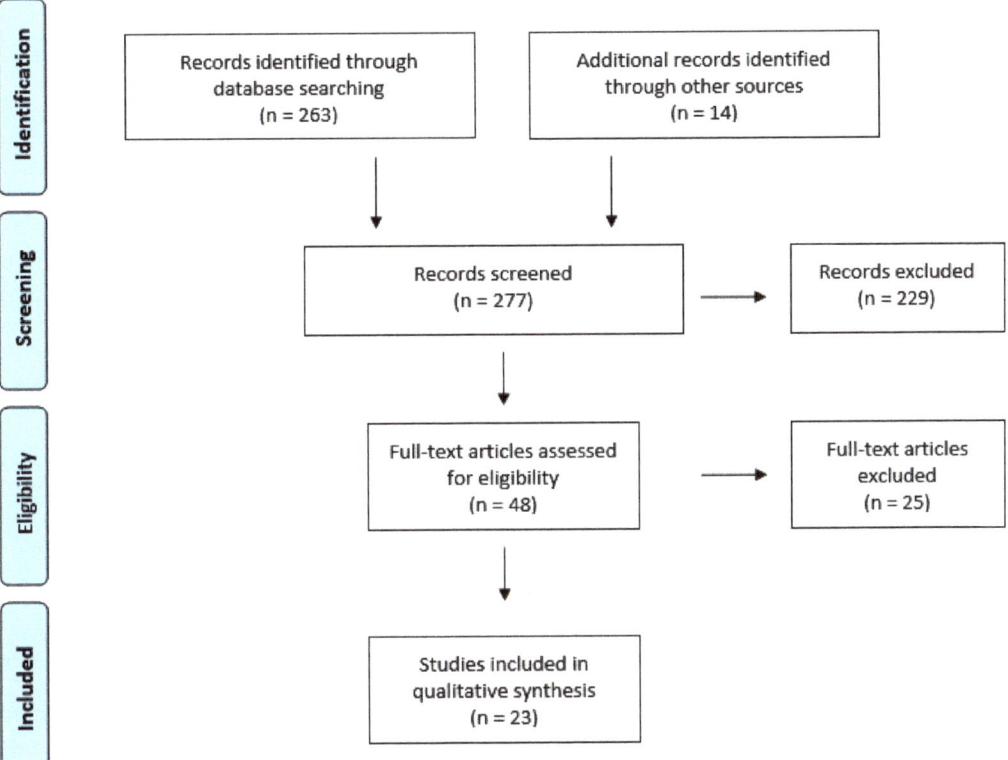

Figure 1. PRISMA Flow Diagram.

Table 1. Study characteristics.

STUDY	Population N, Age/Male	Symptom Evaluation	Ultrasound Evaluation	Main Findings	Other Findings
Depression					
Becker, 1997 [11]	30 PD+. 68,3/25 30 PD− 65/24	DSM-III HDRS CGI-S	TCS, 2.25 MHz. BR echogenicity * Ventricles Width	PD+, D+: ↓BR echogenicity, ↑lateral ventricles. Correlation: BR echogenicity and D severity.	No differences PD+, D− and healthy controls.
Berg, 1999 [12]	31 PD+ 65,5/16	DSM-IV HDRS BDI	TCS, 2.5 MHz. BR echogenicity *	PD+, D+: ↓BR echogenicity	MRI: PD+, D+: hyperintense mesencephalic midline
Walter, 2007a [13]	101 PD+ 66,6/58	DSM IV	TCS, 2.5 MHz. BR echogenicity ^	PD+, D+: ↓ BR echogenicity	N.R.
Walter, 2007b [14]	45 PD+, D+ 45 PD+, D− 55 PD−, D+ 55 PD−, D− 61/84	DSM IV DRS BDI	TCS, 2.5 MHz. SN echogenicity (N < 20 mm^2) BR echogenicity ^.	PD+, D+: ↓BR echogenicity. PD+, D+ vs. D−: No difference in SN. ↑SN, ↓BR: Depression prior to PD diagnosis	PD−, D+: ↑SN
Cho, 2011 [15]	61 PD+ 68/38 41 PD−, D− 58/28	HDRS BDI	TCS, 2.5 MHz. BR echogenicity *	PD+, D+: ↓BR echogenicity, Correlation: ↓ BR echogenicity and ↑Hamilton Depression Scale.	PD + D+: higher motor severity
Stankovic, 2015 [16]	118 PD+ 61/72	HARS Apathy Scale MADRS	TCS, 2.5 MHz SN echogenicity (N < 19 mm^2) BR echogenicity *	PD+, D+: ↓BR echogenicity (> sadness, pessimism, >anxiety)	↓BR echogenicity, ↑L-Dopa motor complications.
Bouwmans, 2016a [17]	72 PD+, 68/N.R. 54 other PK 72/N.R.	HDRS	TCS, 2–4 MHz. SN echogenicity (N < 20 mm^2) BR echogenicity ^ 3rd. ventricle Width	No differences (Only 16 D+)	N.R.
Zhang, 2016 [18]	80 PD+ 40 PD− D+ 40 PD− D− 61/97	HDRS BDI	TCS, 2.5 MHz BR echogenicity †	PD+, D+ and PD−, D+: ↓BR echogenicity. Correlation: ↓ BR echogenicity and ↑HDRS, BDI.	N.R.
Toomsoo, 2017 [19]	266 PD+ 168 PD− 69,7/228	BDI	TCS, 1.8–3.6 MHz SN echogenicity (N < 20 mm^2) BR echogenicity *	PD + D+ and PD− D +: ↓BR echogenicity. Correlation: ↓ BR echogenicity and ↑BDI	Correlation: D and PD duration, motor and cognitive impairment.
Liu, 2018 [20]	30 D+ PD+ 30 D− PD+ 24 D+ PD− 28 D− PD− 55/56	HDRS Platelet serotonin levels	TCS, 2.5 MHz BR echogenicity ^ SN echogenicity (N < 20 mm^2). 3rd. ventricle width	PD+, D+ and PD− D+: ↓BR echogenicity. No association SN and RN echogenicity.	Platelet serotonin. Levels: no differences.
Ritcher, 2018 [21]	31 PD+ 16 ET+ 16 PD−, ET−	Lille apathy rating scale. BDI	TCS, 2.5 MHz. SN echogenicity (N < 20 mm^2) BR echogenicity *	PD+: ↓BR echogenicity. Correlation: ↓ BR echogenicity and ↑Apathy, Beck Scores.	No difference: SN in ET+ and controls.
Bei, 2020 [22]	135 PD+ 63/83	HDRS HARS	TCS, 2.5 MHz SN echogenicity (N < 20 mm^2) BR echogenicity ^	D+, Anxiety+: ↓BR echogenicity. Correlation: ↓ BR echogenicity and ↑Hamilton Scores, PDQ-39	No relation BR and motor symptoms.

Table 1. Cont.

STUDY	Population N, Age/Male	Symptom Evaluation	Ultrasound Evaluation	Main Findings	Other Findings
Dementia					
Walter, 2006a [23]	104 PD+ 14 DLB+ 70/69	MMSE Addenbrooke cognitive examination	TCS, 2.5 MHz SN echogenicity (N < 20 mm^2) Thalami, Caudate, BR echogenicity ^, 3rd. ventricle Width	PD + Dementia+: ↑ lateral frontal (17.3 mm), 3rd ventricle (8.6 mm) widths.	DLB+ vs. PD+ dementia +: Bilateral ↑ SN in DLB+. Similar ventricle widths.
Walter, 2007a [13]	101 PD+ 66,6/58	DSM IV MMSE	TCS, 2.5 MHz. ventricles width	PD + Dementia+: Lateral frontal horn ≥15.4 mm	↑Caudate echogenicity: ↑drug-induced psychosis.
Bouwmans, 2016b [24]	72 PD+ 68/70 54 other PK 72/80	SCOPA-COG: PD cognition Scale.	TCS, 2–4 MHz. SN echogenicity (N < 20 mm^2) BR echogenicity ^, 3rd. ventricle width	Larger 3rd ventricle in PD+ and cognitive impairment. SN: Not related to cognition.	Atypical PK + cognitive symptoms: ↓BR echogenicity (not in PD)
Dong, 2017 [25]	98 PD+ 77/68 40 PD− 65/27	Dementia clinical diagnosis. MMSE MoCA PD-NMSQ	TCS, 2.5 MHz. SN echogenicity (N < 20 mm^2) 3rd. ventricle width (Normal < 7/10 mm under/over 60 y.)	Larger 3rd ventricle in PD+ with dementia. Cutoff 6.8 mm (S: 69.6%, Sp: 61.5%). SN: Not related with cognition.	3rd. ventricle: No differences PD without dementia and controls.
Autonomic dysfunction					
Walter, 2006b [26]	116 PD+ 66,5/65	Overactive bladder symptoms (other causes ruled out)	TCS, 2.5 MHz. BR echogenicity * SN echogenicity, thalamus, 3rd.ventricle width	Overactive bladder: ↓BR echogenicity.	N.R.
Fedtke, 2018 [27]	32 PD+ 30 PD− 70/40	UPDRS I–IV	HRUS Vagus nerve (cervical CSA)	No differences PD+, PD−. No correlation with UPDRS I-IV.	Positive correlation: Right CSA and bradykinesia score.
Pelz, 2018 [28]	35 PD+ 35 PD− 67/34	PD-NMSQ, MoCA	15 MHz HRUS Vagus nerve (cervical CSA)	PD+: Smaller bilateral CSA. No correlation with PD− NMSQ.	N.R.
Walter, 2018 [29]	20 PD+ 73/13 61 PD− 45/23	PD-NMSQ, heart rate variability (R-R)	15 MHz HRUS Vagus, spinal, accessory, phrenic nerves (cervical CSA)	PD+: Smaller bilateral CSA. Negative Correlation: CSA and PD-NMSQ, autonomic items. Heart rate variability and right CSA in PD + and PD−. No differences in other nerves	Left CSA correlates with motor severity.
Restless legs syndrome					
Kwon, 2010 [30]	63 PD+ 65/30 40iRLS+ 53/21 40 controls 69/21	Sleep questionnaire Neurologist assessment	TCS, 2.5 MHz. SN echogenicity (N < 20 mm^2)	SN: No differences in PD + with and without RLS.	iRLS+: ↓↓SN size than PD+ and controls.
Ryu, 2011 [31]	44PD+ 41iRLS+ 35 controls 60–71	RLS Diagnostic criteria	TCS, 2.5 MHz. SN echogenicity (N < 20 mm^2)	SN: No differences in PD + with and without RLS.	iRLS +: ↓↓SN size than PD+ and controls.

Table 1. Cont.

STUDY	Population N, Age/Male	Symptom Evaluation	Ultrasound Evaluation	Main Findings	Other Findings
Hallucinations and psychosis					
Zhou, 2016 [32]	201 PD+ 92 PD− 60/193	PD-NMSQ Odor test RBDSQ SCOPA-AUT MMSE HDRS	TCS, 2.5 MHz. SN echogenicity (N < 18 mm^2)	No correlation SN and non-motor symptoms	Correlation: SN and UPDRS-II score
Li, 2020 [33]	111 PD+ 61 PD− 66;63/110	PD-NMSQ Sleep Scale, Constipation, Fatigue, MMSE HDRS, HARS	TCS, 1.82 MHz. SN echogenicity (N < 23.5 mm^2)	PD with hallucinations: ↑ SN echo-size	No other differences

BDI: Beck's Depression Inventory, BR: Brainstem Raphe, CGI-S: Clinical Global Impression-Severity scale, CSA: cross-sectional area, D+: depression, D−: no depression, DLB+: dementia with Lewy bodies, DSM: Diagnostic and Statistical Manual of Mental Disorders, ET+: essential tremor, ET−: no essential tremor, HARS: Hamilton Anxiety Rating Scale, HDR: Hamilton Depression Rating Scale, HRUS: high resolution ultrasound, iRLS: idiopathic restless legs syndrome, MADRS: Montgomery–Asberg Depression Rating Scale, MMSE: Minimental State Examination, MoCA: Montreal Cognitive Assessment, N: normal reference value, N.R.: not reported, PD+: Parkinson's disease, PD−: No Parkinson's disease, PD-NMSQ: Non-Motor Symptoms Questionnaire for patients with Parkinson's disease, PK: Parkinsonism, RBDSQ: Rapid Eye Movement Sleep Behavior Disorder Screening Questionnaire, iRLS+: idiopathic Restless Leg Syndrome, SCOPA-AUT: Scale for outcomes in PD of autonomic symptoms, SN: Substantia nigra, TCS: transcranial sonography, UPDRS: the Movement Disorder Society-sponsored revision of the Unified Parkinson's Disease Rating Scale. ↑ Increase or improved, ↓ Decreased or worsened. * Three grades semiquantitative scale using the hyperechogenic red nucleus as a reference point: 1 = raphe not visible/isoechogenic raphe compared with adjacent brainstem parenchyma, 2 = slightly echogenic raphe, 3 = normal raphe echogenicity (echogenicity of the raphe is identical to that of the red nucleus). ^ Two grades semiquantitative scale: 1 = not visible or interrupted echogenicity; 2 = continuous echogenicity compared to red nucleus. † Four grades semiquantitative scale: 1 = invisible raphe, echogenic raphe was not visible; 2 = interrupted raphe, echogenic raphe was interrupted compared with the red nucleus; 3 = decreased raphe, echogenic raphe was decreased compared with the red nucleus, but it was continuous; 4 = normal raphe, with the same echogenicity of red nucleus. Grades 1–3 are determined as abnormal.

3.1. Study Characteristics

The included studies were published between 1997 and 2020, with 60% published during the last five years. The articles consisted of cross-sectional, case-control, and cohort prospective studies, including mainly patients with PD, healthy controls, and non-PD patients with depression or other NMS. The mean participant sample size was 133 (SD = 85.2; range = 81–143). The PD participants' ages ranged from 45 to 77, with a majority being male patients. The disease duration varied considerably between studies and within each study, ranging from 30 months to 15 years. Three studies included newly diagnosed PD. The main NMS evaluated was depression (12 articles), followed by dementia (4 studies), and dysautonomic symptoms (4 studies). Standardized clinical scales and neurologist or psychiatrist evaluation were the preferred instrument used for assessing NMS, summarized in Table 1. Main referred structures identified by transcranial ultrasound can be found in Appendix A.

3.2. Quality Assessment

We analyzed the quality of the studies using the QUADAS-2 tool. Most of the observational studies showed a low risk of bias. Regarding patient selection, the main limitations were that the sample was not based in an epidemiological registry and in a few studies, selection criteria were not clearly described. For the index test, most studies were homogeneous, describing the pre-stablished evaluation criteria, with more than one experienced evaluator blinded to the patient diagnosis. In addition, inconsistent application of reference standard and not having a clear time of application were identified (Figure 2).

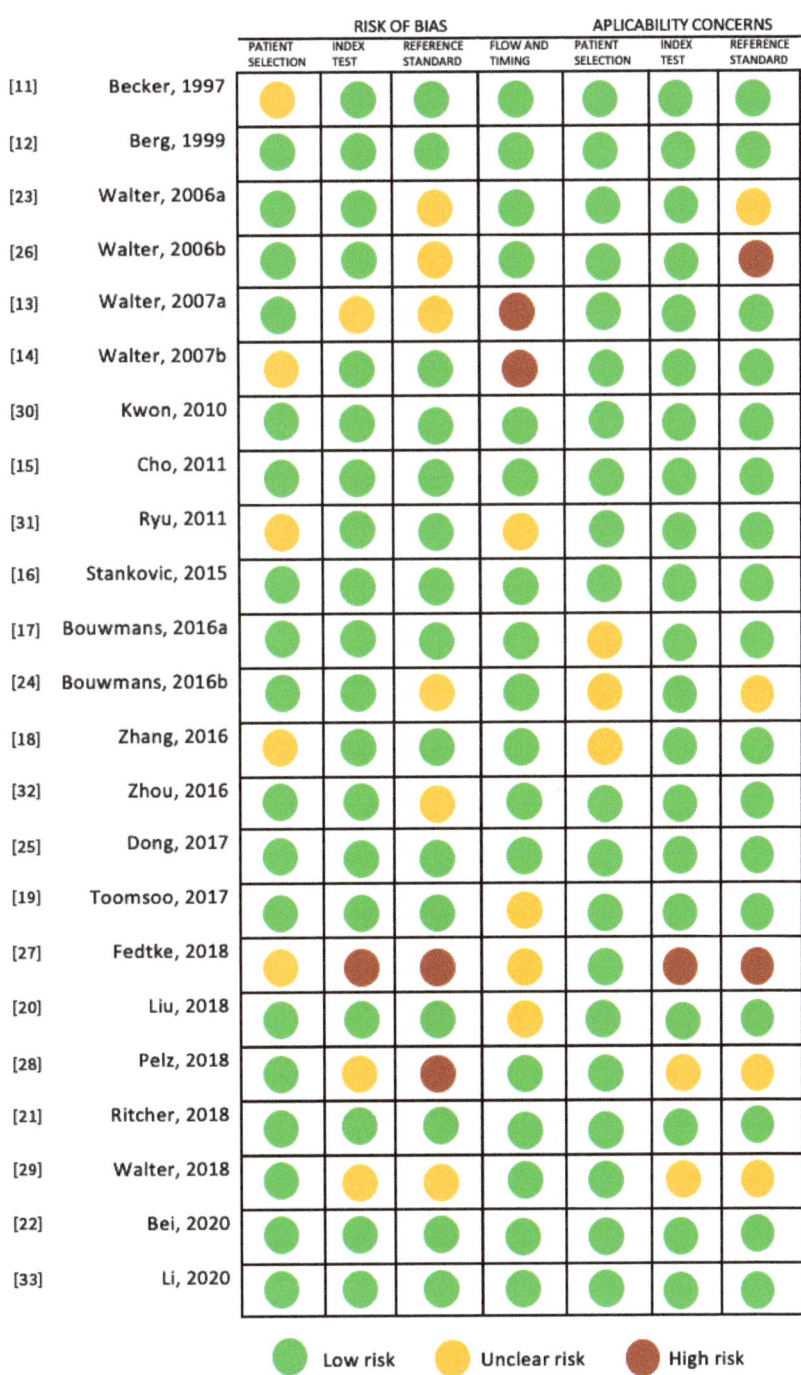

Figure 2. Assessment of risk of bias of studies. QUADAS-2 tool. QUADAS-2, Quality Assessment of Diagnostic Accuracy Studies-2.

3.3. Main Findings

3.3.1. Depression

In 1997, Becker el al. [11] evaluated for the first time ultrasound midbrain changes in depressed PD patients, comparing with non-depressed PD patients and non-PD control subjects. They reported a relationship between BR hypoechogenicity and the presence of depression, with an inverse correlation between the grade of echogenicity and the severity of depression ($\rho = -0.646$, $p < 0.001$). They also found a significant enlargement of the lateral ventricles compared to non-depressed PD patients. In 1999, Berg et al. [12] analyzed RMI and ultrasound midbrain changes in 31 PD patients, they found that BR echogenicity was significantly reduced in depressed PD patients, which was consistent with the findings previously reported. However, no correlation between midbrain intensity in RMI and BR echogenicity was demonstrated. Since then, many authors have studied brain parenchy mal ultrasound characteristics and related them to NMS, especially to the presence of de pression. BR hypoechogenicity, found in 35 to 85% depressed PD patients compared to 6 to 27% in controls, was associated with concomitant depression in PD patients in all revised studies [11–16,18–22], except for one which involved 126 early stage PD patients and compared BR and SN alterations between depressed (only 16 out of the 72 included subjects) and non-depressed patients based on the Hamilton Depression Rating Scale [17]. In addition, BR hypoechogenicity was also more frequent in non-PD patients with unipolar depression [14,18,20]. Interestingly, when compared to healthy controls, non-depressed PD patients showed no differences in BR echogenicity [11,14,15,18–21]. Most of the studies reported a correlation between BR hypoechogenicity and the severity of depressive symp toms independently of age, disease duration, and Hoehn and Yahr stage [11,15,16,18,19,21,22]. One study analyzed platelet serotonin levels as a biomarker of depression and correlated them with the TCS findings, without evidencing a significant relation [20]. Apathy, pessimistic thoughts, and anxiety were also related to BR hypoechogenicity [16,21].

In a study by Walter et al. [14] with 200 patients, 45 PD without depression, 45 PD with a depressive syndrome, and 110 non-PD patients, 55 of them with depression, SN hyperechogenicity was found in 40% non-PD patients with depression, 69% PD without depression and 87% depressed PD subjects, while it was only found in 3% of healthy controls. Non-Parkinsonian subjects with depression had a 3-fold higher frequency of SN hyperechogenicity compared to controls. Moreover, the combination of marked SN hyperechogenicity and reduced raphe echogenicity was significantly associated with a history of depressive disorder prior to onset of PD and with motor asymmetry in non-PD subjects with depression [14].

3.3.2. Dementia

Four studies focused on the link between midbrain ultrasound changes and cognitive impairment or dementia in PD patients. They included a total of 375 PD subjects with and without dementia, 54 patients with other Parkinsonism, 14 patients with dementia with Lewy bodies (DLB), and 40 healthy controls [13,23–25]. Frontal horn dilatation and third ventricle dilatation were associated with dementia and the width of both ventricles corre lated with age but not with PD duration. No differences were identified between PD patients without dementia and controls [13,23–25]. Walter et al. [13] found that PD subjects with dementia had larger third ventricle width (8.7 ± 2.1 vs. 6.9 ± 2.5 mm; $p = 0.002$) and frontal horn width (17.3 ± 3.1 vs. 14.9 ± 3.1 mm; $p = 0.003$) compared to PD patients without dementia. Frontal horn was found to discriminate dementia in PD slightly better (AUC, 0.70; $p = 0.006$) than third ventricle (AUC, 0.69; $p = 0.007$), with a proposed cutoff value ≥ 15.4 mm for 82% sensitivity and 58% specificity [13].

In addition, based on the ROC curve, Dong et al. [25] suggested that a third ventricle width cut-off of 6.8 mm had a 69.6% sensitivity and a 61.5% specificity for discriminating between PD patients with and without dementia.

No differences in SN sizes were found in PD patients with dementia compared to those without dementia, both showing a larger SN than healthy controls [13,24,25]. The study of SN was useful to discriminate between DLB and PD, based on SN asymmetry and echogenic size [23].

Interestingly, in the group of atypical Parkinsonism, a significantly higher frequency of hypoechogenic BR was described in subjects with cognitive impairment compared to atypical Parkinsonisms without cognitive impairment [24].

3.3.3. Autonomic Dysfunction

For the purpose of this review, the term autonomic dysfunction comprises all the symptoms derived from organs mainly dependent on the autonomic nervous system, such as constipation or urinary incontinence, even if the neurological mechanisms responsible for these symptoms in PD patients are not fully clarified and may present a central, peripheral, or combined pathophysiological mechanism.

Regarding urinary symptoms, Walter et al. [26] studied TCS characteristics (SN echogenic size and BR, thalami, lenticular nuclei and heads of caudate nuclei echogenicity, and widths of third ventricle and of frontal horns of lateral ventricles) in 116 PD patients divided into two groups, PD patients with overactive bladder symptoms (OAB) and PD patients without OAB symptoms, assessed by a clinical interview with the neurologist. Alternative etiologies of OAB were ruled out. BR hypoechogenicity was more pronounced in subjects with longer duration of urinary symptoms, with no other differences identified in the rest of the analyzed structures. Other authors evaluated the relation of midbrain transcranial structures and autonomic specific items in the Non-Motor Symptoms Questionnaire for patients with PD (PD-NMSQ), as well as the Scale for Outcomes in PD, autonomic symptoms (SCOPA-AUT) [32,33]. The PD-NMSQ consists of 30 items that address nine domains including gastrointestinal, cardiovascular, and urinary symptoms, sexual function, cognition (apathy, attention, memory), presence of hallucinations, depression or anxiety, sleep disorders, pain, and fatigue [34]. The SCOPA-AUT includes 25 items assessing autonomic symptoms: gastrointestinal, urinary, cardiovascular, thermoregulatory, pupillomotor, and sexual dysfunction [35]. None of the included studies reported any relevant relation between PD-NMSQ and SCOPA-AUT scores and the US findings [32,33].

In recent years, four studies have been published evaluating the vagus nerve diameter and cross-sectional area (CSA) in the cervical region by high resolution ultrasound, comparing between PD patients and healthy subjects [27–29,36]. In three of them, NMS were assessed with the Unified Parkinson's Disease Rating Scale, part I (UPDRS I) [37], which has four questions concerning intellectual impairment, thought disorder, depression, and motivation/initiative [27], and with the PD-NMSQ [28,29]. Electrocardiographic heart rate variability was also analyzed as a marker of vagal cardiac innervation [29]. Walter et al. [29] found significant bilateral atrophy of the vagus nerve without differences in the spinal accessory or the phrenic nerves in PD patients compared to age-matched controls. Moreover, bilateral vagus nerve CSA correlated negatively with the PD-NMSQ total score ($r = -0.51$; $p = 0.001$) and with the sum score of autonomic items of the PD-NMSQ ($r = -0.46$; $p = 0.003$). Heart rate variability correlated only with the right vagus nerve CSA ($r = 0.58$; $p = 0.001$) [29]. Pelz et al. [28] obtained similar results regarding vagus CSA but did not demonstrate correlation with the PD-NMSQ. Contrary to this, Fedtke et al. [27] found no differences in the SCA in both groups.

3.3.4. Restless Leg Syndrome

The TSC findings of 107 PD patients, 81 subjects with idiopathic restless leg syndrome (iRLS) and 75 age- and sex-matched healthy controls were analyzed in two studies [30,31]. SN echogenicity was significantly decreased in iRLS patients and increased in PD− RLS. Likewise, iRLS SN was significantly hypoechogenic compared to healthy controls [30,31]. No differences in SN were found between PD patients with and without RLS [30,31].

3.3.5. Hallucinations and Psychosis

Walter et al. [13] found an association between the caudate nuclei hyperechogenicity and the presence of drug-induced psychosis in a group of 101 PD subjects. This finding was independent from PD duration. More recently, Li et al. [33] compared the TCS findings in a group of 111 PD patients and 61 non-PD controls, evaluating the presence of NMS with the PD-NMSQ, the Parkinson's disease sleep scale, addressing sleep and nocturnal disability [38], the constipation severity instrument [39], and the Parkinson's disease Fatigue Scale [40]. They reported, for the first time, that the SN echogenic area in PD patients with visual hallucinations (VH) was significantly higher than in those without VH. This finding was constant after adjusting by age, disease duration, and Minimental State Examination and UPDRS scores [33].

4. Discussion

The present systematic review aimed to provide a comprehensive analysis of the available literature reporting ultrasound findings in NMS in PD population. Given the expanding awareness of non-motor complaints in PD, we believe that such a review was necessary to better delineate the usefulness of ultrasound in the diagnosis and understanding of those features.

4.1. Brainstem Raphe

In the revised literature, BR hypoechogenicity has been related with depressive states in PD patients [11–16,18–22]. Reduced echogenicity of BR was more frequent in PD patients (25 to 30%) compared to controls (6 to 9%) [13,14], with a 3.5 higher risk of developing depression compared to non-depressed PD population [16]. This alteration had been previously reported for non-Parkinsonian patients with unipolar depression and depressive mood disorders, with a prevalence of 50–70% [41,42] and was confirmed in the studies comparing PD with depression and depressed patients without PD [14,18,20]. The same TCS pattern has been described in depressive patients suffering from other neurological conditions such as Wilson's disease and Huntington disease [43,44], but not in multiple sclerosis [45,46].

There is no consensus about the association between BR hypoechogenicity and the severity of depressive symptoms, although some groups showed a negative significant correlation. In depressed non-PD patients, the presence of BR hypoechogenicity seems to predict a better response to serotonin reuptake inhibitors with 70% sensitivity, 88% specificity, and 88% positive predictive value [42].

The BR sonographic findings could be correlated to an increase in the signal intensity of the brainstem midline (raphe) on T2-weighted images on MRIs performed in depressed patients with and without PD [12], suggesting a structural disruption of the BR. These similarities in depressive patients with and without PD support the hypothesis of a structural alteration of the mesencephalon with a common pathophysiological basis [45].

Anatomically, the echogenic midline represents various nuclei and fiber tracts connecting serotonergic, dopaminergic, and noradrenergic brainstem nuclei with subcortical and cortical brain areas. The dorsal raphe nucleus is one of the BR structures and is considered the major origin for serotonin release in the brain [47]. A reduced echogenic signal of the BR could be due to alterations in the micro-architecture of this region, confirmed by a few histological reports, reflecting a serotonin deficiency which is involved in depression pathophysiology [45]. Depressed PD patients have low concentrations of serotonin, dopamine, and noradrenalin or their metabolites in cerebrospinal fluid [48]; this has been compared to platelet serotonin levels as a peripheral biomarker for depression, without success [21,49].

Serotonergic systems affection has also been proposed as a cause of overactive bladder in PD, activity in the serotonergic pathway generally enhances sympathetic innervation tone and detrusor hyperreflexia [50]. Epidemiological studies in humans have suggested an association between urinary incontinence and depression [51]. In agreement with these reports, Walter et al. [26] found a significant hypogenic BR in PD patients with OAB.

Moreover, there was a greater number of OAB patients suffering from dysthymia or major depressive disorder. In line with these data, in a recent study by Roy et al., mean MRI diffusivity in the ventral brainstem, in areas close to the pontine micturition center and the pontine continence center, correlated significantly with the bladder symptom severity in PD patients [52].

4.2. Substantia Nigra

Not only raphe hypoechogenicity but also SN hyperechogenicity has been related to increased liability of depression, in both PD and non-PD populations [14]. Non-PD depressed patients present a 3-fold increased frequency of presenting SN hyperechogenicity [14]. This finding could be interpreted as a risk marker for PD development, supported by epidemiological studies that evidenced an increased risk of PD development in depressive patients [53–55]. Furthermore, the co-occurrence of SN hyperechogenicity and BR hypoechogenicity in PD patients was associated with history of depression prior to PD onset [14].

Another interesting finding of Li et al. [33] involving SN hyperechogenicity was its relationship with the presence of VH, evaluated with the PD-NMSQ. The exact pathogenesis of VH in PD patients is not clearly understood. Based on brain imaging studies, an abnormality and dysfunction in visual cortex and cholinergic structures such as the SN and pedunculopontine nucleus have been proposed [56], in line with TCS findings. Caudate nucleus hyperechogenicity was also found to be related to drug-induced psychosis. The relation between SN hyperechogenicity and other NMS such as constipation, fatigue, and the presence of restless legs syndrome (RLS) has also been evaluated, without finding any difference between PD patients suffering or not from the evaluated symptom. Interestingly, when comparing RLS in PD and iRLS, a significant reduction of SN was found in iRLS. This suggests that, despite both having a good response to levodopa, a different pathophysiological mechanism may be involved.

4.3. Lateral and Third Ventricle (Width)

Previous reports found that elderly non-PD individuals with enlarged SN performed worse in neuropsychological tests than individuals with normal SN echogenicity; however, that was not confirmed in the analyzed publications [57,58].

The main finding correlated with cognitive impairment was enlarged lateral and third ventricles, not present in PD patients without dementia and healthy controls [13,23–25]. Those changes are not specific of PD and have been reported in other neurodegenerative dementias. Previous studies have described a pattern of brain atrophy which is similar in Alzheimer's disease (AD) and in PD. Nevertheless, the cognitive impairment profile is different in both diseases; while AD predominantly affects memory, PD is characterized by the involvement of executive functions. At a pathological level, dementia in PD is thought to be secondary to Lewy body deposits in the neocortical and limbic system. However, pathological changes normally associated with Alzheimer's disease, such as abnormal deposition of β-amyloid and neurofibrillary tangles, have been additionally proposed to contribute to dementia in some PD patients [59,60].

4.4. Vagus Nerve Atrophy

Finally, the most recently explored neurological structure is the vagus nerve diameter and CSA, assessed at the cervical level with high resolution ultrasound. The interest of this structure is based on the hypothesis that the vagus nerve may represent one major route of disease progression in PD, with an active retrograde transport of α-synuclein originating in the enteric nervous system, ascending the vagus nerve, and eventually reaching the dorsal motor nucleus of the vagus in the lower brainstem [61–63].

Four studies evaluated the vagus nerve in PD and non-PD patients, with inconsistent results [27–29,36] regarding higher susceptibility of this long nerve to α-synucleinopathies. Only one proved a relation between vagus nerve atrophy and the presence of NMS and an increase in hearth rate variability [29]. A few reasons could explain the varying results, including differences in methodology and clinical heterogeneity of the PD group, although age and UPDRS-III scores, addressing motor examination, were similar.

In this review, we found some limitations, such as the possible variability of the ultrasound evaluation protocols between the study groups. Furthermore, TCS is dependent on the examiner's skill and examinations are limited by variables such as the acoustic bone window and angulation of the scanning plane. Moreover, due to the characteristic physical features of PD patients, blindness to diagnosis might be difficult to achieve. Regarding the assessment of NMS, mainly based on scales and anamnesis due to biomarkers scarcity, it is possible that interindividual self-perception variability may have been a limitation.

5. Conclusions

The results of this systematic review support the use of transcranial ultrasound as a valuable complementary tool in the evaluation and diagnosis of the main NMS in PD. Future studies assessing US characteristics in non-PD patients with NMS and evaluating the risk of developing PD as well as the response to medical treatment are needed.

Author Contributions: C.d.T.P., L.A.P. and P.M.-S. conceived and designed the methodology of the systematic review. C.d.T.P. and L.A.P. extracted and collected the relevant information and drafted the manuscript. P.M.-S. supervised the article selection and reviewed and edited the manuscript. A.A.P., J.O.R., M.V.M.O., J.F.P. and M.P.O. reviewed and edited the manuscript. All authors have read and agreed to the published version of the manuscript.

Funding: This research received no external funding.

Conflicts of Interest: The authors declare no conflict of interest.

Appendix A. Trascranial Ultrasound Images Identifying the Main Referred Structures

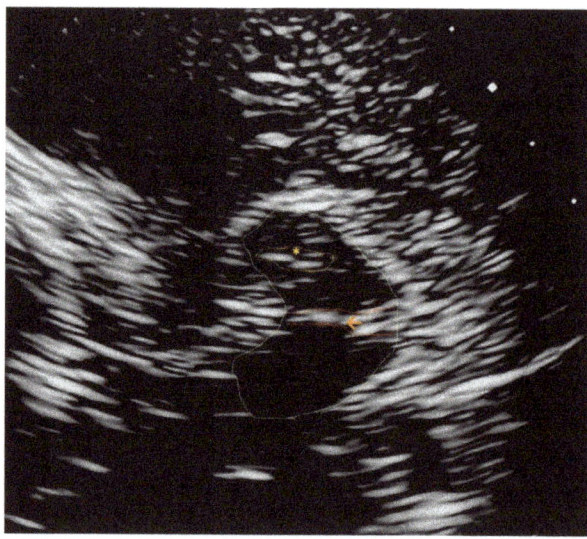

Figure A1. 7 MHz transducer. The silhouette of midbrain is marked with a colored line. Substantia nigra (*) and brainstem raphe (arrow) can be identified.

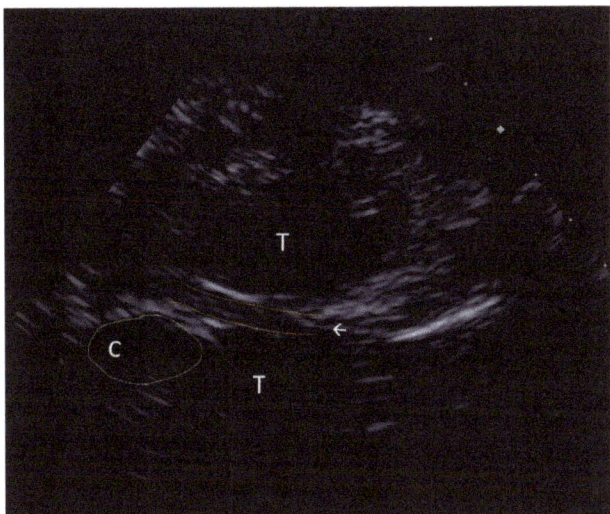

Figure A2. Transcranial ultrasound of a healthy subject performed with a 2.7 MHz transducer, transthalamic axial section. Hypoechoic ovoid silhouettes correspond to normal thalamic nuclei (T) and caudate nucleus (C). The arrow indicates the normal 3rd ventricle, as a hypoechoic tubular structure with hyperechoic margins.

References

1. Pfeiffer, R.F. Non-motor symptoms in Parkinson's disease. *Park. Rela Disord.* **2016**, *22*, S119–S122. Available online: https://pubmed.ncbi.nlm.nih.gov/26372623/ (accessed on 22 May 2021). [CrossRef] [PubMed]
2. Weerkamp, N.J.; Tissingh, G.; Poels, P.J.E.; Zuidema, S.U.; Munneke, M.; Koopmans, R.T.C.M.; Bloem, B.R. Nonmotor symptoms in nursing home residents with Parkinson's disease: Prevalence and effect on quality of life. *J. Am. Geriat. Soc.* **2013**, *61*, 1714–1721. Available online: https://pubmed.ncbi.nlm.nih.gov/24117286/ (accessed on 22 May 2021). [CrossRef] [PubMed]
3. Reijnders, J.S.A.M.; Ehrt, U.; Weber, W.E.J.; Aarsland, D.; Leentjens, A.F.G. A systematic review of prevalence studies of depression in Parkinson's disease. *Mov. Disord.* **2008**, *23*, 183–189. Available online: https://pubmed.ncbi.nlm.nih.gov/17987654/ (accessed on 22 May 2021). [CrossRef] [PubMed]
4. Den Brok, M.G.H.E.; van Dalen, J.W.; van Gool, W.A.; Moll van Charante, E.P.; de Bie, R.M.A.; Richard, E. Apathy in Parkinson's disease: A systematic review and meta-analysis. *Mov. Disord.* **2015**, *30*, 759–769. Available online: https://pubmed.ncbi.nlm.nih.gov/25787145/ (accessed on 22 May 2021). [CrossRef] [PubMed]
5. Alonso-Cánovas, A.; López-Sendón, J.L.; Buisán, J.; DeFelipe-Mimbrera, A.; Guillán, M.; García-Barragán, N.; Corral, I.; Matute-Lozano, M.C.; Masjuan, J.; Martínez-Castrillo, J.C.; et al. Sonography for diagnosis of parkinson disease-From theory to practice: A study on 300 participants. *J. Ultrasound Med.* **2014**, *33*, 2069–2074. Available online: https://pubmed.ncbi.nlm.nih.gov/25425362/ (accessed on 22 May 2021). [CrossRef]
6. Pilotto, A.; Yilmaz, R.; Berg, D. Developments in the Role of Transcranial Sonography for the Differential Diagnosis of Parkinsonism. *Curr. Neurol. Neurosci. Rep.* **2015**, *15*, 1–10. Available online: https://link.springecom/article/10.1007/s11910-015-0566-9 (accessed on 22 May 2021). [CrossRef]
7. Walter, U.; Wittstock, M.; Benecke, R.; Dressler, D. Substantia nigra echogenicity is normal in non-extrapyramidal cerebral disorders but increased in Parkinson's disease. *J. Neural Transm.* **2002**, *109*, 191–196. Available online: https://pubmed.ncbi.nlm.nih.gov/12075859/ (accessed on 22 May 2021). [CrossRef]
8. Walter, U.; Školoudík, D.; Berg, D. Transcranial sonography findings related to non-motor features of Parkinson's diseas. *J. Neurol. Sci.* **2010**, *289*, 123–127. Available online: https://pubmed.ncbi.nlm.nih.gov/19735925/ (accessed on 22 May 2021). [CrossRef]
9. Shamseer, L.; Moher, D.; Clarke, M.; Ghersi, D.; Liberati, A.; Petticrew, M.; Shekelle, P.; Stewart, L.A.; PRISMA-P Group. Preferred reporting items for systematic review and meta-analysis protocols (prisma-p) 2015: Elaboration and explanation. *BMJ* **2015**, *349*, 1–25. [CrossRef]
10. Whiting, P.F.; Rutjes, A.W.S.; Westwood, M.E.; Mallett, S.; Deeks, J.J.; Reitsma, J.B.; Shekelle, P.; Stewart, L.A.; PRISMA-P Group. Quadas-2: A revised tool for the quality assessment of diagnostic accuracy studies. *Ann. Intern. Med. Am. Coll. Physicians* **2011**, *155*, 529–536. Available online: https://pubmed.ncbi.nlm.nih.gov/22007046/ (accessed on 4 May 2021). [CrossRef]

11. Becker, T.; Becker, G.; Seufert, J.; Hofmann, E.; Lange, K.W.; Naumann, M.; Lindner, A.; Reichmann, H.; Riederer, P.; Beckmann, H.; et al. Parkinson's disease and depression: Evidence for an alteration of the basal limbic system detected by transcranial sonography. *J. Neurol. Neurosurg. Psychiatry* **1997**, *63*, 590–596. Available online: https://jnnp.bmj.com/content/63/5/590 (accessed on 4 May 2021). [CrossRef]
12. Berg, D.; Supprian, T.; Hofmann, E.; Zeiler, B.; Jäger, A.; Lange, K.W.; Reiners, K.; Becker, T.; Becker, G. Depression in Parkinson's disease: Brainstem midline alteration on transcranial sonography and magnetic resonance imaging. *J. Neurol.* **1999**, *246*, 1186–1193. Available online: https://pubmed.ncbi.nlm.nih.gov/10653314/ (accessed on 4 May 2021). [CrossRef]
13. Walter, U.; Dressler, D.; Wolters, A.; Wittstock, M.; Benecke, R. Transcranial brain sonography findings in clinical subgroups of idiopathic Parkinson's disease. *Mov. Disord.* **2007**, *22*, 48–54. [CrossRef]
14. Walter, U.; Hoeppner, J.; Prudente-Morrissey, L.; Horowski, S.; Herpertz, S.C.; Benecke, R. Parkinson's disease-like midbrain sonography abnormalities are frequent in depressive disorders. *Brain* **2007**, *130*, 1799–1807. Available online: https://pubmed.ncbi.nlm.nih.gov/17329323/ (accessed on 22 May 2021). [CrossRef]
15. Cho, J.W.; Baik, J.S.; Lee, M.S. Mesencephalic midline change on transcranial sonography in early Parkinson's disease patients with depression. *J. Neurol. Sci.* **2011**, *310*, 50–52. Available online: https://pubmed.ncbi.nlm.nih.gov/21862038/ (accessed on 22 May 2021). [CrossRef] [PubMed]
16. Stanković, I.; Stefanova, E.; Žiropadja, L.; Mijajlović, M.; Pavlović, A.; Kostić, V.S. Transcranial midbrain sonography and depressive symptoms in patients with Parkinson's diseas. *J. Neurol.* **2015**, *262*, 689–695. Available online: https://pubmed.ncbi.nlm.nih.gov/25557281/ (accessed on 22 May 2021). [CrossRef]
17. Bouwmans, A.E.P.; Weber, W.E.J.; Leentjens, A.F.G.; Mess, W.H. Transcranial sonography findings related to depression in parkinsonian disorders: Cross-sectional study in 126 patients. *PeerJ* **2016**, *2016*, e2037. Available online: https://peerj.com/articles/2037 (accessed on 22 May 2021). [CrossRef]
18. Zhang, Y.C.; Hu, H.; Luo, W.F.; Sheng, Y.J.; Chen, X.F.; Mao, C.J.; Xiong, K.P.; Yu, L.F.; Zhang, Y.; Liu, C.F. Alteration of brainstem raphe measured by transcranial sonography in depression patients with or without Parkinson's disease. *Neurol. Sci.* **2016**, *37*, 45–50. Available online: https://europepmc.org/article/med/26253340 (accessed on 22 May 2021). [CrossRef]
19. Toomsoo, T.; Randver, R.; Liepelt-Scarfone, I.; Kadastik-Eerme, L.; Asser, T.; Rubanovits, I.; Berg, D.; Taba, P. Prevalence of depressive symptoms and their association with brainstem raphe echogenicity in patients with Parkinson's disease and non-PD controls. *Psychiatry Res. Neuroimaging* **2017**, *268*, 45–49. Available online: https://europepmc.org/article/med/28865346 (accessed on 22 May 2021). [CrossRef] [PubMed]
20. Liu, X.J.; Zhang, L.; Zhang, Y.F.; Xu, W.; Hu, Y.; Liu, Y.; Bai, J. Echogenic alteration in the raphe nuclei measured by transcranial sonography in patients with Parkinson disease and depression. *Medicine* **2018**, *7*, e13524. [CrossRef] [PubMed]
21. Richter, D.; Woitalla, D.; Muhlack, S.; Gold, R.; Tönges, L.; Krogias, C. Brainstem raphe alterations in TCS: A biomarker for depression and apathy in parkinson's disease patients. *Front. Neurol.* **2018**, *9*, 645. Available online: https://www.frontiersin.org/articles/10.3389/fneur.2018.00645/full (accessed on 22 May 2021). [CrossRef]
22. Bei, H.Z.; Chen, J.P.; Mao, C.J.; Zhang, Y.C.; Chen, J.; Du, Q.Q.; Xue, F.; He, P.C.; Jin, H.; Wang, F.Y.; et al. Echogenicity Changes in Brainstem Raphe Detected by Transcranial Parenchymal Sonography and Clinical Characteristics in Parkinson's Disease. *Front. Neurol.* **2020**, *11*, 821. Available online: www.frontiersinorg (accessed on 22 May 2021). [CrossRef] [PubMed]
23. Walter, U.; Dressler, D.; Wolters, A.; Wittstock, M.; Greim, B.; Benecke, R. Sonographic discrimination of dementia with Lewy bodies and Parkinson's disease with dementia. *J. Neurol.* **2006**, *253*, 448–454. Available online: https://pubmed.ncbi.nlm.nih.gov/16267638/ (accessed on 22 May 2021). [CrossRef] [PubMed]
24. Bouwmans, A.E.; Leentjens, A.F.; Mess, W.H.; Weber, W.E. Abnormal echogenicity of the substantia nigra, raphe nuclei, and third-ventricle width as markers of cognitive impairment in parkinsonian disorders: A cross-sectional study. *Parkinsons Dis.* **2016**, *2016*, 4058580. [CrossRef]
25. Dong, Z.F.; Wang, C.S.; Zhang, Y.C.; Zhang, Y.; Sheng, Y.J.; Hu, H.; Luo, W.F.; Liu, C.F. Transcranial sonographic alterations of substantia Nigra and third ventricle in Parkinson's disease with or without dementia. *Chin. Med. J.* **2017**, *130*, 2291–2295. Available online: https://pubmed.ncbi.nlm.nih.gov/28937033/ (accessed on 22 May 2021).
26. Walter, U.; Dressler, D.; Wolters, A.; Wittstock, M.; Benecke, R. Overactive bladder in Parkinson's disease: Alteration of brainstem raphe detected by transcranial sonography. *Eur. J. Neurol.* **2006**, *13*, 1291–1297. Available online: https://pubmed.ncbi.nlm.nih.gov/17116210/ (accessed on 22 May 2021). [CrossRef]
27. Fedtke, N.; Witte, O.W.; Prell, T. Ultrasonography of the vagus nerve in Parkinson's disease. *Front. Neurol.* **2018**, *9*, 525. [CrossRef] [PubMed]
28. Pelz, J.O.; Belau, E.; Fricke, C.; Classen, J.; Weise, D. Axonal degeneration of the vagus nerve in Parkinson's disease-a high-resolution ultrasound study. *Front. Neurol.* **2018**, *9*, 951. Available online: https://pubmed.ncbi.nlm.nih.gov/30483212/ (accessed on 22 May 2021). [CrossRef]
29. Walter, U.; Tsiberidou, P.; Kersten, M.; Storch, A.; Löhle, M. Atrophy of the Vagus Nerve in Parkinson's Disease Revealed by High-Resolution Ultrasonography. *Front. Neurol.* **2018**, *9*, 805. Available online: https://pubmed.ncbi.nlm.nih.gov/30319534/ (accessed on 22 May 2021). [CrossRef]
30. Kwon, D.Y.; Seo, W.K.; Yoon, H.K.; Park, M.H.; Koh, S.B.; Park, K.W. Transcranial brain sonography in Parkinson's disease with restless legs syndrome. *Mov. Disord.* **2010**, *25*, 1373–1378. Available online: https://pubmed.ncbi.nlm.nih.gov/20544813/ (accessed on 22 May 2021). [CrossRef]

31. Ryu, J.H.; Lee, M.S.; Baik, J.S. Sonographic abnormalities in idiopathic restless legs syndrome (RLS) and RLS in Parkinson's disease. *Park. Relat. Disord.* **2011**, *17*, 201–203. Available online: https://pubmed.ncbi.nlm.nih.gov/21183393/ (accessed on 22 May 2021). [CrossRef] [PubMed]
32. Zhou, H.Y.; Sun, Q.; Tan, Y.Y.; Hu, Y.Y.; Zhan, W.W.; Li, D.H.; Wang, Y.; Xiao, Q.; Liu, J.; Chen, S.D. Substantia nigra echogenicity correlated with clinical features of Parkinson's disease. *Park. Relat. Disord.* **2016**, *24*, 28–33. Available online: https://pubmed.ncbi.nlm.nih.gov/26842545/ (accessed on 22 May 2021). [CrossRef] [PubMed]
33. Li, T.; Shi, J.; Qin, B.; Fan, D.; Liu, N.; Ni, J.; Zhang, T.; Zhou, H.; Xu, X.; Wei, M.; et al. Increased substantia nigra echogenicity correlated with visual hallucinations in Parkinson's disease: A Chinese population-based study. *Neurol. Sci.* **2020**, *41*, 661–667. Available online: https://link.springer.com/content/pdf/10.1007/s10072-019-04110-z.pdf (accessed on 22 May 2021). [CrossRef] [PubMed]
34. Chaudhuri, K.R.; Martinez-Martin, P.; Schapira, A.H.V.; Stocchi, F.; Sethi, K.; Odin, P.; Brown, R.G.; Koller, W.; Barone, P.; MacPhee, G.; et al. International multicenter pilot study of the first comprehensive self-completed nonmotor symptoms questionnaire for Parkinson's disease: The NMSQuest study. *Mov. Disord.* **2006**, *21*, 916–923. [CrossRef]
35. Visser, M.; Marinus, J.; Stiggelbout, A.M.; van Hilten, J.J. Assessment of autonomic dysfunction in Parkinson's disease: The SCOPA-AUT. *Mov. Disord.* **2004**, *19*, 1306–1312. Available online: https://pubmed.ncbi.nlm.nih.gov/15390007/ (accessed on 23 May 2021). [CrossRef]
36. Laucius, O.; Balnytė, R.; Petrikonis, K.; Matijošaitis, V.; Jucevičiūtė, N.; Vanagas, T.; Danielius, V. Ultrasonography of the Vagus Nerve in the Diagnosis of Parkinson's Disease. *Park. Dis.* **2020**, *2020*, 2627471. Available online: https://www.frontiersin.org/articles/10.3389/fneur.2018.00525/full (accessed on 22 May 2021). [CrossRef]
37. Goetz, C.C. The Unified Parkinson's Disease Rating Scale (UPDRS): Status and recommendations [Internet]. Vol. 18, Movement Disorders. *Mov. Disord.* **2003**, *18*, 738–750. Available online: https://pubmed.ncbi.nlm.nih.gov/12815652/ (accessed on 23 May 2021).
38. Chaudhuri, K.R.; Pal, S.; Dimarco, A.; Whately-Smith, C.; Bridgman, K.; Mathew, R.; Pezzela, F.R.; Forbes, A.; Högl, B.; Trenkwalder, C. The Parkinson's disease sleep scale: A new instrument for assessing sleep and nocturnal disability in Parkinson's disease. *J. Neurol. Neurosurg. Psychiatry* **2002**, *73*, 629–635. Available online: www.jnnp.com (accessed on 27 May 2021). [CrossRef] [PubMed]
39. Varma, M.G.; Wang, J.Y.; Berian, J.R.; Patterson, T.R.; McCrea, G.L.; Hart, S.L. The constipation severity instrument: A validated measure. *Dis. Colon Rectum* **2008**, *51*, 162–172. Available online: https://link.springecom/article/10.1007/s10350-007-9140-0 (accessed on 27 May 2021). [CrossRef]
40. Brown, R.G.; Dittner, A.; Findley, L.; Wessely, S.C. The Parkinson fatigue scale. *Park. Relat. Disord.* **2005**, *11*, 49–55. Available online: https://pubmed.ncbi.nlm.nih.gov/15619463/ (accessed on 27 May 2021). [CrossRef]
41. Becker, G.; Struck, M.; Bogdahn, U.; Becker, T. Echogenicity of the brainstem raphe in patients with major depression. *Psychiatry Res. Neuroimaging* **1994**, *55*, 75–84. Available online: https://pubmed.ncbi.nlm.nih.gov/10711796/ (accessed on 22 May 2021). [CrossRef]
42. Walter, U.; Prudente-Morrissey, L.; Herpertz, S.C.; Benecke, R.; Hoeppner, J. Relationship of brainstem raphe echogenicity and clinical findings in depressive states. *Psychiatry Res. Neuroimaging* **2007**, *155*, 67–73. Available online: https://pubmed.ncbi.nlm.nih.gov/17391931/ (accessed on 22 May 2021). [CrossRef]
43. Walter, U.; Krolikowski, K.; Tarnacka, B.; Benecke, R.; Czlonkowska, A.; Dressler, D. Sonographic detection of basal ganglia lesions in asymptomatic and symptomatic Wilson disease. *Neurology* **2005**, *64*, 1726–1732. Available online: https://pubmed.ncbi.nlm.nih.gov/15911799/ (accessed on 22 May 2021). [CrossRef]
44. Krogias, C.; Strassburger, K.; Eyding, J.; Gold, R.; Norra, C.; Juckel, G.; Saft, C.; Ninphius, D. Depression in patients with Huntington disease correlates with alterations of the brain stem raphe depicted by transcranial sonography. *J. Psychiatry Neurosci.* **2011**, *36*, 187–194. Available online: https://pubmed.ncbi.nlm.nih.gov/21138658/ (accessed on 22 May 2021). [CrossRef]
45. Becker, G.; Berg, D.; Lesch, K.P.; Becker, T. Basal limbic system alteration in major depression: A hypothesis supported by transcranial sonography and MRI findings. *International Journal of Neuropsychopharmacology. Int. J. Neuropsychopharmacol.* **2001**, *4*, 21–31. Available online: https://pubmed.ncbi.nlm.nih.gov/11343670/ (accessed on 22 May 2021). [CrossRef] [PubMed]
46. Berg, D.; Supprian, T.; Thomae, J.; Warmuth-Metz, M.; Horowski, A.; Zeiler, B.; Magnus, T.; Rieckmann, P.; Becker, G. Lesion pattern in patients with multiple sclerosis and depression. *Mult. Scler. J.* **2000**, *6*, 156–162. Available online: https://pubmed.ncbi.nlm.nih.gov/10871826/ (accessed on 22 May 2021). [CrossRef] [PubMed]
47. Brooks, D.J.; Piccini, P. Imaging in Parkinson's Disease: The Role of Monoamines in Behavior. *Biol. Psychiatry* **2006**, *59*, 908–918. Available online: https://pubmed.ncbi.nlm.nih.gov/16581032/ (accessed on 22 May 2021). [CrossRef]
48. Mayeux, R.; Stern, Y.; Sano, M.; Williams, J.B.W.; Cote, L.J. The relationship of serotonin to depression in Parkinson's disease. *Mov. Disord.* **1988**, *3*, 237–244. Available online: https://pubmed.ncbi.nlm.nih.gov/2461509/ (accessed on 22 May 2021). [CrossRef] [PubMed]
49. Zhuang, X.; Xu, H.; Fang, Z.; Xu, C.; Xue, C.; Hong, X. Platelet serotonin and serotonin transporter as peripheral surrogates in depression and anxiety patients. *Eur. J. Pharmacol.* **2018**, *834*, 213–220. Available online: https://europepmc.org/article/med/30031795 (accessed on 22 May 2021). [CrossRef] [PubMed]

50. Andersson, K.E.; Pehrson, R. CNS Involvement in Overactive Bladder: Pathophysiology and Opportunities for Pharmacological Intervention Drugs. *Drugs* **2003**, *63*, 2595–2611. Available online: https://pubmed.ncbi.nlm.nih.gov/14636079/ (accessed on 22 May 2021). [CrossRef] [PubMed]
51. Cheng, S.; Lin, D.; Hu, T.; Cao, L.; Liao, H.; Mou, X.; Zhang, Q.; Liu, J.; Wu, T. Association of urinary incontinence and depression or anxiety: A meta-analysis. *J. Int. Med. Res.* **2020**, *48*, 300060520931348. Available online: https://pubmed.ncbi.nlm.nih.gov/32552169/ (accessed on 22 May 2021). [CrossRef]
52. Roy, H.A.; Griffiths, D.J.; Aziz, T.Z.; Green, A.L.; Menke, R.A.L. Investigation of urinary storage symptoms in Parkinson's disease utilizing structural MRI techniques. *Neurourol. Urodyn.* **2019**, *38*, 1168–1175. Available online: https://pubmed.ncbi.nlm.nih.gov/30869824/ (accessed on 22 May 2021). [CrossRef]
53. Nilsson, F.M.; Kessing, L.V.; Bolwig, T.G. Increased risk of developing Parkinson's disease for patients with major affective disorder: A register study. *Acta Psychiatr. Scand.* **2001**, *104*, 380–386. Available online: https://pubmed.ncbi.nlm.nih.gov/11722320/ (accessed on 22 May 2021). [CrossRef]
54. Schuurman, A.G.; Van den Akker, M.; Ensinck, K.T.J.L.; Metsemakers, J.F.M.; Knottnerus, J.A.; Leentjens, A.F.G.; Buntinx, F. Increased risk of Parkinson's disease after depression: A retrospective cohort study. *Neurology* **2002**, *58*, 1501–1504. Available online: https://pubmed.ncbi.nlm.nih.gov/12034786/ (accessed on 22 May 2021). [CrossRef]
55. Leentjens, A.F.G.; Van den Akker, M.; Metsemakers, J.F.M.; Lousberg, R.; Verhey, F.R.J. Higher incidence of depression preceding the onset of parkinson's disease: A register study. *Mov. Disord.* **2003**, *18*, 414–418. Available online: https://pubmed.ncbi.nlm.nih.gov/12671948/ (accessed on 22 May 2021). [CrossRef] [PubMed]
56. Lenka, A.; Jhunjhunwala, K.R.; Saini, J.; Pal, P.K. Structural and functional neuroimaging in patients with Parkinson's disease and visual hallucinations: A critical review. *Parkinsonism Relat. Disord.* **2015**, *21*, 683–691. Available online: https://pubmed.ncbi.nlm.nih.gov/25920541/ (accessed on 22 May 2021). [CrossRef]
57. Liepelt, I.; Wendt, A.; Schweitzer, K.J.; Wolf, B.; Godau, J.; Gaenslen, A.; Bruessel, T.; Berg, D. Substantia nigra hyperechogenicity assessed by transcranial sonography is related to neuropsychological impairment in the elderly population. *J. Neural. Transm.* **2008**, *115*, 993–999. Available online: https://pubmed.ncbi.nlm.nih.gov/18368284/ (accessed on 22 May 2021). [CrossRef] [PubMed]
58. Yilmaz, R.; Behnke, S.; Liepelt-Scarfone, I.; Roeben, B.; Pausch, C.; Runkel, A.; Heinzel, S.; Niebler, R.; Suenkel, U.; Eschweiler, G.W.; et al. Substantia nigra hyperechogenicity is related to decline in verbal memory in healthy elderly adults. *Eur. J. Neurol.* **2016**, *23*, 973–978. Available online: https://onlinelibrary.wiley.com/doi/full/10.1111/en12974 (accessed on 22 May 2021). [CrossRef] [PubMed]
59. Lucero, C.; Campbell, M.C.; Flores, H.; Maiti, B.; Perlmutter, J.S.; Foster, E.R. Cognitive reserve and β-amyloid pathology in Parkinson disease. *Park. Relat. Disord.* **2015**, *21*, 899–904. Available online: https://pubmed.ncbi.nlm.nih.gov/26037458/ (accessed on 22 May 2021). [CrossRef]
60. Armstrong, R.A. Laminar degeneration of frontal and temporal cortex in Parkinson disease dementia. *Neurol. Sci.* **2017**, *38*, 667–671. Available online: https://pubmed.ncbi.nlm.nih.gov/28181068/ (accessed on 22 May 2021). [CrossRef]
61. Braak, H.; Rüb, U.; Gai, W.P.; Del Tredici, K. Idiopathic Parkinson's disease: Possible routes by which vulnerable neuronal types may be subject to neuroinvasion by an unknown pathogen. *J. Neural Transm.* **2003**, *110*, 517–536. Available online: https://pubmed.ncbi.nlm.nih.gov/12721813/ (accessed on 22 May 2021). [CrossRef] [PubMed]
62. Holmqvist, S.; Chutna, O.; Bousset, L.; Aldrin-Kirk, P.; Li, W.; Björklund, T.; Wang, Z.Y.; Roybon, L.; Melki, R.; Li, J.Y. Direct evidence of Parkinson pathology spread from the gastrointestinal tract to the brain in rats. *Acta Neuropathol.* **2014**, *128*, 805–820. Available online: https://pubmed.ncbi.nlm.nih.gov/25296989/ (accessed on 22 May 2021). [CrossRef]
63. Svensson, E.; Horváth-Puhó, E.; Thomsen, R.W.; Djurhuus, J.C.; Pedersen, L.; Borghammer, P.; Sørensen, H.T. Vagotomy and subsequent risk of Parkinson's disease. *Ann. Neurol.* **2015**, *78*, 522–529. Available online: https://pubmed.ncbi.nlm.nih.gov/26031848/ (accessed on 22 May 2021). [CrossRef] [PubMed]

MDPI
St. Alban-Anlage 66
4052 Basel
Switzerland
www.mdpi.com

Brain Sciences Editorial Office
E-mail: brainsci@mdpi.com
www.mdpi.com/journal/brainsci

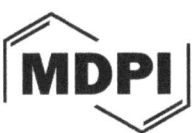

Disclaimer/Publisher's Note: The statements, opinions and data contained in all publications are solely those of the individual author(s) and contributor(s) and not of MDPI and/or the editor(s). MDPI and/or the editor(s) disclaim responsibility for any injury to people or property resulting from any ideas, methods, instructions or products referred to in the content.

www.ingramcontent.com/pod-product-compliance
Lightning Source LLC
LaVergne TN
LVHW070151120526
838202LV00013BA/913